NURSING EXCELLENCE FOR CHILDREN AND FAMILIES

About the Editors

MARTHA CRAFT-ROSENBERG, PhD, RN, FAAN, is professor and chair of the Parent, Child, and Family Area of Studies at The University of Iowa College of Nursing. She has studied siblings of hospitalized children and siblings of ill children for 25 years. Dr. Craft-Rosenberg has been an investigator on 17 funded studies focused on siblings of ill children and families of critically ill adults, with awards from the American Association of Critical Care Nurses and the Midwest Nursing Research Society for research on children and families. Dr. Craft-Rosenberg has coedited two previous books with Janice Denehy on interventions for infants, children, and families. Her language classification research includes intervention classification since 1987 and diagnoses classification for a decade as principal investigator for the Nursing Diagnosis Extension and Classification (NDEC) team.

Dr. Craft-Rosenberg has served two terms on the NANDA Taxonomy Committee and participated in the consensus conference for development of the Taxonomy of Nursing Practice. She is president of NANDA International, and codirector with Sue Moorhead on a T32 grant for "Training in Nursing Effectiveness Research."

MARILYN J. KRAJICEK, EdD, RN, FAAN, is professor of nursing at the University of Colorado at Denver and Health Sciences Center (UCDHSC) School of Nursing, and assistant clinical professor, Department of Pediatrics, School of Medicine.

In addition to her faculty teaching roles, Dr. Krajicek is director of the National Resource Center for Health and Safety in Child Care (NRC) and Nursing Leadership: Pediatric Special Needs. These programs are funded by the Maternal and Child Health Bureau, Health Resources and Services Administration, U.S. Public Health Service. As director of the NRC, Dr. Krajicek worked with project faculty and staff to copublish the second edition of *Caring for Our Children: National Health and Safety Standards: Guidelines for Out-of-Home Child Care* in collaboration with the American Academy of Pediatrics (AAP), the American Public Health Association (APHA), and the Maternal and Child Health Bureau in 2002. In 2003, she directed the work of the NRC in publishing *Stepping Stones to Using Caring for Our Children*, developed to identify those standards most necessary to prevent disease, disability, and death (morbidity and mortality) in child care settings. She is also coeditor of the recently published *Student Handbook, First Start: Care of Infants, Toddlers, and Young Children with Disabilities and Chronic Conditions* (2004, 2nd ed.).

Nursing Excellence for Children and Families

Edited by
Martha Craft-Rosenberg, PhD, RN, FAAN
Marilyn J. Krajicek, EdD, RN, FAAN

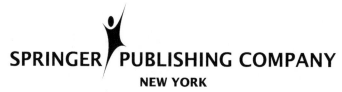

SPRINGER PUBLISHING COMPANY
NEW YORK

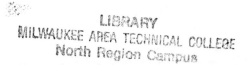

Springer Publishing Company, Inc.
11 West 42nd Street
New York, NY 10036

Acquisitions Editors: Ruth Chasek and Sally J. Barhydt
Production Editor: Jeanne Libby
Cover design by Joanne Honigman
Typeset by Daily Information Processing, Churchville, PA

06 07 08 09 10 / 5 4 3 2 1

Library of Congress Cataloging-in-Publication Data

Nursing excellence for children and families / [edited] by Martha
    Craft-Rosenberg and Marilyn J. Krajicek.
        p. ; cm.
    Includes bibliographical references and index.
    ISBN 0-8261-8815-X
    1. Pediatric nursing—Standards. 2. Family nursing—
Standards. I. Craft-Rosenberg, Martha. II. Krajicek, Marilyn J.
    [DNLM: 1. Pediatric Nursing—standards. 2. Family
Nursing—standards. WY 159 N973967 2006]
    RJ245.N876 2006
    618.92'00231—dc22

2005031309

Printed in the United States of America by Bang Printing.

Contents

Contributors

Cecily Betz, PhD, RN, FAAN
Associate Professor
University of Southern California
University Excellence for
  Developmental Disabilities
Children's Hospital of Los Angeles
Los Angeles, CA

Julia Muennich Cowell, PhD,
  RNC, FAAN
Professor and Chair Community
  and Mental Health Nursing
Rush University
College of Nursing
Chicago, IL

Janet A. Deatrick, PhD, RN,
  FAAN
Associate Professor
University of Pennsylvania
School of Nursing
Philadelphia, PA

Shelly Eisbach, RN, MSN
Graduate Student
The University of Iowa
College of Nursing
Iowa City, IA

Roxie Foster, PhD, RN, FAAN
Associate Professor
University of Colorado at Denver
  and Health Sciences Center
  School of Nursing
Denver, CO

Barbara U. Hamilton, MA
Professional Research Assistant
University of Colorado at Denver
  and Health Sciences Center
  School of Nursing
National Resource Center for
  Health Safety and Child Care
Aurora, CO

Judith B. Igoe, RN, BSN, FAAN
Associate Professor
University of Colorado at Denver
  and Health Sciences Center
  School of Nursing
Denver, CO

Charmaine Kleiber, PhD, RN,
  CPNP, FAAN
Associate Professor
The University of Iowa Hospitals
  and Clinics
Iowa City, IA

Kathleen Knafl, PhD, RN, FAAN
Professor and Acting Associate
    Dean for Academic Affairs
Yale University
School of Nursing
New Haven, CT

Marie L. Lobo, PhD, RN, FAAN
Professor
University of New Mexico
College of Nursing
Albuquerque, NM

**Margaret M. Mahon, PhD, RN,
    CRNP, FAAN**
Associate Professor
George Mason University
College of Nursing and Health
    Science
Fairfax, VA

Rose M. Mays, PhD, RN, FAAN
Professor and Associate Dean
    Office of Community Affairs
Indiana University Purdue
    University Indianapolis
School of Nursing
Indianapolis, IN

**Ann Marie McCarthy, PhD, RN,
    FAAN**
Professor
The University of Iowa
College of Nursing
Iowa City, IA

**Wendy M. Nehring, PhD, RN,
    FAAMR, FAAN**
Associate Professor; Associate
    Dean for Academic Affairs;
    and Director, Graduate Program
Rutgers, The State University
    of New Jersey
College of Nursing
Newark, NJ

Ann M. Rhodes, RN, MA, JD
Assistant to the Vice President
The University of Iowa
Office of the Provost
Iowa City, IA

**Kathryn Swartwout, MS, RN,
    DNSc, APN-CNP**
Doctoral Student and Teaching
    Assistant
Rush University
College of Nursing
Chicago, IL

**Martha K. Swartz, PhD, APRN,
    BC, PNP**
Assistant Professor and Assistant
    Dean for Academic Affairs
Yale University
School of Nursing
New Haven, CT

**Judith Vessey, PhD, MBA, PNP,
    FAAN**
Professor, Carroll Chair
    in Nursing
Boston College
William F. Connell School
    of Nursing
Chestnut Hill, MA

**Janet K. Williams, PhD, RN, PNP,
    FAAN**
Professor
The University of Iowa
College of Nursing
Iowa City, IA

Preface

Although nurses caring for infants, children, and families strive for excellence, the core elements of nursing excellence remain unclear. These elements, or indicators, are presented as chapter titles in the book. Through systematic consensus building led by the Expert Panel on Children and Families from the American Academy of Nursing (AAN) over a 4-year period, leaders of nursing organizations with members who share expertise in the care of infants, children, youth, and families identified elements, or indicators, of nursing excellence using their organizational standards. Leaders who participated in this consensus represented organizations including the Society of Pediatric Nurses (SPN), National Association of Pediatric Nurse Associates and Practitioners (NAPNAP), National Association of Neonatal Nurses (NANN), Association of Women's Health, Obstetric, and Neonatal Nurses (AWHONN), National Association of School Nurses (NASN), American Association on Mental Retardation (AAMR), American Nurses Association (ANA), Pediatric Endocrinology Nursing Society (PENS), Northeast Pediatric Cardiology Nurses Association (NPCNA), Children's Hospice International, International Association of Newborn Nurses, the Expert Panel on Children and Families from the American Academy of Nursing, and the International Society of Nursing Genetics.

We believe that *Nursing Excellence for Children and Families* will provide the gold standard of pediatric nursing care because the content integrates elements or indicators of nursing excellence from organizational standards supported by national leaders. These elements are interchangeable with indicators. They belong in undergraduate and graduate educational programs. In practice, they should be a part of orientation and evaluation for nurses, and be viewed as central for communication with members of other disciplines. Families, too, may find these standards useful as guidelines in the selection of health care for their infants and children. They can also help families more effectively assess the quality of the care they receive and advocate for improved services.

The text is organized around the identified indicators of nursing excellence. Experts on each nursing element or indicator serve as chapter authors. These authors define and describe elements of nursing excellence and discuss appropriate nursing care. Each chapter concludes with a case study illustrating use of the element or indicator. The following are the elements or indicators of nursing excellence:

1. Children and youth have an identified health care home.
2. The families of children and youth are partners in decisions, planning, and delivery of care.
3. Family values, beliefs, and preferences are part of care.
4. Family strengths and main concerns are obvious in the care of children and youth.
5. Children, youth, and families will have accessible health care.
6. Pregnant women will have accessible health care.
7. Family needs are identified and services are offered.
8. Children, youth, and families are directed to community services when needed.
9. Children, youth, and families receive care that promotes and maintains health and prevents disease.
10. Pregnant women, children, youth, and families have access to genetic testing and advice.
11. Children and youth receive care that is physically and emotionally safe.
12. Privacy and rights of children, youth, and families are protected.
13. Children and youth who are very ill receive the full range of needed services.
14. Children and youth with disabilities and/or special health care needs receive the full range of services.
15. Children, youth, and families receive comfort care.
16. Health and risky behaviors and problems of children, youth, and families are identified and addressed.
17. Children, youth, and families receive care that supports development.
18. Children, youth, and families are fully informed of the outcomes of care.

Acknowledgments

The editors of this book wish to thank Linda Curran from The University of Iowa College of Nursing, Office for Nursing Research, Development and Utilization, who is the project coordinator for our book. Her expertise, patience, and competence have made the development of our book systematic and paced. We also wish to thank Ginny Torrey, program specialist at the University of Colorado at Denver and Health Sciences Center School of Nursing who assisted in communication.

This book would not have been possible without the willingness of all authors to volunteer their writing for the good of the Expert Panel on Children and Families from the American Academy of Nursing. Words are inadequate to express our gratitude for their encouragement, suggestions, and their gifts of knowledge and writing.

A special thank-you goes to Ruth Chasek, our editor at Springer Publishing. She had the vision to see the product of our work as more than a monograph describing the process, but as a book including a chapter for each element or indicator.

MARTHA CRAFT-ROSENBERG, PhD, RN, FAAN
MARILYN J. KRAJICEK, EdD, RN, FAAN

Foreword

For many years, health care and specialty organizations have engaged in developing assessment tools and measurement methods to get at the essence of "quality" health care and recognize the distinction of "excellence" from the sea of "adequate." Child health professionals from a variety of constituencies have contributed to the discussions and development of general tools on the grounds that children present unique problems and circumstances that warrant careful differentiation from the larger population of consumers. Pediatric and child health nurses from a wide range of organizations and special interest groups have participated in a variety of efforts aimed at developing standards of clinical practice and markers of quality care. From the masses of products that establish yardsticks against which care can be measured in general, child health professionals have longed for a definitive subset of quality indicators that can be recognized within their respective memberships in order to know what distinguishes quality health care for children at the individual patient and family level to the organization and system level.

In the early months of 1998, plans for convening an invitational conference for pediatric and child health nurses were launched by the Expert Panel on Children and Families from the American Academy of Nursing (AAN). Select nursing organizations would be invited to share their expertise and contribute toward an integrated effort that would develop, through consensus, a collection of standards or guidelines to inform leaders in health care and assist consumers in their pursuit of quality services. The vision evolved over the years to acknowledge the key elements that would identify quality in child health care to be disseminated widely to professionals and policy makers with a usable terminology, shared set of assumptions and evidence-based tools. Noble as this vision was, as Lang and Mitchell (2004) ponder, "[if] quality measures have been used largely to evaluate quality rather than to improve it, [then] what is needed to cause a shift from merely judging quality . . . to striving for excellence of care?" (p. 2). Fast forward 7 years and several meetings later and the culmination is the book *Nursing Excellence for Children and Families,* coedited by Martha Craft-Rosenberg and Marilyn Krajicek.

The literature on quality, performance, and standards to inform the development of child health quality measures is both rich and confusing with vague nomenclature and paradigm overlap (Solloway, 1997). Nonetheless, quality has become a highly visible public issue, catapulted to national attention by the Institute of Medicine's (IOM) quality initiative in the late 1990s and substantiated by evidence of a large "quality gap." Concurrently, increased interest throughout government is being given to the effectiveness of monitoring, performance measures, and expected standards of care. Thus, in an effort to empower consumers and facilitate choice, there has been a growing demand for objective, comparative information about performance of providers and relevant practice guidelines with data-driven evaluation that includes outcomes measures.

It was for this reason that the Expert Panel on Children and Families from the American Academy of Nursing sought to develop a list of elements or indicators that could be used to identify excellence in child health care. These quality health care and outcome elements or indicators with their associated assumptions and values represent a landmark effort of communication among multiple pediatric and child health nursing organizations. The consensus on these elements or indicators of excellence was achieved through collaboration and with mutual respect, the process as important in the quest for excellence as the product. The elements or indicators go beyond the theoretical, supplemented with a translation for consumers into specific questions. This book presents for nursing and health care professionals a practical structure for developing methods to differentiate between acceptable levels of care and excellence. The scholarly chapters, written by some of the most notable leaders in pediatric and child health nursing, put substantive knowledge onto the frame. It will serve clinicians and providers, administrators, researchers, and policy makers in their continuous efforts to strive for excellence in pediatric nursing care.

VERONICA D. FEEG, PhD, RN, FAAN
AAN/ANF Institute of Medicine
Scholar-in-Residence (2004–2005)

REFERENCES

Lang, N. M., & Mitchell, P. H. (2004). Guest Editorial: Quality as an enduring and encompassing concept. *Nursing Outlook, 52*(1), 1–2.

Solloway, M. (1997, August). *Developing a framework for pediatric measures of accountability.* Report prepared for the Foundation of Accountability (FACCT), Department of Health Management and Policy. Durham, NH: University of New Hampshire.

CHAPTER ONE

Background

Martha Craft-Rosenberg
Marilyn J. Krajicek

Beginning in 1999, the Expert Panel on Children and Families from the American Academy of Nursing worked with other nursing organizations representing more than 60,000 nurses who provide care to women, children, youth, and their families. Together, they developed *Health Care Quality and Outcome Guidelines,* which was published as a journal article in *Nursing Outlook* (Betz, Cowell, Lobo, & Craft-Rosenberg, 2004). The vision of these early panel leaders was to develop subsequent quality and outcome indicators/guidelines, or essential nursing elements for use by consumers (parents) in the selection of health care for their children. These statements will assist families to assess more effectively the quality of care received and to advocate for improved services.

The long-range goal for dissemination includes plans to place these statements on a Web site for easy access by parents and other health care consumers. It is our hope that they will also be used by families for the selection and evaluation of the health care for their children.

The chapter authors for this book are recognized nationally and internationally as authorities in their subspecialties in nursing of infants, children, youth, and families. All of them are members of the AAN, with the exception of a nurse lawyer. These scholars were selected for their expertise in their respective fields and their ability to communicate their knowledge of our science and discipline to audiences that include students, practicing nurses, and researchers.

This book is the culmination of thinking and organizational leadership beginning in the mid 1990s by Drs. Marion Broome, Veronica Feeg, Marie Lobo, Cecily Betz, Julia Cowell, and other members of the AAN

1

Expert Panel on Children and Families. For this reason, this book is considered an AAN Expert Panel on Children and Families project. The royalties will be donated by the editors to the AAN Expert Panel on Children and Families to continue our work.

Craft-Rosenberg and Krajicek called an invitational meeting at the annual AAN meeting in Washington, DC, in 1999. The purpose of the invitational meeting was to begin a process of developing a conceptually organized and easily accessible collection of concepts drawn from nursing standards to identify and link quality indicators and measures. The objectives were to (a) discuss standards and guidelines of organizations represented; (b) compare similarities and differences; (c) evaluate presented standards for concept clarity and comprehensiveness in scope; (d) determine indicators and measures for concepts; and (e) prioritize standards and guidelines (Craft-Rosenberg, Krajicek, & Shin, 2002). The 1999 invitational conference formed a framework for integrating documents and for subsequent discussions related to influencing the quality of children's health in public policy and service arenas.

This first meeting of organizational leaders included leaders from following organizations:

- The Society of Pediatric Nurses (SPN)
- National Association of Pediatric Nurse Associates and Practitioners (NAPNAP)
- National Association of Neonatal Nurses (NAN)
- International Association of Newborn Nurses (IANN)
- Pediatric Endocrinology Nursing Society (PENS)
- National Pediatric Cardiology Nurse Association (NPCNA)
- Children's Hospice International (CHI)
- Maternal and Child Health Bureau (MCH)
- American Nurses Association (ANA)
- Association of Women's Health, Obstetric and Neonatal Nurses (AWHONN)
- National Association of School Nurses (NASN)
- American Association of Mental Retardation
- American Nurses Association
- Members of the AAN Expert Panel on Children and Families.

The assumptions and values of the working group guiding our thinking and planning were identified at the first meeting on November 17, 1999, and they are listed below (Betz et al., 2004).

Assumptions:

1. All children, youth, and families should have the assurance their providers are competent.

2. All children, youth, and families should have access to affordable health care.
3. The child, youth, and family health include their social, physical, mental, and spiritual aspects of living.
4. The home and community environments significantly impacts children, youth, and families.
5. Optimal health care is a continuous health team effort.
6. Health care is affected by economic factors.

Values:

1. Mother's health directly impacts the health of the children, youth, and families.
2. Holistic health care is integrated into the range of services offered.
3. Care is provided from preconception to a peaceful death.
4. The health care provider is responsible for quality care. Quality care is based on scientific evidence, is ethical, safe, and economically reasonable. Quality care is health care that meets family needs and wishes.

The outcome of our process was a synthesis of documents on standards and outcome indicators in matrix (Shin, 1999) and electronic forms (see Table 1.1). These outcomes were reached during our meeting: (a) discussion of standards of organizations represented; (b) comparison of similarities and differences in standards presented; and (c) development of schemata showing the relationship of nursing care concepts with nursing context, as reported in the 2002 article written by the authors (Craft-Rosenberg et al., 2002).

This second invitational meeting in 2001 was planned and chaired by Cecily Betz and Julia Cowell, the new panel cochairs. The commitment to move this work forward continued on the part of the editors Craft-Rosenberg and Krajicek as new cochairs assumed leadership. At the 2001 meeting, the 1999 draft was reviewed by a similar group of leaders representing organizations of nurses with expertise in care of infants, children, youth, and families, as well as members of the Expert Panel on Children and Families from the AAN. During the 2001 second invitational conference, participants reviewed the work of 1999 for readability and clarity and expanded the list from 11 to 18 guidelines/elements (Betz et al., 2004). The group increased the specificity of the original statements by placing them in the form of questions that parents can ask when selecting or evaluating health care for their children.

The dissemination of the guidelines/indicators includes the development of this book. It is our hope that this book has far-reaching effects in developing a consistent and high level of quality in pediatric nursing practice.

TABLE 1.1 Example of Standards Submitted for Discussion and Utilized in the Matrix at the 1999 Invitational Meeting for the American Academy of Nursing Expert Panel on Children and Families

Expert Panel: School Nursing (1998)*

I. Assessment

1. Data collection involves the student, family, school staff, community, and other providers, as necessary.
2. The priority of data collection is determined by the nursing diagnosis and the client's immediate condition and/or needs.
3. Pertinent individual and aggregate data are collected, using appropriate assessment techniques, and reviewed in light of relevant supporting information.
4. Relevant data are documented in a retrievable form.
5. The data collection process is systematic, organized, and ongoing.

II. Diagnosis

1. Nursing diagnoses, individual and aggregate, are derived from the evaluation of assessment data.
2. Nursing diagnoses, individual and aggregate, are validated with the student, family, school staff, community, and other providers, when appropriate.
3. Nursing diagnoses, individual and aggregate, are documented in a manner that facilitates the determination of expected outcomes and the plan of care/action.

III. Outcomes

1. Outcomes are derived from the nursing diagnoses.
2. Outcomes are mutually formulated with the student, family, school staff, community, and other providers, as appropriate.
3. Outcomes are culturally appropriate and realistic in relation to the client's present and potential capabilities.
4. Outcomes are obtained in relation to resources necessary and attainable.
5. Outcomes include a reasonable timeline.
6. Outcomes provide direction for continuity of care and the plan of care/action.
7. Outcomes are documented as measurable goals.

IV. Planning

1. The plan is individualized to the student's diagnosis/nursing diagnosis.
2. A plan is a component of the individual program for students with special health care needs. The plan is developed in compliance with local, state, and federal regulations, as needed.
3. The plan is collaboratively developed with the student, family, school staff, community, and other providers, as appropriate.
4. The plan reflects current standards of school nursing practice.

(continued)

TABLE 1.1 (*Continued*)

5. The plan provides for continuity of care and plan of action to be taken.
6. Priorities for care/action and timeline for interventions are established.
7. The plan is documented in a retrievable form.

V. Implementation

1. Interventions are consistent with the established plan of care/action.
2. Interventions are implemented in a safe, timely, and appropriate manner.
3. Interventions are documented in a retrievable form.
4. Interventions reflect current standards of school nursing practice.

VI. Evaluation

1. Evaluation is systematic, continuous, and criterion based.
2. The student, family, school staff, community, and other providers are involved in the evaluation process as appropriate.
3. Ongoing assessment data, including incremental goal attainment in achieving the expected outcomes, are used to revise diagnoses and outcomes, and the plan of care/action, as needed.
4. Revisions in nursing diagnoses, outcomes, and the plan of care/action are documented in a retrievable form.
5. The client's responses to interventions are documented in a retrievable form.
6. The effectiveness of interventions is evaluated in relation to outcomes.

*These standards were the ones used in the 1999 meeting. Since that time, the National Association of School Nurses (NASN) has revised their standards in 2001 and a 2005 revision is in process at the time of writing.

REFERENCES

Betz, C. L., Cowell, J. M., Lobo, M. L., & Craft-Rosenberg, M. (2004). American Academy of Nursing Child-Family Expert Panel health care quality and outcome guidelines for nursing of children and families: Phase II. *Nursing Outlook, 52,* 311–316.

Craft-Rosenberg, M., Krajicek, M., & Chin, D-S. (2002). Report of the American Academy of Nursing Child-Family Expert Panel: Identification of quality and outcome indicators for maternal child health nursing. *Nursing Outlook, 50,* 57–60.

Shin, D-S. (1999). *Matrix for the comparison of practice standards across organizations.* Unpublished report. The University of Iowa College of Nursing, Iowa City, Iowa.

CHAPTER TWO

Access to Health Care

Marie L. Lobo

INTRODUCTIONS, DEFINITIONS, AND THEIR MEASUREMENT

Access to health care is a critical factor in the health and well-being of children. It has been a key factor for influencing morbidity and mortality in children. Access to care issues differ for infants, young children, school-aged children, and adolescents, including mental health care, vision health care, and dental health care. Nurses long have been advocates for children in the health care system and need to be viewed as an integral partner in helping families and children to access care.

Children's health has not been defined well. Most literature uses the definitions applied to individuals of all ages. The Committee on Evaluation of Children's Health (2004) of the National Research Council and Institute of Medicine (IOM) has proposed the following definition:

> Children's health should be defined as the extent to which individual children or groups of children are able or enabled to a) develop and realize their potential, b) satisfy their needs, and c) develop the capacities that allow them to interact successfully with their biological, physical, and social environments. (p. ES-3)

The committee recognized that there are multiple influences on a child's health and that these all need to be considered in examining children's health and well-being.

The term *access to care* is poorly defined in the health care literature and not used consistently. In the Oxford English Dictionary (2004) *access* is defined as the "the action of going or coming to or into; coming into the presence of, or into contact with; approach, entrance." In much of the health literature, access to care implies access to medical care and is often defined by what is *not* available. For example, "health insurance" is used as a proxy to indicate someone has access to medical or health care because having insurance is known to improve a child's access to care (IOM, 2002). Access to care also does not imply access to nursing care, but may only mean traditional medical care. According to the IOM, access means the timely use of personal health services to achieve the best possible health outcomes (U.S. Department of Health and Human Services [USDHHS], 2000a).

Access to care is often discussed in terms of the barriers to patients and families receiving care. According to *Healthy People 2010* (USDHHS, 2000a), these barriers include patient, health provider, and system components. Patient barriers include any mental, physical, or psychosocial conditions that prevent an individual from accessing needed health care. Examples include attitudes or biases, mental disorders or illnesses, behavioral disorders, physical limitations, cultural or linguistic factors, sexual orientation, and financial constraints. Health provider barriers include any mental, physical, psychosocial, or environmental condition that prevent or discourage health care providers from offering services. Examples of provider barriers include a poor practice environment, lack of knowledge, and lack of efficacy studies. System barriers can include conditions within a health care system that prevent people from accessing needed services or prevent health care providers from delivering those services. System barriers include physical, cultural, linguistic, and financial barriers, as well as the availability of health care facilities or providers with special skills, a particular problem in impoverished neighborhoods or frontier states (USDHHS, 2000a).

The lack of access to quality health care and primary care is so great that one of the first goals of *Healthy People 2010* is to increase the proportion of persons who have a specific source of ongoing care. In the year 1998, 93% of children age 17 or younger had a source of ongoing care. The goal is to that 97% of all children have a specific source of care by 2010 (USDHHS, 2000a).

Definitions

A *health home* is defined as a specific agency or provider that provides continuity for a child and family receiving primary care and care for uncomplicated illnesses. *Healthy People 2010* looks at this as a "usual source of care"—a particular doctor's office, clinic, health center, or other health care facility to which an individual usually would go to obtain health care services. Having a usual source of care is associated with improved access both preventive services and follow-up care.

In the care of children, the American Academy of Pediatrics (AAP) uses the term *medical home* for a child and supports provision of health care only under the direction of a physician, preferably a pediatrician. A medical home, as defined by the AAP, should be

> accessible, continuous, comprehensive, family centered, coordinated, compassionate and culturally effective. It should be delivered or directed by well-trained physicians who provide primary care and help to manage and facilitate essentially all aspects of pediatric care. The physician should be known to the child and family and should be able to develop a partnership of mutual responsibility and trust with them. (AAP, 2002, p. 429)

The AAP position is that any physician, regardless of specialty type, is a "better" provider than a nonphysician primary care specialist such as a pediatric nurse practitioner.

Historical Overview

During the early part of the twentieth century, the Maternal and Child Health Bureau (MCHB) began pressing for more services for children and women. The belief was that if you could improve the health of mothers, you would improve the health of their children. Although clinics were begun for immunizations and other aspects of well-child care, they were usually focused on only the poorest and most vulnerable families and no child was "guaranteed" access to well-child care.

The Maternal and Child Health Bureau has set three goals for children in the twenty-first century (van Dyck, 2003):

> 1) to eliminate disparities in health status outcomes through the removal of economic, social, and cultural barriers to receiving comprehensive, timely and appropriate health care;
> 2) to ensure the highest quality of care through the development of practice guidelines and data monitoring and evaluation tools; the use of evidence-based research; and the availability of a culturally diverse workforce; and
> 3) to facilitate access to care through the development and improvement of the maternal and child health infrastructure and systems of care to enhance the provision of necessary, coordinated, quality health care. (p. 727)

Although these goals are laudable, they do little to assist the 27% of children ages 0 to 17 who are uninsured (Leatherman & McCarthy, 2004, p. 61).

The first use of the term *medical home* appeared in the 1967 *Standards of Child Health Care*, a book published by the AAP (Sia, Tonniges, Osterhus, & Taba, 2004). However, the focus was initially on the importance of centralized medical records for children with special health care needs. The fact that children received care from multiple sources increased the fragmentation of records and inefficient delivery of care. For example, some children were receiving duplicate immunizations and others were receiving none, simply because the records were so fragmented. In the late 1970s, North Carolina developed the concept of a "health home," which delineated the expectations of both the provider and the child and family (Sia et al., 2004). However, the AAP chose to focus on a "medical home" for the child and family.

The AAP expanded the original definition of the medical-home concept as follows:

> The AAP believes that the medical care of infants, children, and adolescents ideally should be accessible, continuous, comprehensive, family centered, coordinated and compassionate. It should be delivered or directed by well-trained physicians who are able to manage or facilitate essentially all aspects of pediatric care. The physician should be known to the family and should be able to develop a relationship of mutual responsibility and trust with them. (Sia et al., 2004).

This definition, created in 1992, completely focuses on only one member of the health care team.

In 2002, the 1992 statement was amended to include the terms "accessible, continuous, comprehensive, family centered, coordinated, compassionate, and culturally effective" (Sia et al., 2004). Although this movement has garnered the AAP much support from MCHB and other national and state family organizations, other professional groups have been asked to agree or support the concept after the fact. In 2003, the AAP published a policy statement on the *Scope of Practice Issues in the Delivery of Pediatric Health Care* (AAP Committee on Pediatric Workforce, 2003). Although the document speaks to the fact that the "provision of optimal pediatric health care depends on a team based approach" (AAP Committee on Pediatric Workforce, 2003, p. 426) they also advocate that the coordination must be by a physician leader, "preferably a pediatrician." This approach does not consider the best interest of the child. As care coordination with children with special needs has shown, the health professional in the coordination role is determined most appropriately by the child's needs.

In the *Scope of Practice* document, the AAP attempts to define the scope of practice of pediatric nurse practitioners (PNPs) and other providers (AAP Committee on Pediatric Workforce, 2003). This document states that nonphysician providers should be under the supervision of a "physician leader," preferably a pediatrician. Patient care responsibilities can be "delegated" to other providers. This document links PNPs with massage therapists, homeopaths, naturopaths, and other alternative-care providers. This model is advocated as the only approach to care, regardless of community resources. "The AAP believes it is ill advised, even in underserved areas, to create a system of care that allows for the independent practice of nonphysician clinicians" (AAP Committee on Pediatric Workforce, 2003, p. 427).

Care by other members of the team would be "delegated" as the physician sees the need. This hierarchical model does not let parents participate in selecting the optimum provider for their child. Additionally, because the AAP asserts that it is "ill-advised" to allow for the independent practice of nonphysician clinicians—even in underserved areas, many children would be denied the most basic access to a competent and safe provider. For frontier states such as New Mexico, Montana, Wyoming, and Alaska, this position is tantamount to denying health care to many of the children living outside of the metropolitan areas in those states. In some sparsely populated counties, care may be available only through a single nurse practitioner.

Although the goal for every child to have a health home is laudable, there are still major gaps in access to care. Children living in rural communities, particularly in sparsely populated frontier states; children above the poverty line, yet uninsured and ineligible for State Children's Health Insurance Programs because their families make too much money, or because the program slots are filled; and children with special needs often have difficulty accessing care. Disparities in access to care are also evident in children of color, with African American and Hispanic children having lower rates of access to care than White children (Leatherman & McCarthy, 2004).

The State Children's Health Insurance Program (SCHIP) was developed in the 1990s. Initially this program enrolled children who were above the poverty line, with each state having varying entry criteria. The concept of SCHIP was to provide affordable health insurance to those families who did not meet Medicaid criteria for care. These families usually did not have employer-supported health insurance programs. For example, in a study in California it was found that children of working low-income parents were more likely to be uninsured than children of nonworking low-income parents and the non-poor (Guendelman, Wyn, & Tsai, 2000). Keane, Lave, Ricci, and LaVallee (1999) found that after being covered by SCHIP there was a decrease in delayed care and an increase in utilization and access for all ages, particularly for preteens and adolescents. The increase in access to care after SCHIP also has been supported by data from New York State (Holl et al., 2000). One of the major barriers to SCHIP is the application process, which has been described as "onerous" by one author (Davidoff, Garrett, Makuc, & Schirmer, 2000). Again, however, this varies by state, with some states having simple one-page applications and others having lengthy, complex applications that require verification of income. SCHIP has a great possibility of increasing family resources for access to health care. The question will be whether state and federal governments are willing to pay the price of these programs, even though they have been proven cost-effective over time.

INFLUENCE OF ACCESS TO HEALTH CARE FOR INFANTS, CHILDREN AND FAMILIES

The quality of life for children and families is influenced by access to health care. Children without access to health care have more emergency department visits, are less likely to be healthy and ready to learn when they enter school, and are more likely to have vision and dental problems. The challenges and consequences of lack of access to care are discussed in this section.

Access to Mental Health Services

Mental health services for children are also limited. First, there is a shortage of providers, particularly child psychiatrists (Semansky & Koyanagi, 2004). Second, the system is crisis oriented, which means preventive care or early intervention is not available (Semansky & Koyanagi, 2004). Because of limited resources through Medicaid and SCHIP, a choice may be made to cover more children but with less intensity. TennCare (Tennessee's Medicaid managed-care program) served more youths in their behavioral health system, but provided less intense treatment (Saunders & Heflinger, 2003). There also was a trend away from inpatient treatment during those years. Overall, there was "a shift from treatment to support services" (Saunders & Heflinger, 2003, p. 1369). According to Leatherman and McCarthy (2004), 79% of children with insurance, 73% of children with public insurance (Medicaid, SCHIP), and 87% of the uninsured children who needed mental health services did not receive it (p. 63). Only one study was found showing that school-based mental health services were effective when compared to traditional clinic care (Armbruster & Lichtman, 1999). These findings may reflect the lack of mental health services in the schools, as school psychologists are usually focused on testing rather than interventions and few school systems have mental health workers to provide services. Using schools as the base for mental health services could increase the accessibility for children and families and decrease the stigma of receiving mental health services, which still exists in some communities.

Disparities in mental health services occur with poor children and children of color and are also affected by geography. Hispanic children have the highest unmet needs. Using a sample of 13 states, Sturm, Ringel, and Andreyeva (2003) demonstrated the variation in availability of mental health services. As an example, children in California are three times more likely to have unmet needs as a child with a similar problem in Massachusetts. Sturm and colleagues concluded that the disparities that emerge from unmet needs were a result of state-driven factors rather than the demographic characteristics of the state. Much more information is needed to determine the most important precursors of service in a state that increases the quality of mental health services.

Access to Dental Care

Unmet dental needs are currently being addressed through various programs; however, the area is not as well developed as general health care. The data describing unmet dental needs are from the National Health Interview Survey. The question: "During the past 12 months, was there any time when [child's name] needed any of the following but didn't get it because you couldn't afford it: Dental care (including check-ups)?" This question has been used to determine where and how much dental care is needed.

Although tooth decay is recognized as one of the most prevalent chronic illnesses facing children in the United States today, there are many gaps in prevention and treatment, particularly for poor children (Casamassimo, 1996; Kenney, Ko, & Ormond, 2000; Seale & Casamassimo, 2003). There are many disparities in access to care based on such factors as age, race, family income, and access to health and dental insurance (Edelstein, 2002). Children living under 100% of the federal poverty level have twice the decay rate as children over the poverty level (Edelstein, 1998). In 2002, 16% of children without health insurance needed dental care but did not get it for financial reasons ("Unmet dental needs," n.d.).

The *Surgeon General's Report on Oral Health* (USDHHS, 2000b) identifies dental and oral diseases as a major threat to public health. Even with private insurance, 4% of the children have dental care needs as did 7% of those covered by Medicaid ("Unmet dental needs," n.d.). Children of color are even less likely to have their dental needs met with 31% of non-Hispanic Black children and 38% of Hispanic children between 2 to 17 years not having seen a dentist in the past year. Additionally, in 2002, 37% of children from poor families and 34% of children from non-poor families had not been to a dentist in a year, compared to 20% of children from non-poor families.

Part of the solution to the lack of access to care is the establishment of "dental homes" that are funded through private insurance and Medicaid or other public funds. However, there are also barriers to Medicaid dental care. They include provider participation, with only 1 in 6 dentists participating in Medicaid receiving $10,000 or more in Medicaid, indicating that few dentists participate in Medicaid for a great part of their practice. Reimbursement rates by Medicaid do not meet the costs of providing the service. Low reimbursement rates are confounded with the red tape of enrollment forms, billing forms, prior authorization requirements, eligibility determination problems, and other administrative problems. Medicaid patients have a greater number of broken appointments or no shows. Geographical barriers can be a major factor, with children living in rural states and low-income neighborhoods the least likely to have access to a dentist. Families where parents do not include dental hygiene as a part of their personal behaviors, as well as a lack of valuing of dental care, also may influence decisions not to enroll. Additionally, many dentists may elect not to enroll as providers of Medicaid Managed Dental Care, which also contributes to a lack of dental homes (Edelstein, n.d.).

The American Academy of Pediatric Dentistry (AAPD) policy on the dental home states the dental home should provide the following:

1. Comprehensive oral health care, including acute care and preventive series in accordance with AAPD periodicity schedules.
2. A comprehensive assessment for oral diseases and conditions.
3. An individualized preventive dental health program based upon a caries-risk assessment and a periodontal disease risk assessment.
4. Anticipatory guidance about growth and development issues (i.e., teething, digit or pacifier habits).
5. A plan for acute dental trauma.
6. Information about proper care of the child's teeth and gingivae. This would include the prevention, diagnosis, and treatment of disease of the supporting and surrounding tissues and the maintenance of health, function, and esthetics of those structures and tissues.
7. Dietary counseling.
8. Referrals to dental specialists when care cannot be provided directly within the dental home.
9. Education regarding future referral to a dentist knowledgeable and comfortable with adult oral health issues for continuing oral health care; referral at an age determined by patient, parent and pediatric dentist. (AAPD, Oral Health Policy on the Dental Home, 2004).

This comprehensive approach to dental care has not been made available to many children.

Access to Vision Care

Access to vision care has not been as well researched as access to dental care. The current issue of *Bright Futures* (Green & Palfrey, 2000) does not have a statement on vision care. Good epidemiological data on vision impairments in children are virtually nonexistent (Kemper, Cohn, & Dombkowski, 2004), although it is estimated that 2% to 5% of preschoolers have vision impairment. Universal vision screening for preschoolers has been recommended through the Project Universal Preschool Vision Screening (PUPVS) advisory body (AAP, n.d.). Kemper, Bruckman and Freed (2004) found that the incidence of corrective lenses increased as the child became older. They also found that boys were less likely to have corrective lenses than girls were and Hispanic children and Black children were less likely to have corrective lenses than White children were. Children with family incomes less than 200% of federal poverty level were also less likely to have corrective lenses. There are major gaps in knowledge about access to vision care and adequacy of the care that currently is implemented. There have been no proposals for a "vision home" similar to dental home or health care home. However the American Academy of Ophthalmology (2001) has developed a policy statement on vision screening for infants and children.

In discussing the issues of lack of access to medical, dental, vision, and mental health services, little concern is shown for the parents of children needing those services. Parents are rarely consulted by those who are developing standards or recommendations for care. Issues around companies that change insurance providers yearly, thus changing the eligibility of the primary care provider, are never addressed. Parents often are left out of the discussion when they need to be key members of the team making the decisions.

NURSING CARE EXCELLENCE

Access to health care is a challenging area for nurses to address. The health care systems vary by state and the child's eligibility may differ by state. Much of the literature on access to health care for children is from medical and health services literature. The focus on access to "health care" has been primarily a focus on access to medical care. Little attention has been given to a child's access to nursing care, vision care, dental care, or mental health services. To give children and families access to comprehensive health care takes a commitment of time, energy, and resources by the government as well as the providers. Nurses must become more visible as both providers of, and advocates for, access to health care for children. A model was developed, using the Health Care Quality guidelines or elements developed by AAN as a guide for developing comprehensive access to care.

With the many issues that children have in accessing health care, it is imperative that we develop new models of access to care for children and families. These models must insure that children and families have access to health care beyond the medical care and medical model implemented currently. The guidelines developed by the Expert Panel on Children and Families from the American Academy of Nursing can serve as the structure for a new model of access to care that is based on a family's strengths instead of identifying their deficits. This approach should encourage families to confide in their health care providers rather than fear them.

1. Children and youth have an identified health care home, which is selected by the parents and, if appropriate developmentally, the child. The parent and child (when appropriate) will select the health care provider. This provider includes pediatric nurse practitioners as the primary care provider. Parents and children will also have the freedom to select their vision, dental, and mental health care providers. This allows parents the option of identifying providers with whom they are satisfied and who address their questions and concerns.

2. Providers will establish a partnership with parents and children in decisions, planning, and delivery of care. A major consideration will be given to providers who give the parents and children sufficient information about the child's needs for health care.

3. A family's values, beliefs, and preferences are part of the care. This includes recognition of the cultural or religious rituals that may be unfamiliar to a provider with a Western medicine approach to health care.

4. Innovative approaches to the design of health care systems will improve accessibility to health care. The innovative approaches will include not only the physical placement of the facility, but also the types of providers accessible in those facilities. Children and families would have access to nursing, medical, dental, vision, social, and mental health services in a central location that is clean and safe. Although it is not reasonable to think that this will happen in all sparsely populated areas of the United States, centers can be set up within a reasonable drive from those isolated communities. Incentives could be given to providers who develop mobile approaches to serving isolated communities.

5. A commitment will be made to the concept that well-child care begins before conception. Improving preconception care and nutrition will lead to healthier babies, which leads to healthier children.

6. Health promotion and risk reduction will be included as a part of well-child care. This includes anticipatory guidance about growth and development and potential risk behaviors based on the child's developmental level. As the child moves into adolescence, this means having interactions with the provider to address activities such as drug usage, sexual activity, and mental health problems that may not emerge if the parents are in the room with the child and provider.

MULTIDISCIPLINARY INTEGRATION AND PARTNERSHIP: CASE STUDY

There are two major challenges to accessing health care that families in the United States face. First, transportation may be a challenge for families living in cities as well as in rural areas. In the city, it may be the lack of public transportation or bureaucratic rules that impede access to transportation, whereas in the rural areas, the challenge may be lack of transportation or distances so great that transportation is difficult and expensive. The second challenge is the lack of financing of health care for individuals above the poverty lines who have jobs that do not include health insurance. Two case studies are presented to illustrate these problems.

Case Study 1

Rosemary lives in a suburb of a small, southern, metropolitan town. She has three children—Rachel, 4; Jimmy, 2; and Susie, 6 months old. Susie has a congenital heart defect. She receives her care at the local children's hospital specialty clinic. All three children receive primary care at a teaching clinic staffed by nurse practitioners and their students, residents, and medical students. Rosemary was almost always late for Susie's well-child visits, as well as for her cardiac clinic visits. Appointments were usually made for Rosemary and her children without consultation about whether she had transportation or child care for the other children on the day of the appointment. As Rosemary seemed to be a very attentive and concerned parent, her lateness to appointments was difficult for the staff to understand. Rosemary agreed to work with a graduate nursing student, Teresa, who was learning case management skills.

Teresa decided that the way to find out what was causing Rosemary to be late was to go to her home and to go with her as she traveled to the clinic. Teresa found that although Rosemary could take the Medicaid van, it came early in the morning (around 7 a.m.) and even if her appointment was at 11 a.m. that was the only time she could be picked up by the van. The van would only take Rosemary and the child or children who had an appointment, meaning she had to find costly child care for her other children. It also meant Rosemary and her children were at the clinic for 4 to 5 hours at a time, requiring her either to pack snacks in addition to formula and diapers, or to purchase food with scarce resources. The system was not cooperative in scheduling multiple appointments for her children at the same time. Further investigation showed that Rosemary needed to walk six blocks with all three children to the nearest bus line. She then would have to take a bus to a central location where she changed buses to one that would take her to the university. If all connections were made in a timely manner, it averaged 2 hours on public transportation with three children under the age of 4. This trip would take 15 minutes in a car, which Rosemary did not have available to her. Difficulty in accessing adequate transportation is often viewed as a problem for individuals living in rural communities; however it can also be a problem for urban and suburban residents.

Case Study 2

Another form of difficulty in accessing care is the lack of family resources to pay for health care, yet having resources or income above the state cutoff line for Medicaid or SCHIP eligibility. The Smith family had health insurance through Mr. Smith's employment until 4 months ago when his company shifted production to China and he was laid off. Mr. Smith could buy COBRA at a cost of $839 a month. However, his unemployment benefits and severance pay brought in approximately $2000 monthly for the first 6 months of unemployment. The Smiths had owned their own home for 10 years and had equity in the home. With a projected annual income of $24,000 and the equity in the house, the Smiths made too much money for the local SCHIP program, although they placed their name on the waiting list. (It was estimated that when their benefits ran out they would still have a 12- to 18-month wait for space to become available in the program). If the Smiths purchased insurance under the COBRA plan, they would not have the money to make their house payment. The dilemma for the Smith family was to make the house payment or pay for health insurance. The Smiths had never received any type of what they considered government assistance in the past and were reluctant to attempt to enroll their children in SCHIP. Even if they could qualify, they believed they would have to "swallow their pride" in going on the waiting list for the program. Although they knew that their children should have regular checkups and worried about a catastrophic event like a major injury, they believed the best choice for their family was to keep their home.

Both of these case studies illustrate common difficulties in accessing health care for children in the United States. There are many issues around transportation and availability, both from the urban and suburban environment and the rural environment, and as noted previously, in frontier states transportation problems may be related to the total absence of roads, or the need to travel by boat, ferry, or airplane to access health care, including dental, eye, and specialty care for specific conditions. In frontier states, weather can also become a major problem, with some communities isolated by snow or ice for long periods of time in the winter. There may also be a lack of communication equipment in rural and frontier communities. Many areas of the United States still lack landline telephone service, much less cell phone access. In these areas, an emergency health need cannot be addressed in a timely manner.

Family finances are troublesome as a cause of lack of access to care. The United States is one of the wealthiest countries in the world. Children are our future, and their health and well-being should be a critical goal for the country. As a group, children are among the poorest individuals in the U.S. Insuring access to care is the beginning of insuring healthy and productive adult citizens.

SUMMARY

Providing safe and effective health care to children is a complex societal issue. First, our society needs to value children and their well-being. Second, resources must be made available to facilitate access to care. Third, recognition of the quality of care provided by diverse providers must be acknowledged. Finally, parents, children, and family members must be integral parts of the health care process and decision making if optimum quality health care is to be provided to children.

REFERENCES

American Academy of Ophthalmology. (2001). *Vision screening for infants and children: AAO policy statement*. Retrieved July 20, 2004, from http://www.medem.com

American Academy of Pediatrics. (n.d.). *Project Universal Preschool Vision Screening Fact Sheet*. Retrieved September 1, 2004, from http://www.medicalhomeinfo.org/screening/vision.html

American Academy of Pediatrics. (2002). Policy statement: The medical home. *Pediatrics, 110,* 184–186.

American Academy of Pediatrics, Committee on Pediatric Workforce. (2003).

Scope of practice issues in the delivery of pediatric health care. *Pediatrics, 111,* 426–435.

American Association of Pediatric Dentists. (2004). *Oral health policy on the dental home.* [Rev.] Retrieved July 16, 2004, from http://www.aapd.org/members/referencemanual/pdfs/02-03/P_DentalHome.pdf

Armbruster, P., & Lichtman, J. (1999). Are school based mental health services effective? Evidence from 36 inner city schools. *Community Mental Health Journal, 35,* 493–504.

Casamassimo, P. (1996). *Bright futures in practice: Oral health.* Arlington, VA: National Center for Education in Maternal and Child Health. Retrieved July 20, 2004, from http://www.brightfutures.org/oralhealth/pdf/index.html

Committee on Evaluation of Children's Health. (2004). *Children's health, the nation's wealth: Assessing and improving child health.* Prepublication copy retrieved September 3, 2004, from http://www.nap.edu/books/0309091187/html

Davidoff, A. J., Garrett, A. B., Makuc, D. M., & Schirmer, M. (2000). Medicaid-eligible children who don't enroll: Health status, access to care, and implications for Medicaid enrollment. *Inquiry, 37,* 203–218.

Edelstein, B. L. (2002). Disparities in oral health and access to care: Findings of national surveys. *Ambulatory Pediatrics, 2*(Suppl. 2), 141–147.

Edelstein, B. L. (June 1998). *Racial and income disparities in pediatric oral health.* Children's Dental Health Project. Retrieved July 19, 2004, from http://www.cdhp.org/downloads/Publications/Disease/racialdisparities.pdf

Edelstein, B. L. (n.d.). *At a glance disparities in access to pediatric dental care.* Retrieved July 19, 2004, from http://www.cdhp.org/downloads/factsheets/factsheet4.pdf

Green, M., & Palfrey, J. S. (Eds.). (2000). *Bright futures: Guidelines for health supervision of infants, children and adolescents* (2nd ed.). Arlington, VA: National Center for Education in Maternal and Child Health.

Guendelman, S., Wyn, R., & Tsai, Y. (2000). Children of working low-income families in California: Does parental work benefit children's insurance status, access, and utilization of primary health care? *HSR: Health Services Research, 35,* 417–441.

Holl, J. L., Szilagyi, P. G., Rodewald, L. E., Shone, L. P., Zwanziger, J., Mukamel, D. B., et al. (2000). Evaluation of New York State's Child Health Plus: Access, utilization, quality of health care, and health status. *Pediatrics, 105,* 711–718.

Institute of Medicine. (2002). *Report brief: Health insurance is a family matter.* Retrieved September 3, 2004, from http://www.iom.edu/file.asp?id=4161

Keane, C. R., Lave, J. R., Ricci, E. M., & LaVallee, C. P. (1999). The impact of children's health insurance program by age. *Pediatrics, 104,* 1051–1058.

Kemper, A. R., Bruckman, D., & Freed, G. L. (2004). Prevalence and distribution of corrective lenses among school-age children. *Optometry and Vision Science, 81,* 7–10.

Kemper, A. R., Cohn, L. M., & Dombkowski, K. J. (2004). Patterns of vision care among Medicaid-enrolled children. *Pediatrics, 113,* e190–e196.

Kenney, G. M., Ko, G., & Ormond, B. A. (April, 2000). *Gaps in prevention and treatment: Dental care for low-income children: A pre-CHIP baseline.*

Urban Institute, Series B, No. B-15. Retrieved July 20, 2004, from http://www.urban.org

Leatherman, S., & McCarthy, D. (April, 2004). *Quality of health care for children and adolescents: A chartbook.* New York: Commonwealth Fund.

Oxford English dictionary. [Online] (2004). Access. Retrieved November 19, 2004, from http://www.askoxford.com/concise_oed/access?view=uk

Saunders, R. C., & Heflinger, C. A. (2003). Access to and patterns of use of behavioral health services among children and adolescents in TennCare. *Psychiatric Services, 54,* 1364–1371.

Seale, N. S., & Casamassimo, P. S. (2003). Access to dental care for children in the United States: A survey of general practitioners. *Journal of the American Dental Association, 134,* 1630–1640.

Semansky, R. M., & Koyanagi, C. (2004). Child and adolescent psychiatry: Obtaining child mental health services through Medicaid: The experience of parents in two states. *Psychiatric Services, 55,* 24–25.

Sia, C., Tonniges, T. F., Osterhus, E., & Taba, S. (2004). History of the medical home concept. *Pediatrics, 113*(5 Suppl.), 1473–1478.

Sturm, R., Ringel, J. S., & Andreyeva, T. (2003). Geographic disparities in children's mental health care. *Pediatrics, 112,* e308–e315.

Unmet dental needs. (n.d.). Retrieved July 15, 2004, from http://www.childtrends-databank.org

U.S. Department of Health and Human Services. (2000a). *Healthy people 2010.* Washington, DC: U.S. Department of Health and Human Services. Retrieved July 19, 2004, from http://www.healthypeople.gov/

U.S. Department of Health and Human Services. (2000b). *Oral health in America: A report of the Surgeon General.* Washington, DC: U.S. Department of Health and Human Services. Retrieved July 19, 2004, from http://www.surgeongeneral.gov/library/oralhealth/

van Dyck, P. C. (2003). A history of child health equity legislation in the United States. *Pediatrics, 112*(3 pt. 2), 727–730.

CHAPTER THREE

Health Care Home: Ensuring Access to a Regular Health Care Provider

Julia Muennich Cowell
Kathryn Swartwout

INTRODUCTION, DEFINITIONS AND THEIR MEASUREMENT

The concept of *health care home* refers to a logical approach to assure access to care and elimination of health disparities. The reality of the health care home for children and families is yet to be achieved, as was described in the previous chapter. The challenges we face are related to provider issues, including competition, quality issues and coverage, and consumer choice. The concept is new in the literature and, in what literature there is, is typically referred to as "medical home." Despite the emergence of the term *medical home,* the term *health care home* was unanimously agreed upon by the Expert Panel on Children and Families from the American Academy of Nursing, rather than "medical home," which the panel felt was not inclusive of the disciplines or broad care required for comprehensive, continuous care of children and families. Despite the panel's resolve to utilize a broad, inclusive term, guidelines from agencies (Health Resources and Services Administration and Title V funders) are promulgating guidelines that have broad interdisciplinary input. For this chapter the term *health care home* is utilized whereas the literature usually refers to "medical home."

The enabling legislation of Title V of the Social Security Act (§§701-710, subchapter V, chapter 7, Title 42) provided funding to improve the health of mothers and children through the assurance of health care across the levels of prevention. Although the health and health care of all mothers and children is referenced, Title V underscores attention to maternal and child health services with special health care needs and to low-income families. The concept of health care home is implied through definitions related to care coordination and case management (Social Security Online, 2004).

HISTORICAL OVERVIEW

American Academy of Pediatrics (AAP)

In 1992, the AAP first proposed a definition for the medical home in a policy statement. But, according to Sia, Tonniges, Osterhus, and Taba (2004), the concept had been in the making since as early as 1967. Multiple AAP initiatives followed the 1992 statement including the Community Access to Child Health (CATCH) program, the Medical Home Training Program, and the establishment of the National Center of Medical Home Initiatives for Children with Special Needs (Sia et al., 2004). In 2002, a new AAP policy statement expanded and clarified the definition of the medical home. Presently, the AAP definition of the medical home includes medical care for all pediatric ages that is "accessible, continuous, comprehensive, family centered, coordinated, compassionate, and culturally effective" (AAP, 2002a). A 2004 AAP policy statement includes an operational definition of the medical home, including that all care given in the medical home be led by a designated primary care physician and provide 24-hour availability (AAP, 2004). The AAP believes the promotion of the medical home concept, when implemented correctly, will improve both quality and cost-effectiveness of medical care.

National Association of Pediatric Nurse Practitioners (NAPNAP)

NAPNAP agrees with and supports the medical home policy of the AAP, but with some exceptions. In a 2002 position statement, NAPNAP advocates for a pediatric health care home that is "accessible, comprehensive, coordinated, culturally sensitive and focused on the overall well-being of the child within the family" (NAPNAP, 2002). NAPNAP asserts that the pediatric nurse practitioner (PNP), working collaboratively with other providers, is an appropriate leader in a pediatric health care home. Recognizing the important role of PNPs in the provision of a health care home recognizes their professional expertise and promotes access to health care for all children.

Public Health Nursing

The concept of a health care home is not a new one although it is a contemporary label. Public health nursing has its roots in providing just such care for the medically underserved with guidelines spelled out for anticipatory guidance to primary care (American Public Health Association, 1955; Caplan, 1961; Pridham, 1993). However, decline in funding for public health has resulted in shrinking services provided by public health departments. Now, most public health organizations strive to maintain a safety net for services rather than provide direct nursing services or primary care services (Hawryluk, 2002).

School-Based Health Centers (SBHC)

The recent expansion of SBHC's throughout the United States is a direct response to the need to make high-quality health care more accessible to children and families. SBHCs have the following important components: "location within a school building, provision of comprehensive primary and mental health care, and interrelation of family, school and community" (Brellochs, Zimmerman, Zink, & English, 1996). Many SBHCs meet the NAPNAP criteria for a pediatric health care home. Schools are often the heart of a community. Usually conveniently located, schools are familiar to families, who frequent them regularly. Placing health care in a school building allows health care providers to work collaboratively with school personnel as well as other community resources that are frequently available in schools. Other common features of SBHCs include multidisciplinary teams of providers; links to local hospitals, health departments, or other medical practices; and the presence of an advisory board with broad community representation (National Assembly on School-Based Health Care, n.d.).

Community Health Centers

Community health centers are privately operated, not-for-profit entities that have been delivering primary care to medically underserved groups since the 1960s. Community health centers must meet certain federal requirements provided in the U.S. Public Health Service Act (U.S. Public Health Service, 1994) that include having a board of directors comprised of health-center users by at least 51% and thus representing the voice of the community. Community health centers are also referred to as

Federally Qualified Health Centers (FQHCs). According to the National Association of Community Health Centers, FQHCs are currently medical home to 15 million people in the United States, with about half of these residing in rural areas (National Association of Community Health Centers, 2004).

Managed Care

Many insurance plans such as health maintenance organizations (HMOs) and preferred provider organizations (PPOs) may promote the health care home concept to their enrollees by requiring their subscribers to select a primary care provider within a specified provider network and promoting preventive care while discouraging only episodic care (Hughes & Luft, 1998). Often the provider is then mandated to act as a "gatekeeper" for all other health services the subscriber needs to access. This gatekeeper role includes initiating consultations and approving referrals.

Health care delivery models of managed care have been in existence since the nineteenth century. Before the 1970s, various physicians and employer groups throughout the U. S. experimented successfully with managed care. The modern HMO movement began in 1971 with the support of federal grants and loans from the Nixon Administration. Employers with 25 or more employees were required to offer an HMO option to their employees at the HMO's request. In the 1990s, Medicaid added a managed care choice (Tufts Managed Care Institute, 1998). Currently 184.7 million Americans are enrolled in a managed care insurance program (MCOL, 2004).

State Child Health Insurance Plans

The Balanced Budget Act of 1997, signed by President Clinton, created a new program called the State Children's Health Insurance Program (SCHIP). SCHIPs provide health insurance for medically uninsured families with incomes too high to qualify for Medicaid, thus expanding the number of families that can gain access to a health care home. As of the end of the first fiscal quarter of 2004, there were 3.7 million enrollees in state child health insurance programs (Centers for Medicare and Medicaid Services [CMS], 2004).

Looking Towards the Future

Health care home as a nursing concept has been evolving for at least 20 years. Innovative models of primary care delivery and modern health insurance initiatives are indicative of endeavors toward making the health care home concept viable. Nursing, with its strong history of public health involvement and advocacy for all, can and will be integral in creating the reality of a health care home for every American.

INFLUENCES OF CORE ELEMENT FOR INFANTS AND CHILDREN

Related Theoretical Framework

A variety of frameworks provide direction for studying health care access related to health care homes (Aday, 2001; Green & Kreuter, 1999). Common concepts among the models are the concepts of reinforcing and enabling factors. Reinforcing factors refer to those feedback factors that encourage or discourage health care utilization and ultimately the identification of a health care home. They include provider attitudes and behaviors that foster a positive patient/provider relationship. Enabling factors include structural factors such as access, policies related to practice, and office hours that indicate openness to patients and families. Theoretically, those factors suggest that service delivery that is responsive to the needs of the population should provide adequate assurance of a health care home. The results of efforts to increase access through system changes are mixed, as evaluated by a number of measures including immunization rates, satisfaction, and emergency room use.

Synthesis of Literature in the Area

Research utilizing the health care home concept is in its fledgling stages. A computer search using the Ovid Web Gateway of both the MEDLINE and CINAHL databases (1996 and onward) conducted in August 2004, found no pertinent literature related to the "health care home" concept. The same search of the "medical home" concept resulted in 87 hits, 72 of which had relevance to the AAP medical home concept.

Does Having a Health Care Home Improve Health?

A recent literature review (Starfield & Shi, 2004) reports evidence of improved health in a variety of population groups with access to a medical home. However, this is not consistently the case. Childhood immunizations rates are frequently used as one childhood health indicator. Using an operational definition of the AAP medical home concept, Ortega and colleagues (2000a) found that young children (aged 6 to 48 months) with a medical home did not necessarily have better immunization coverage rates than those who did not have a medical home. Among the study's limitations, the authors acknowledge the difficulties in operationalizing the definition of the medical home and the need to test further the performance of the medical home measure used in the study. In another study, Cunningham and Trude (2001) reported that having a "usual physician" reduced the number of unmet health needs. However, the effect was inconsistent between population groups being less for the uninsured than for the insured.

Does Having a Health Care Home Improve Access?

Many barriers exist to health care access for children. Ortega and colleagues (2000b) studied the perceptions of children's caregivers, all of whom had structural access to a group of children's clinics located in Delaware that were specifically designed as medical homes. Using the 5-item Short Medical Home Index as a measure of the medical home concept, they found that insurance status and race were significantly associated with access perceptions. Specifically, Whites people and those with private insurance had higher perceptions of perceived access to a medical home than did Black individuals and those who were uninsured or on Medicaid.

Do State Insurance Programs Have an Impact on Medical Home Utilization?

State child health insurance plans (SCHIPs) allow uninsured children from low-income families that do not financially qualify for Medicaid to obtain health insurance. Each state manages its own plan. One retrospective study of a state health insurance plan found that enrollment in the plan increased health maintenance visits, shifted immunization location to the medical home, and increased utilization of the medical home rather than emergency room services (Kempe et al., 2000). Similarly, in a recent literature review of studies related to costs and effectiveness of a medical home, Starfield and Shi (2004) conclude that having insurance is not a guarantee that a child will have a medical home, but certainly increases that probability.

Special Needs or Vulnerable Populations

It makes sense that children with special needs or from vulnerable population groups would particularly benefit from a health care home model. This includes children of low-income families, children in foster care, and children with chronic illness or disability. Much of the published research on medical homes focuses on children with special health care needs.

Kempe and colleagues (2000) found that children enrolled in a state managed care plan for children of low income utilized their medical care home for most acute care needs rather than emergency rooms and had a higher mean number of health maintenance visits (1.2 visits) than did children with traditional Medicaid (0.8 visits) or private insurance (1.0 visits).

Using an operational definition of medical home based on five essential medical home elements, McPherson and colleagues (2004) found that 52.6% of children with special health care needs met all the outcome criteria for having received care in a medical home. Antonelli and Antonelli (2004) examined the cost to a medical home for unreimbursable care coordination services for children with special health care needs. They found that children with special health care needs consumed 4 times more staff time than other patients and that most of this time was spent in nontypical medical care such as working with educational programs. Gupta, O'Connor, and Quezada-Gomez (2004) report that in their random mailed survey of AAP members, fewer than one fourth report always contacting the school as part of care coordination for children with special health care needs.

One goal of *Healthy People 2010* (U. S. Department of Health and Human Services [DHHS], 1999) is for all children with special needs to have a medical home. The AAP National Center of Medical Home Initiatives for Children with Special Needs provides support and training to enable the provision of medical homes to children with special needs. The AAP also especially advocates for the designation of a medical home for children in foster care whose needs are often complex (AAP, 2002b).

INFLUENCES OF CORE ELEMENT FOR THE FAMILY

Related Theoretical Framework

A variety of family theories address family functioning and adaptation. Further family models usually identify the functioning and adaptation in the face of stress. For example, the Resiliency Model of Family Adjustment and Adaptation (McCubbin, Thompson, & McCubbin, 1996) provides a view of family functioning in the face of stress and directs attention to a broad system of interpersonal relationships, development, well-being and spirituality, and community relationships in the context of family structure and function. Such a framework would direct an analysis of the effect of the health care home on family functioning. Another approach might be to explore system gaps that inhibit resilience in family functioning.

Synthesis of Literature in the Area

Do Providers Want to Provide the HealthCare Home Model to Families?

In recent years, some patients receiving Medicaid have been moved into managed care programs that promote provision of primary care services from one medical provider source (CMS, 2004). This model of care was designed to improve access and quality of care, and to lower costs by increasing Medicaid patients' utilization of a primary care provider and avoiding the higher cost of specialty and emergency room care. One study of this type of Medicaid managed care program found that implementation of the program was associated with a reduction in the number of participating physicians in certain regions of Alabama and Georgia (Adams, Bronstein, & Florence, 2003). Multiple reasons might exist for physician providers to avoid participating in a program of this sort, including low reimbursement rates and the lack of knowledge, systems, or other resources necessary to provide a health care home.

Does Having a Health Care Home Improve Access for all Families?

Managed care insurance plans play a predominant force in the provision of medical care in the United States today. A major concept behind most managed care plans is the selection of a primary care provider who then coordinates all care for that member. The good intentions of a managed care plan—to improve quality of care while keeping high costs at bay—are similar to the AAP's medical care concept. Litaker and Cebul (2003) investigated a large sample of adults residing in Ohio and report "an important trend in the prevalence of access problems across all insurance categories as managed care activity increases" (p. 1093). Similarly, a study of a national cross-sectional sample of U.S. households found that communities with higher rates of managed care activity were associated with lower rates of uninsured persons reporting a usual source of care or a usual physician, thus concluding that managed care may have unintended effects on the uninsured (Cunningham & Trude, 2001).

NURSING CARE EXCELLENCE

Nurses, at all levels of preparation, play an important role in the creation and maintenance of the health care home concept. School nurses play a central role in assuring continuity of care, and partner in the provision of the health care home for children through the coordination of services (National Association of School Nurses, 2001). School nursing services are not universal; however, children in schools without school nurses are at risk for inconsistent services. Because of their advanced training in primary care, nurse practitioners can provide ideal leadership for delivering the health care home. Similarly, clinical nurse specialists in most specialties provide for continuity of care and, by definition of coordination of services, contribute to the identification and support of the health care home.

In all roles, nurses need to assure that care is culturally competent and focused on closing the gap of health disparities. The Office of Minority Health (OMH) refers to culturally competent care as *culturally and linguistically appropriate services* (CLAS). In their final report on Standards for Culturally and Linguistically Appropriate Services (OMH, 2001), experts outline factors referring to the delivery of services and how services are received. Underlying the delivery of services, the experts call attention to organizations' and their employees' sensitivity to consumers who are diverse both culturally and linguistically. From the consumer perspective, needs and preferences are diverse and must be recognized.

Advocating for Care

Nurses must advocate for and identify a health care home for all family members, regardless of insurance status. Nurses are cognizant of the fact that the health of every member of the family impacts the health of the children. All nurses should be aware of the resources in their communities, particularly those that are accessible to the uninsured or underinsured. Nurses interact with consumers at various entry points in the health care system. Regardless of entry point, nurses should assess the family for evidence of a health care home for every member. If homes do not exist, the nurse can assist the family in connecting each member with an appropriate home. If homes are identified, the nurse can make sure that pertinent information about the present encounter is relayed back to that home.

Supporting the Delivery of Care via Multidisciplinary Teams

The needs of families are often complex and varied, and one provider type cannot meet every need a family may present with. Likewise, the health care home concept cannot be carried out by a single individual or provider type. The ideal cost-effective team includes a nurse practitioner and physician working collaboratively. A social worker should also be readily accessible, if not immediately available. Registered nurses (RNs), dieticians, and health educators are other helpful additions to the team. Links to specialists, mental health workers, physical and occupational therapists, and academic experts are essential.

Creating Effective Communication Systems and Partnerships for Each Family

The health care home should provide each family with a designated "care partner." This person partners with the family in facilitating access to appropriate services and making choices about health care treatment options. The partnership aspect of this relationship is emphasized. The care partner should not mandate a certain scenario of care, but rather support the family in decision-making processes. The credentials of the designated care partner may vary depending on the health care home setting. The care partner must be someone who is easily accessible and known to the family. The care partner should be familiar with the family's medical and social history and capable of making and carrying out medical decisions so as not to hamper efficiency of care. Ideally, but not necessarily, the care partner is a primary care provider. Multiple means for communicating with the care partner should be offered to families: phones with voice-mail boxes, e-mail, fax, and the postal system.

Enabling a Central Location for Medical Records

The health care home must be proactive in assisting the family in gathering records. This often proves to be a major hurdle for families for a myriad of reasons. At times, families are too overwhelmed with other priorities to keep track of essential records or they have simply gotten lost in frequent moves. Children are sometimes moved from one household to another and their current caregivers have no knowledge of where the children previously received care. Nurses can act as "detectives," sleuthing out old medical records by calling previously attended schools or clinics in the neighborhoods where children lived. Pharmacies can be excellent sources for finding out what medications a child has previously received. When doing so, nurses should obtain written consents for requesting medical records in accordance with HIPAA regulations.

Involving Family Members and Individualizing Care

Nontraditional family structures are pervasive in today's society. Only about half (51.7%) of U.S. households are traditional married-couple households (U.S. Census Bureau, 2001). Single-parent families, grandparenting families, same-gender parents, and involvement of nonrelatives in a child's care are not uncommon. About 12% of U.S. households are families maintained by single women (U.S. Census Bureau, 2001). It is important to ascertain who makes up the entire child's family and involve those people. The health care home must also recognize that no two families are alike, and thus no one system of care will meet the needs of every family.

Being an Expert at Knowing Community Resources

Community programs and resources are in a constant state of flux particularly in the present day environment where funding priorities come and go. It is important for the providers in the health care home to be knowledgeable about community resources and the logistics for accessing them. Many communities have networks of local agencies that meet regularly. The optimally functioning health care home will be an active part of such a network. It is helpful to maintain a current list of contacts at agencies in the community that is readily available to all staff in the health care home.

Being an Expert on State and Federal Policies, Regulations, and Programs

State and federal policies affect practically every aspect of medical care. Confidentiality, reporting of abuse, dispensing of medications, and laboratory licensure are just a few examples of areas where laws regulate practice. State funding for programs such as childhood immunizations and sexually transmitted infection testing may be available. The health care home must develop systems for keeping abreast of legal and regulatory changes that impact practice or that may have benefits for their clientele.

Inclusion of Quality Monitoring

The health care home needs an organized system in place for monitoring the provision of quality care. In such a system, a systematic review process regularly generates recommendations for the improvement of care. All staff, both clerical and professional, can actively participate in the process. Minimally, indicators representing accessibility of appointments and providers, customer satisfaction, and basic health indicators (such as immunization rates) are measured annually.

Tracking Preventive Care

The health care home has systems in place for assisting families in tracking preventive care. There are many systems available for tracking physical exams, immunizations, and routine testing. Growth and academic and behavioral developments are also indicators that ideally are tracked.

Providing Comprehensive Primary Care

The health care home must be able to provide comprehensive primary care services for children of all ages. These services include preventive care plus assessment and treatment for uncomplicated acute and chronic illnesses. Preferably, basic lab testing facilities and mental health services are available on-site. Comprehensive care for adolescents should be available and teens should not be referred to other providers for basic reproductive health issues such as pregnancy and sexually transmitted infections (STI) testing, which fragments care and follow-up.

Working With the Schools

A health care home for children needs to include a relationship with the child's school. Schools that provide school nursing services expect the school nurse to partner with the families to ensure communication of essential health information in order to maximize learning potential. In schools without school nursing services, families can be encouraged to share any academic or behavioral concerns with the health care home. When concerns are expressed, the health care home should request a partnering meeting with school nurses or designated school personnel and family members. If appropriate, older children should be present at the meeting to include their input.

Providing Creative Solutions for Those Who Are Uninsured

In 2002, 11.4% of all children in the United States were uninsured (DeNavas-Walt, Proctor, & Mills, 2004). Many of these children come from families that do not receive child state health insurance coverage due to nonqualifying family income levels, illegal immigrant status, or personal choice. Parents or guardians frequently move in and out of insurance coverage due to changes in employment status. COBRA coverage (an extension of health care benefits made available after leaving a place of employment) is often unaffordable when a family becomes unemployed. Nurses working in health care homes must think creatively to assist families in maintaining their relationship with the health care home during uninsured periods. Nurses can advocate for sliding scale fee-for-service and deferred monthly payment plans. Nurses can seek external funds through federal, state, and private-program grants to assist in covering costs incurred in providing services to uninsured families. Foundations such as Blue Cross Blue Shield and Robert Wood Johnson prioritize funding to programs for uninsured Americans. Private local businesses or community foundations may be willing to respond to requests for funds to assist local families in maintaining their health care home. Nurses can assist families in identifying health insurance options for which they may qualify, such as state child health insurance. Families are often unaware that many state plans offer multiple options, including rebates for traditional plan costs and coverage for the adult caregivers. Nurses can arrange for money-management seminars to assist families in budgeting for health care coverage. Families are frequently simply unaware of the options available to them, and when provided with the correct information can find the means at least to purchase catastrophic coverage.

Providing Support During Periods of Transition

Families face multiple transitional periods during normal development. Examples include marriage, the birth of a child or death of a family member, a move to a new geographical location, and the transition of a teen to adulthood. These transitions often include changes in the health care needs of family members. The pediatric health care home must continually be aware of the repercussions these transitions have for all family members. The health care home should be responsive to and supportive of these transitional periods.

Nurses should ask about the status of all family members at routine well-child visits. Information and resources can be provided when necessary. For example, a new mother can be screened in the pediatric office for postpartum depression and connected with local parenting support groups. "Sandwich generation" adults who are caring for aging parents as well as their own children can be referred to organizations that offer caregiver support or respite services. College-bound teens can be assisted in transitioning to an existing college health service or appropriate medical provider in their new locale. Records can be proactively sent to the new provider rather than waiting for an urgent request at the time the records are actually needed.

Working With Families With Special Needs

The AAP specifically addresses the need for medical homes for children with special needs in order to meet the goal of *Healthy People 2010* that "all children with special health care needs will receive regular ongoing comprehensive care within a medical home" (DHHS, 1999). To this end, the AAP has established a National Center of Medical Home Initiatives for Children with Special Needs to advocate for medical homes and provide education and networking.

Assisting Families in Becoming Independent, Informed Health Care Consumers

Pediatric health care providers often complain about the lack of involvement and lack of decision-making abilities of the families they serve. There are many reasons why families may appear unconcerned with their children's welfare including time constraints, lack of knowledge, lack of resources, poor communication skills, and lack of trust.

Nurses recognize that families do care about their children's health and find solutions to allow families to become proactively involved in their care. Nurses can assist families by advocating for family-friendly office hours and easy-access office locations. Free parking, on-site lab testing, and nearby pharmacies all increase convenience and compliance. Important prescriptions may not get filled simply because a family has no means of transportation or a parent does not want to sit and wait in the pharmacy with a sick child in tow.

All families are capable of making choices. Even small choices increase feelings of importance and involvement. Choices promote self-efficacy. The health care home involves parents as partners in care. A parent with a child with mild iron-deficiency anemia can be given the choice of taking a supplement versus a month's trial of a higher-iron diet. Parents can be given choices about the timing of immunizations so long as they stay within recommended standards. Teens can be given choices about rewards and consequences in the treatment of behavior problems such as chronic school tardiness; they can be offered choices in treatment modalities for medical issues such as acne or in choosing a smoking cessation program.

Putting trust in the health care home can be difficult for families who have experienced years of mistreatment from the heath care system. These experiences may include waiting for hours (sometimes an entire day) in public health institutions only to receive a cursory exam and referral to another clinic. Stories abound of lost medical, x-ray, or lab records, disrespectful office staff, and unreturned phone messages. The health care home must consistently eliminate these barriers to care in order to build trust. Office staff must be trained in public relations and a policy formulated that allows easy phone access and the timely return of phone calls. Family members may be very amenable to waiting a day or two for a return phone call or for an appointment for a nonurgent problem if they are simply given a reasonable explanation for why the provider is currently unavailable.

Last, nurses can help families develop appropriate skills for communicating with their primary providers. Parents can be encouraged to bring lists of questions and concerns to appointments or be given checklists by the reception staff that are completed while waiting for appointments. Nurses should directly address children of all ages, encouraging them to describe their symptoms. Nurses can hold seminars or give out printed materials that teach families how to make the most of a primary care visit despite time constraints.

Generating Nursing Research Related to Health Care Home Concept

Research is necessary to support the adoption and expansion of the health care home concept. Nurses need continually to seek health-enhancing solutions for all population groups. In relation to the health care home, there are many questions still to be answered. What is the best service delivery model for a health care home? Will the health care home concept work for all population groups? What cultural issues must be considered in designing and implementing a health care home?

MULTIDISCIPLINARY INTEGRATION AND PARTNERSHIP: CASE STUDY

DJ, 14 years old, presented in a school-based health center (SBHC) for a school entry physical after the boy's grandmother came in mid school-year to register him for classes. He was medically uninsured and had no immunization or other medical records. DJ was currently living with his grandmother after getting thrown out of his aunt's home. He had no knowledge of his parents' whereabouts. He had lived at other times with various family members and had attended five different schools. He had never been in state care. His grandmother was running a home day-care.

DJ stated he had a history of ADHD. He took Ritalin "when he could get it" and felt it really helped. His aunt had taken him to a local pediatrician recently for a medication refill. Unfortunately, DJ was unable to fill the medication due to the cost, and no assistance was offered. On physical exam, DJ was friendly and well groomed. His physical exam was normal with the exception of his being overweight, a mildly elevated blood pressure, and decreased visual acuity.

Working with DJ and his grandmother, the nurse practitioner seeing DJ coordinated a prioritized problem list and plan. Phone calls were made to previous schools, and immunization records obtained. School entry requirements were completed the same day. A social worker immediately began the process of obtaining state child health insurance for both DJ and his grandmother (who also qualified for the insurance in this particular state because she was DJ's caregiver). His medication was filled by using an emergency fund for that purpose. Arrangements were made for academic consultation with school officials, ongoing counseling, an urgent optometry exam, and a dental referral. His grandmother was referred to a grandparents' parenting support group. At subsequent visits, a health-promotion plan for weight loss and blood pressure control was created.

The SBHC provided a health care home for DJ. Medical, psychological, social, and academic issues were addressed in a coordinated comprehensive plan. Knowledgeable staff assisted the family in navigating the school system and utilizing local community resources.

SUMMARY

This chapter has highlighted the origins of the concept of medical home by the American Academy of Pediatrics and the subsequent adoption of the health care home concept by the Expert Panel on Children and Families from the American Academy of Nursing. Both approaches are directed to maximizing the care of children and family and can be viewed as complementary. Although much current work is focused on children with special needs, ultimately the concept of health care home will be available to all children. The research for the future should not only analyze the outcomes of care for those with a health care home, but also identify the barriers to developing a health care home.

REFERENCES

Adams, E. K., Bronstein, J. M., & Florence, C. S. (2003). The impact of Medicaid primary care case management on office-based physician supply in Alabama and Georgia. *Inquiry, 40,* 269–282.

Aday, L. A. (2001). *At risk in America* (2nd ed.). San Francisco: Jossey-Bass.

American Academy of Pediatrics Medical Home Initiatives for Children with Special Needs Project Advisory Committee. (2002a). The medical home (pt. 1). *Pediatrics, 110,* 184–186.

American Academy of Pediatrics. (2002b). Health care of young children in foster care. *Pediatrics, 109,* 536–541.

American Academy of Pediatrics Medical Home Initiatives for Children with Special Needs Project Advisory Committee. (2004). Policy statement: Organizational principles to guide and define the child health care system and/or improve the health of all children. *Pediatrics, 113*(Suppl. 5), 1545–1547.

American Public Health Association, Inc. (1955). *Health supervision of young children.* New York: Author.

Antonelli, R. C., & Antonelli, D. M. (2004). Providing a medical home: The cost of care coordination services in a community-based, general pediatric practice. *Pediatrics, 113*(Suppl. 5), 1522–1528.

Brellochs, C., Zimmerman, D., Zink, T., & English, A. (1996). School-based primary care in a managed care environment: Options and issues. *Adolescent Medicine, 7,* 197–206.

Caplan, G. (1961). *An approach to community mental health.* New York: Grune & Stratton.

Centers for Medicaid and Medicare Services. (2004). *Medicaid managed care.* Retrieved October 13, 2004, from http://www.cms.hhs.gov/medicaid/managedcare/default.asp

Centers for Medicare and Medicaid Services. (2004). *SCHIP enrollment report.* Retrieved July 7, 2004, from http://www.cms.hhs.gov/schip/enrollment

Cunningham, P. J., & Trude, S. (2001). Does managed care enable more low income persons to identify a usual source of care? Implications for access to care. *Medical Care, 39,* 716–726.

DeNavas-Walt, C., Proctor, B. D., & Mills, R. J. (2004). *Income, poverty, and health insurance coverage in the United States: 2003.* Retrieved November 4, 2004, from http://www.census.gov/prod/2004pubs/p60-226.pdf

Green, L., & Kreuter, M. (1999). *Health promotion planning: An educational and ecological approach* (3rd ed.). Mountain View, CA: Mayfield.

Gupta, V. B., O'Connor, K. G., & Quezada-Gomez, C. (2004). Care coordination services in pediatric practices. *Pediatrics, 113*(Suppl. 5), 1517–1521.

Hawryluk, J. (2002). *Legislation authorizes spending for community health centers and the National Health Service Corps.* Retrieved July 21, 2004, from http://www.ama-assn.org/amednews/2002/11/11/gvsa1111.htm

Hughes, D. C., & Luft, H. S. (1998). Managed care and children: An overview. *Future of Children, 8,* 25–38.

Kempe, A., Beaty, B., Englund, B. P., Roark, R. J., Hester, N., & Steiner, J. F. (2000). Quality of care and use of the medical home in a state-funded capitated primary care plan for low-income children. *Pediatrics, 105,* 1020–1028.

Litaker, D., & Cebul, R. D. (2003). Managed care penetration, insurance status, and access to health care. *Medical Care, 41,* 1086–1095.

McCubbin, H., Thompson, A., & McCubbin, M. (1996). *Family assessment: Resiliency, coping and adaptation.* Madison: University of Wisconsin Press.

MCOL. (2004). *Managed care national statistics.* Retrieved July 11, 2004, from http://www.mcareol.com/factshts/factnati.htm

McPherson, M., Weissman, G., Strickland, B. B., van Dyck, P. C., Blumberg, S. J., & Newacheck, P. W. (2004). Implementing community-based systems of services for children and youths with special health care needs: How well are we doing? *Pediatrics, 113*(Suppl. 5), 1538–1544.

National Assembly on School-Based Health Care (n.d.). *About SBHC.* Retrieved June 13, 2004, from http://www.nasbhc.org

National Association of Community Health Centers. (2004). *About health centers.* Retrieved June 20, 2004 from http://www.nachc.com/about/aboutcenters.asp

National Association of Pediatric Nurse Practitioners. (2002). *NAPNAP position statement on the pediatric health care home.* Retrieved June 13, 2004, from http://www.napnap.org/practice/positions/healthcarehome.html

National Association of School Nurses. (2001). *Scope and standards of professional school nursing practice.* Washington, DC: American Nurses Publishing.

Office of Minority Health. (2001). *National standards for culturally and linguistically appropriate services in health care: Final report.* Retrieved July 26, 2004, from http://www.omhrc.gov/inetpub/wwwroot/omh/programs/2pg-program   38s/cultural4.htm

Ortega, A. N., Stewart, D. C., Dowshen, S. A., & Katz, S. H. (2000a). The impact of a pediatric medical home on immunization coverage. *Clinical Pediatrics, 39,* 89–96.

Ortega, A. N., Stewart, D. C., Dowshen, S. A., & Katz, S. H. (2000b). Perceived access to pediatric primary care by insurance status and race. *Journal of Community Health, 25,* 481–493.

Pridham, K. F. (1993). Anticipatory guidance of parents of new infants: Potential contribution of the internal working model construct. *Image: Journal of Nursing Scholarship, 25,* 49–56.

Sia, C., Tonniges, T. F., Osterhus, E., & Taba, S. (2004). History of the medical home concept. *Pediatrics, 113*(Suppl. 5), 1473–1478.

Social Security Online. (2004). *Authorization of appropriations.* Retrieved October 27, 2004, from http://www.ssa.gov/OP_Home/ssact/title05/0501.htm

Starfield, B., & Shi, L. (2004). The medical home, access to care, and insurance: A review of evidence. *Pediatrics, 113*(Suppl. 5), 1493–1498.

Tufts Managed Care Institute. (1998). *A brief history of managed care.* Retrieved June 13, 2004, from http://www.thci.org/downloads/BriefHist.pdf

U.S. Census Bureau. (2001). *Households and families: 2000.* Retrieved October 13, 2004, from http://www.census.gov/prod/2001pubs/c2kbr01-8.pdf

U.S. Department of Health and Human Services. (1999). *Healthy people 2010.* Retrieved July 24, 2004, from http://www.healthypeople.gov

U.S. Public Health Service. (1994). *U.S. Public Health Services Act. Bethesda:* U.S. Department of Health and Human Services.

CHAPTER FOUR

Family Partnerships in Nursing Care

Janet A. Deatrick

INTRODUCTION, DEFINITIONS, AND THEIR MEASUREMENT

Although the ideal of family-centered care has existed for many years, nurses who are engaged in clinical practice, research, teaching, and policy initiatives with families often lack the evidence, organizational support, and standards for research or science policy to fully realize its potential contribution to their work (Biester & Velsor-Friedrich, 1998; Meister, 1998). Current ideas about family partnerships promise to operationalize family-centered care more fully. The purposes of this chapter are to provide a working definition of partnering with families; describe the potential outcomes of family partnerships; describe an example of a nursing care model that can form the basis for partnerships with families; and illustrate one example of partnering with families using a case study.

Society became concerned about the health of children in the United States by the 1880s because of industrialization, urbanization, and massive immigration. The suffering and death of high-risk infants and children stemmed from contagion and infectious diseases and influenced the development of the modern child-health movement. Throughout the years, nurses translated complex clinical knowledge and scientifically based evidence into practical solutions for these problems in community, school, home, outpatient, and hospital settings.

Today's social and health care agenda for families is being sparked by complex clinical and scientific evidence concerning genetics, health disparities, poverty, environmental degradation, and terrorism. Nurses are increasingly turning to interdisciplinary models of research and clinical practice in order to find solutions for many of these problems. Family partnerships are an important building block for these family-centered initiatives (Brodie, 1998; National Institutes of Health, n.d.).

Partnering with families has been promoted as an ideal for nurses and health care professionals, yet the term is not usually defined. Most broadly defined, partnering with families means that nurses and other health care professionals are engaged in a process with children and their families that is oriented toward promoting the mutual trust between the provider and the family in order to achieve health for the family as well as its individual members. Therefore, the emphasis is on an evolving process and an outcome of health not only for individuals but also for the family as a unit.

The paradigm shift inherent in this process is that the family is seen as an active partner or collaborator in the process, not as a passive recipient of the professional's expertise. This process is facilitated by federal, state, and local community policies that enable families to survive and thrive; social and health care organizations that support employees and volunteers to provide family-centered care; positive working relationships between health care professionals, children, and their families; and research that is designed to further our understanding of related processes and outcomes. Partnerships between health care professionals and families are important for all families and especially crucial for at-risk and potentially vulnerable families and their children, including those children with special health care needs (CSHCN). Such partnerships are built on concordance between the health care provider and the family, including assumptions regarding the need for an egalitarian relationship, reality, understanding, trust, and transparency. In fact, one could make the case that discourse about family partnerships is a profound change of rhetoric that has certainly been part of nursing's agenda, but now is firmly embedded in our national health care agenda and in the international policy agenda (Bissell, May, & Noyce, 2004).

Federal, State, and Local Community Policies

Families with children who are seriously or chronically ill are subject to many emotional, social, physical, and financial difficulties. Federal, state, and local communities are constantly challenged to create, implement, and evaluate policies and programs designed to enable families not only to survive these difficulties, but also to thrive. The Institute of Medicine's (IOM) report entitled *Crossing the Quality Chasm* in fact makes many recommendations about the health care system that can be related to fostering family partnerships and ameliorating these difficulties, including (a) access to care on a continuous basis; (b) care customized to family needs and values; (c) control resides in the patient/family; (d) knowledge is shared and communication freely flows; (e) decision making, performance, and satisfaction/dissatisfaction are transparent; and (f) needs are anticipated rather than only reacting to them (IOM, 2003). Related national health policy initiatives include the dissemination of guidelines for child and family health supervision and the financing of health and social programs for vulnerable populations of children and their families.

The U.S. Department of Health and Human Services (DHHS) Maternal and Child Health Bureau (MCHB) now defines CSHCN as those with chronic physical, developmental, behavioral, and emotional conditions that result in an increased need or use of health and related services. *Healthy People 2010* charges states and territories to put in place service systems for all CSHCN by 2010 (McPherson et al., 2004).

Although such policy initiatives are promising, poor and marginalized children and their families lack a political voice and, therefore, are vulnerable to changes in health and social programs linked to entitlements. For instance, a new definition of disability and eligibility for Social Security Income (SSI) and Medicaid health care benefits resulted in many children with special health care needs being disallowed eligibility for SSI and Medicaid because they are no longer deemed to have marked or severe functional limitations (Doolittle, 1998). Even if children meet the new eligibility requirements, the determination process may discourage the parents of eligible children from applying and use of appropriate and needed services to decrease.

In addition, many families with children who qualify for state Title V CSHCN Programs are also enrolled in state Medicaid plans that are increasingly based in managed care. Although such programs promise to decrease care fragmentation and increase access to a medical home/primary health care, families may be required to re-navigate the health care system in terms of providers, receive services from non-specialist providers who are not familiar with children who have complex health care needs, and be hindered by the need for authorizations. In addition, stringent policies and procedures regarding access to care differ state to state, which can be frustrating, ethically questionable, and impractical to families living close to state boundaries (Mentro, 2003).

Social and Health Care Organizations

Social and health care organizations are mandated by health and social policy groups to be organized to provide care not only for the identified client (child), but also to do so within in a family-centered context

(Mentro, 2003). Standards regarding family-centered care models are based on the idea that family members and professionals become integral members of the child's health care team through the sharing of their own perspectives (Shelton & Stepanek, 1994). Family-centered care is generally described as having eight elements that both promote and support the partnership (see Box 4.1).

These elements are very similar to the aforementioned IOM recommendations regarding health care and to ideas about family partnerships. Although these elements have long been at the forefront of pediatric care, they are now being included in recommendations for care across the life span as well across the continuum of care from home, community, and hospital settings.

BOX 4.1 Eight Elements of Family Centered Care

1. The family is at the center of care because they are the constant in the child's life.
2. Family-professional collaboration is important at all levels of hospital, home, and community care for care of the individual child, program development, and policy formation.
3. Family-professional communication involves the exchange of complete and unbiased information between families and professionals in a supportive manner at all times.
4. Policy and practice needs to recognize and honor cultural diversity, strengths, and individuality within and across all families, including ethnic, racial, spiritual, social, economic, educational, and geographic differences.
5. Comprehensive policies and programs need to recognize different ways of coping and include developmental, educational, emotional, spiritual, environmental, and financial supports to meet the diverse needs of families.
6. Family-to-family support and networking also needs to be encouraged and facilitated.
7. Hospital, home, and community service and support systems for children needing specialized health and developmental care and their families need to be flexible, accessible, and comprehensive in order to respond to diverse family-identified needs.
8. And finally, the family should be appreciated as a family and children as children, recognizing a range of strengths, concerns, emotions, and aspirations beyond their special health and developmental needs.

Note: Adapted from *Family-Centered Care: Putting It Into Action,* by L. Lewandowski & M. D. Tesler (Eds.), 2003, Washington, DC: Society of Pediatric Nursing and American Nurses Association.

Professional Initiatives

Many professional groups are active in initiatives to promote standards and programs regarding partnerships with clients or patients (Lewandowski & Tesler, 2003). Many of these, however, are focused on the individual patient. For instance, the American College of Physicians provided leadership to the development of a statement of ethics for managed care that focuses on the provider-patient relationship; patient rights and responsibilities; confidentiality and privacy; resource allocation and stewardship; the obligation of health plans to foster an ethical environment for the delivery of care; and the clinician's responsibility to individual patients, the community, and public health. Families are not included or considered (Povar et al., 2004). The Society of Pediatric Nursing provided leadership to the development of a guide to family-centered care in order to encourage integration of current policy and research into practice. The guide is organized around the eight aforementioned elements of family-centered care (Lewandowski & Tesler, 2003).

The American Academy of Pediatrics (AAP) has been advocating since the early 1990s for the concept of a "medical home," which is closely akin to ideas about developing family partnerships. A medical home is not a building, house, or hospital, but rather a concept for providing services in a high-quality and cost-effective manner to CSHCN through recognition and support of families as the central caregivers for their child, effective community-based coordination and communication, and improved primary care. A medical home is defined by five criteria: (a) health care that includes a usual source for sick/well care; (b) a personal doctor or nurse; (c) no difficulty in obtaining needed referrals; (d) needed care coordination; and (e) a family-centered approach (AAP, 2004). A telephone survey of 38,866 households with CSHCN determined whether or not the children received care that meets all of these five criteria; criteria were met if *all* indicators were met. Findings indicate that approximately 50% of CSHCN receive care that meets all five criteria. Most have a usual source of care and a personal doctor or nurse, but other components of a medical home are lacking, especially elements of care coordination and family-centered care. Access to a medical home is significantly affected by race/ethnicity, poverty, and the limitations imposed on daily activity by the child's special health care need. Parents of children who do have medical home report significantly less delay or forgone care, significantly fewer unmet health care needs, and significantly fewer unmet needs for family support services (Strickland et al., 2004). Therefore, children and their families who may be most vulnerable may not have a medical home or the potential to form partnerships with members of the health care community.

Providers and Families

Family-centered care cannot be accomplished without mutual respect and trust on the level of the providers and families. Regardless of patient age or condition, the setting, the situation of care or type of provider, research has identified the key characteristics of trust between the provider and family. They include mutual intention, time, process, varying levels, reciprocity, boundaries, and expectations. The provider must gain the family's trust through a process that changes over time, depending on development of the family and its members and the presenting issues. This is done through the providers' competence in performing their roles, the respect that is given to the family and its members, and communication skills that are used in interactions. In addition, providers also need to show that they are trustworthy and reliable and will be flexible and negotiate with family members. Finally, establishment of interpersonal boundaries are important to both providers and family members as they develop mutual knowledge of each other and understand what is expected of each other and their roles (Barnsteiner & Gillis-Donovan, 1990; Barnsteiner, Gillis-Donovan, Knox-Fischer, & McKlindon, 1994; McKlindon, & Barnsteiner, 1999; McKlindon & Schlucter, 2004). Likewise, lack of intention, lack of time, lack of movement through the process, superficiality, or nonreciprocal behavior can create distrust. Health care providers are ethically responsible for building and maintaining trust; however, the process of establishing partnerships with families is reciprocal and must also involve willingness on the part of the family and its members.

INFLUENCES OF FAMILY PARTNERSHIPS ON INFANT, CHILD, AND FAMILY OUTCOMES

Outcomes of family partnerships have been documented. First, core outcomes of the medical home/CSHCN initiative given below have been used to ascertain a baseline measure of the proportion of U.S. children who meet the MCH Bureau's core outcomes for the medical home/CSHCN. As noted above, two nationwide telephone surveys ($n = 38,866$; $n = 13,579$) gathered data to calculate the proportion of U.S. children who met each of the six core outcomes. Success rates ranged from 6% (services enable successful transition to adulthood, e.g., adult health care, work, and independence) to 74% (community services organized so that families can use them easily). Proportions of success for other outcomes, include (a) 37% (families receive coordinated ongoing comprehensive case within a medical home); (b) 52% (children screened early and continuously for special health care needs); (c) 53% (child received family-centered care); (d) 58% (families partner in decision making and are satisfied with services received); and (e) 60% (families have adequate public or private insurance to pay for the services they need). Follow-up measures will be done in at midpoint (2005–2006) and with a final assessment in 2010. As an added impetus for action, the six core outcomes have been incorporated as performance measures and benchmarks for state Title V programs (McPherson et al., 2004).

Outcomes of establishing mutual trust have also been explored. They include building a relationship between the family and the provider, enhancing communication, involving the family in treatment guidelines and engaging their commitment to them, and benefiting the client and his or her family (Lynn-McHale & Deatrick, 2000). Because trust is so important to establishing family partnerships, it is surprising that in a study that described the development of the nursing-family relationship in the ICU, critical care nurses did not mention developing or displaying trust or the importance of the family developing or displaying trust. Instead, critical care nurses identified commitment, perseverance, and involvement as important (Hupcey, 1998). Perhaps trust is not unimportant to health care providers; rather, they may perceive that families should and will trust them because of their roles and that there is no need to build trust with families, explicitly learn to trust families, or show their trust in families. Thus, research regarding family trust in health care providers has been helpful in understanding one side of the equation.

Less emphasis in research has been placed on health care providers' trust in families. Both perspectives must be included in research regarding various clinical situations in order to understand the preconditions, characteristics, and level of provider and family trust. For instance, situations where families may loose trust in a health care provider (failed intervention) may be an innovative situation to learn about the process of gaining, losing, and reestablishing trust (Lynn-McHale & Deatrick, 2000).

NURSING CARE EXCELLENCE IN FAMILY PARTNERSHIPS IN NURSING CARE

In order to build partnerships with families, nurses and other health care providers need standardized guidelines regarding family-centered care and medical homes. They also need specific direction in order to individualize their approach to each family. The Family Management Styles (FMS) Framework, developed over the past 20 years through qualitative research and conceptual reviews, describes various ways in which families define and manage illness-related demands and the resulting consequences for family life (Deatrick & Knafl, 1990; Knafl & Deatrick, 2003; Knafl, Breitmayer, Gallo, & Zoeller, 1994). Thus, the FMS framework is potentially useful in both clinical practice and research to understand families who have CSHCN.

The FMS framework describes how a family manages both family life and a child's serious health care problems using a "pattern" approach. A pattern approach usually uses qualitative methods to identify dimensions of typical family types, organize the description of each type, and arrange them in a typology. The FMS framework is a family typology that systematically considers patterns or types of family management, including issues common to all families in a particular situation and how the issue is typically manifested within certain types of families. The dimensions that are common to all families are configured in Table 4.1 with examples of themes and subthemes for two of the five FMS. This framework, therefore, can be used as the basis for planning both standard supportive care (common or general issues/dimensions) and individualized

TABLE 4.1 Dimensions of FMS with Example Themes and Subthemes for Selected Styles

Dimensions	Examples Of Themes*	Examples of Two Family Management Styles and Subthemes	
		Thriving FMS	Floundering FMS
Defining	Child identity: parent's views of the child and the extent to which those views focus on illness or normalcy and capabilities or vulnerabilities	Normal	Tragic, problem
Management	Parenting philosophy: parent's goals, priorities, and values that guide the overall approach and specific strategies for illness management	Accommodative	Usually missing/ inconsistent
Consequences	Future expectation: parent's assessment of the implications of the illness for their child's and family's future	No future dread expressed	Future dread usually expressed

*A total of 8 themes have been identified to date (Knafl & Deatrick, 2003).

care (those issues specific to certain types of families) according to various types of *family management styles* (Knafl, Breitmayer, Gallo, & Zoeller, 1996) (see Figure 4.1).

The general issues or dimensions common to all families comprise the major interacting dimensions of the FMS model, including how family members *define* and *manage* their situation, as well what *consequences they perceive* for family life. FMS are related to *outcomes* concerning individual and family functioning. For example, children in families with a Thriving management style had significantly higher social competence scores as measured by the Social Competence Scale of the CBCL than did children in families with an Enduring, Struggling, or Floundering management styles (Knafl et al., 1994). Families in the Floundering group were characterized by significantly lower satisfaction with family life (Feetham Family Functioning Survey [FFFS]) than those in the other styles. It is assumed that having data from multiple family members, as depicted in Figure 4.1, contributes to a more valid representation of the family's response to the illness.

Considerable specification of the three dimensions of the FMS is included in the framework, including themes and subthemes that comprise definition of the situation, management behaviors, and perceived consequences. To illustrate, in Table 4.1 Child Identity is one of the themes that comprise the Definition of the Situation dimension, Parenting Philosophy is one of the themes comprises the Management dimension, and Future Expectations is one of the themes that comprises the Perceived Consequences dimension. The approach to building family partnerships would be very different, depending on the family's style of managing. A family who has a Thriving FMS sees their child as essentially normal, works to accommodate the child's differences into everyday life, and does not express overwhelming concern for the future of the child and family.

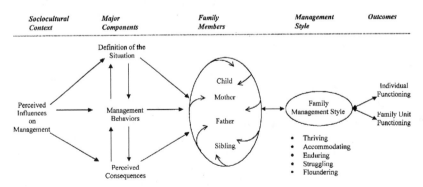

FIGURE 4.1 Family management style framework.

On the other hand, a family with a Floundering FMS sees their child as a tragic figure that has a problematic existence, does not have an overall philosophy for accommodating their child's differences into everyday life, and usually expresses dread about the future of the child and the family (Knafl & Deatrick, 2003; Knafl et al., 1996).

The five FMS (Thriving, Accommodating, Enduring, Struggling, Floundering) were identified in research with CSHCN. The content of these themes and subthemes is described elsewhere (Knafl & Deatrick, 2003; Knafl et al., 1996). They were found to develop and change over time and to reflect a continuum of difficulties that families experience in managing a child's chronic illness and the extent to which the experiences of individual family members were similar or discrepant.

Illness and developmental and family characteristics make less possible a return to family life as it was before the illness, meaning there is less chance for a "thriving" FMS. In particular, illness situations marked by intense uncertainty (Santacroce, 2003), and family situations—including those dominated by the illness, changed parenting style, conflict, and burden (Knafl & Deatrick, 2002) such as those in pediatric oncology—have been found to be most troublesome. These families are probably no less capable of successfully managing the situation than other families if they are given the psychosocial supportive care that matches their psychosocial profiles. Further research is needed not only to confirm these profiles but also to test interventions tailored to them.

MULTIDISCIPLINARY INTEGRATION
AND PARTNERSHIP: CASE STUDY

In order to integrate the aforementioned components of family partnerships, a case study will be analyzed. The analysis will be organized around a family ecological perspective, including the microsystem (family and the disease); the mesosystem (health care providers); the exosystem (preschool); and the macrosystem (health and social policy) levels (Kazak & Simms, 1996).

> Four-year-old Tommie was diagnosed with acute lymphoblastic leukemia (ALL) one year ago. Following a year of intensive chemotherapy, he will begin routine "maintenance therapy" within the next week, thereby reducing the complexity, strength, and frequency of his treatment regimen. While his family is very glad to have the past months behind them, they are now becoming anxious about Tommie's attending preschool. His mother is going to visit several possible preschools and is considering what questions she needs to ask regarding Tommie's special needs. The family describes

Tommie as a tragic figure, family life unlike before Tommie was diagnosed with ALL, and dread about the future. The parents do not describe underlying goals or ideas about how to best guide Tommie toward the future.

Health and Social Policy

The Individuals with Disabilities Education Act requires every public school system to provide free and appropriate education in the least restrictive environment to all handicapped individuals between the ages of 3 and 21. This includes special education programs, physical therapy, occupational therapy, and psychiatric services. In addition, children on and off treatment for childhood cancer may also be eligible for services and accommodations under §504 of the Rehabilitation Act. This law applies when the child does not meet the eligibility requirements for specially designed instruction, but still needs accommodations to perform successfully (Keane, Hobbie, & Ruccione, 2000).

Family and Disease

In the case study, the nature of Tommie's disease is marked by intense uncertainty and is negatively influencing the family's attempts at living life as they did before cancer. They were proud of their spontaneous lifestyle and strove to live "life in the moment" while staying very self-sufficient. They now find themselves dependent on the advice and support of relative strangers in order to keep their son alive and to hopefully cure him of his disease. They are very anxious about the possibility of his relapsing and dying of his disease.

Health Care Providers

Although most health care providers would routinely approach the family and focus on the positive aspects of (less intense) treatment, an approach sensitized by FMS might acknowledge the burden the family has experienced due to Tommie's illness and the fears they might now be experiencing. In order to strengthen the partnership with the family, you might help them establish short-term goals to help decrease the burden they associate with disease management, as well as management strategies that are acceptable to them. These interventions will help them reframe their situation and help move them through their journey as a family, instead of being trapped with strategies based on beliefs about their situation that are more adaptive to a different phase of treatment (Knafl & Deatrick, 2002; Knafl, Deatrick, & Kirby, 2001).

Of equal importance is reinforcing the importance of Tommie's medical home. During continued treatment, the oncology team is undoubtedly coordinating his care and can be supportive with issues such as preschool and other concerns of Tommie and his parents. How will that change over time? Helping the family see the "road map" for the treatment in terms of the medical home is important. Eventually, the child's medical home can transition back to a primary care provider and his "cancer survivorship" can be followed in a comprehensive follow-up program whose staff can act as advocates for Tommie in school and later with insurance agencies and employers.

Preschool

In terms of achieving psychosocial milestone and intellectual development, Tommie's preschool experience will be important in providing a transition between his illness and attending elementary school. It will be important to assist his mother and father in assessing preschools as far as any special accommodations that may be needed, as well as how to best prepare Tommie for elementary school.

SUMMARY

This chapter provided a working definition of partnering with families; described the potential outcomes of family partnerships; described an example of a nursing care model that can form the basis for partnerships with families; and illustrated one example of partnering with families, using a case study. Most broadly defined, partnering with families means that nurses and other health care professionals are engaged in a process with children and their families that is oriented toward promoting the mutual trust between the provider and the family in order to achieve health for the family as well as its individual members. Therefore, the emphasis is on an evolving process and the outcome of health not only for individuals but also for the family as a unit.

Outcomes on the system level concerning family partnerships have been documented. First, core outcomes of the medical home/CSHCN initiative have been used to ascertain a baseline measure of the proportion of U.S. children who meet the MCH Bureau's core outcomes for the medical home/CSHCN. Second, outcomes of establishing mutual trust have been explored. They include building a relationship between the family and the provider, enhancing communication, involving the family in treatment guidelines and engaging their commitment to them, and benefiting the client and his or her family.

The FMS framework was used as an example of a nursing care model that is potentially helpful to clinicians and researchers regarding family partnerships and for CSHCN. More research is needed to further develop and test this model regarding the establishment, implementation, and ongoing assessment of family partnerships.

Finally, a case example was used to further explore the issues presented by CSHCN in terms of integration of the aforementioned relationships, settings, and contexts (Kazak & Simms, 1996). Interventions sensitive to all levels of concern are needed to operationalize the ideals and ideas inherent in building family partnerships.

REFERENCES

American Academy of Pediatrics Medical Home Initiatives for Children with Special Needs Project Advisory Committee. (2004). The medical home: A policy statement. *Pediatrics, 113,* 1545–1547.

Barnsteiner, J. H., & Gillis-Donovan, J. (1990). Being related and separate: A standard for therapeutic relationships. *MCN: American Journal of Maternal Child Nursing, 15,* 223–228.

Barnsteiner, J. H., Gillis-Donovan, J., Knox-Fischer, C., & McKlindon, D. D. (1994). Defining and implementing a standard for therapeutic relationships. *Journal of Holistic Nursing, 12,* 35–49.

Biester, J. D., & Velsor-Friedrich, B. (1998). Historical overview of health care delivery models for children and their families. In M. Broome, K. Knafl, K. Pridham, & S. Feetham (Eds.), *Children and families in health and illness* (pp. 251–267). Thousand Oaks, CA: Sage.

Bissell, P., May, C. R., & Noyce, P. R. (2004). From compliance to concordance: Barriers to accomplishing a re-framed model of health care interactions. *Social Science and Medicine, 58,* 851–862.

Brodie, B. (1998). Historical overview of health promotion for children and families in late 19th and 20th-century America. In M. Broome, K. Knafl, K. Pridham, & S. Feetham (Eds.), *Children and their families in health and illness* (pp. 3–14). Thousand Oaks, CA: Sage.

Deatrick, J. A., & Knafl, K. A. (1990). Management behaviors: Day-to-day adjustments to childhood chronic conditions. *Journal of Pediatric Nursing, 5,* 15–22.

Doolittle, D. K. (1998). Welfare reform: Loss of Supplemental Security Income (SSI) for children with disabilities. *Journal of the Society of Pediatric Nurses, 3,* 33–44.

Hupcey, J. E. (1998). Establishing the nurse-family relationship in the intensive care unit. *Western Journal of Nursing Research, 20,* 180–194.

Institute of Medicine. (2003). *Crossing the quality chasm.* Washington, DC: National Academy Press.

Kazak, A., & Simms, S. (Eds.). (1996). *Children with life-threatening illness:*

Psychological difficulties and interpersonal relationships. New York: Wiley.

Keane, N., Hobbie, W., & Ruccione, K. (2000). *Childhood cancer survivors: A practical guide to your future.* Cambridge, MA: O'Reilly.

Knafl, K., & Deatrick, J. (2002). The challenge of normalization for families of children with chronic conditions. *Pediatric Nursing, 28,* 48–53, 56.

Knafl, K., & Deatrick, J. (2003). Further refinement of the Family Management Style Framework. *Journal of Family Nursing, 9,* 232–256.

Knafl, K., Breitmayer, B., Gallo, A., & Zoeller, L. (1994). *Final report: How families define and manage childhood chronic illness (R01594).* Bethesda, MD: National Institute of Nursing Research.

Knafl, K., Breitmayer, B., Gallo, A., & Zoeller, L. (1996). Family response to childhood chronic illness: Description of management styles. *Journal of Pediatric Nursing, 11,* 315–326.

Knafl, K., Deatrick, J., & Kirby, A. (2001). Normalization promotion. In M. Craft-Rosenberg & J. Dennehy (Eds.), *Nursing interventions for childbearing and childrearing families* (pp. 373–388). Thousand Oaks, CA: Sage.

Lewandowski, L., & Tesler, M. D. (Eds.). (2003). *Family-centered care: Putting it into action.* Washington, DC: Society of Pediatric Nursing and American Nurses Association.

Lynn-McHale, D. J., & Deatrick, J. A. (2000). Trust between family and healthcare provider. *Journal of Family Nursing, 6,* 210–230.

McKlindon, D., & Barnsteiner, J. (1999). Therapeutic relationships: Evolution of The Children's Hospital of Philadelphia Model. *The Journal of Maternal-Child Nursing, 24,* 237–243.

McKlindon, D., & Schlucter, J. (2004). Parent and nurse partnership model for teaching therapeutic relationships. *Pediatric Nursing, 30,* 418–420.

McPherson, M., Weissman, G., Strickland, M., van Dyck, P., Blumberg, S., & Newacheck, P. (2004). Implementing community-based systems of services for children and youths with special health care needs: How well are we doing? *Pediatrics, 113,* 1538–1544.

Meister, S. B. (1998). Community infrastructures: Principles and strategies for improving child health services. In M. Broome, K. Knafl, K. Pridham, & S. Feetham (Eds.), *Children and families in health and illness* (pp. 268–279). Thousand Oaks, CA: Sage.

Mentro, A. (2003). Health care policy for medically fragile children. *Journal of Pediatric Nursing, 18,* 225–232.

National Institutes of Health. (n.d.). *Overview of the NIH roadmap.* Retrieved February 13, 2004, from http://nihroadmap.nih.gov/overview.asp

Povar, G., Blumen, H., Daniel, J., Daub, S., Evans, L., Holm, R. P., et al. (2004). Ethics in practice: Managed care and the changing health care environment; Medicine as a Profession Managed Care Ethics Working Group Statement. *Annals of Internal Medicine, 141,* 131–136.

Santacroce, S. (2003). Parental uncertainty and posttraumatic stress in serious childhood illness. *Journal of Nursing Scholarship, 35,* 45–51.

Shelton, T. L., & Stepanek, J. S. (1994). *Family-centered care for children needing specialized health and developmental services.* Bethesda, MD: Association for the Care of Children's Health.

Strickland, B., McPherson, M., Weissman, G., van Dyck, P., Huang, Z., & Newacheck, P. (2004). Access to the medical home: Results of the national survey of children with special health care needs. *Pediatrics, 113,* 1485–1492.

CHAPTER FIVE

Culturally
Responsive Care

Rose M. Mays

INTRODUCTION, DEFINITIONS,
AND THEIR MEASUREMENT

The ethnic/racial makeup of the United States population is growing increasingly diverse. It is projected that by 2050 non-Hispanic Whites will make up only 53% of the population and that the proportion of Black or African American individuals will be 15% and Asian and Pacific Islanders 9% (Day, 1996). This expanding diversity challenges our health care system to deliver care that accommodates a variety of cultural perspectives. Culture is "the integrated pattern of human behavior that includes thoughts, communications, action, customs, beliefs, values, and institutions of a racial, ethnic, religious, or social group" (Cross, Bazron, Dennis, & Isaacs, 1989). Because these patterns are incorporated into various aspects of life, they have the capacity to affect health in numerous ways.

The increased recognition of the health impact of diverse cultural values, beliefs, and preferences has led to the nation's affirming culturally competent services as a standard of care (Office of Minority Health [OMH], 2001). This chapter addresses one of the Health Care Quality and Outcome Guidelines for nursing of children and families, set forth by the Expert Panel on Children and Families from the American Academy of Nursing: *"family values, beliefs and preferences are part of care"* (Betz et al., 2004). Campinha-Bacote's (2002) model describes the way through which clinicians develop competence. This model posits that cultural competence is not a state but an ongoing, developmental process in which one endeavors to become competent in serving clients within their cultural contexts. This process consists of the intersection of five major, interdependent constructs: cultural awareness, cultural knowledge, cultural skill, cultural encounters, and cultural desire. To determine the degree to which one is developing competence in delivering culturally responsive care, Campinha-Bacote (2003) advises asking oneself the following questions, which correspond to the five constructs of the model:

1. Am I aware of my personal biases and prejudices toward cultural groups different from mine?
2. Do I have the skill to conduct a cultural assessment and perform a culturally based physical assessment in a sensitive manner?
3. Do I have knowledge of the patient's worldview and the field of biocultural ecology?
4. How many face-to-face encounters have I had with patients from diverse cultural backgrounds?
5. What is my genuine desire to "want to be" culturally competent.

Although there are a multitude of cultures that make up the fabric of our country, this chapter will focus on racial/ethnic groups found to have significant health and health care disparities (Smedley, Stith, & Nelson, 2003). Culturally responsive clinical care is seen as one strategy for decreasing or eliminating such inequities. For purposes of this chapter, culturally responsive care is defined as nursing care that is respectful and takes into consideration the values, beliefs, and preferences of the family being served. For illustration, the chapter will discuss the influence of culturally responsive care and its principles as applied to promoting health with adolescents of color. This population is at risk for a number of negative health outcomes and warrants the attention of nurses who care for children and families.

Health Promotion for Adolescents as a Focus for Care

The adolescent period is viewed as a transitional stage during which one enters as a dependent child and emerges as mature, independent adult. This dynamic period entails changes in the biological, psychological, and social arenas. Although families remain influential in the lives of adolescents, responsibility or oversight for health increasingly shifts away from parents as progression through the period unfolds. This change in responsibility brings adolescents into contact more directly with health care providers and concomitantly warrants that providers be cognizant of cultural influences beyond the family such as neighborhoods, schools, peers, and the media.

Historically, health care policy pronouncements for adolescents have received relatively less attention when contrasted with those for younger children, because the adolescent population overall was deemed comparatively healthy on measures of mortality, prevalence of chronic diseases, and health care utilization. However, improved life expectancies for children with chronic conditions and the growing awareness of the links between adolescent behavior and illness or injury and adult chronic conditions has brought greater emphasis to this age group's health needs, particularly those involving health promotion. As one illustration of this trend, the federal government has identified 21 *Healthy People 2010* Critical Objectives (Centers for Disease Control [CDC], 2004) as targeted priorities for adolescents aged 10 to 24 years (Table 5.1). For several of the 21 objectives there are considerable disparities between White and ethnic minority adolescents on the baseline indicators. These disparities are notable for the areas of violence, reproductive health, and antecedent behaviors for chronic disease, such as smoking, inadequate physical activity, and nutrition (Grunbaum et al., 2004). Achievement of these key objectives would reduce death, injury, disease, premature pregnancy, and obesity, which is a precursor of later adult chronic disease.

INFLUENCES OF CORE INDICATORS FOR ADOLESCENTS AND THEIR FAMILIES

Regard for clients' cultural perspectives has been an accepted hallmark of quality nursing practice for more than a decade (Dienemann & Dienemann, 1997; Meleis, 1992). Accordingly, several models, guides, and resources are presently available to inform culturally responsive care. (For a recent annotated compilation, consult Shen, 2004.) Of late, this facet of nursing care has been further energized by the nation's interest in eliminating racial and ethnic health care disparities. The Institute of Medicine's landmark report, *Unequal Treatment: Confronting Racial and Ethnic Disparities in Healthcare* (Smedley et al., 2003), focuses principally on adult health inequalities; however, notable racial and ethnic health care disparities exist for children and adolescents as well. For example, disparities have been documented for the quality of well-child care (Ronsaville & Hakim, 2000); for primary care experiences (Stevens & Shi, 2003); for immunization rates, (Chu, Barker, & Smith, 2004), for access to care, (Borders, Brannon-Goedeke, Arif, & Xu, 2004; Newacheck, Hung, & Wright, 2002), and for asthma treatment (Ortega et al., 2002), just to highlight a few. The precise mechanisms and pathways that produce health and health care disparities for racial/ethnic minority children and adolescents are only beginning to be fully understood; however, culturally

TABLE 5.1 21 Critical Health Objectives for Adolescents and Young Adults*

The 21 Critical Health Objectives represent the most serious health and safety issues facing adolescents and young adults (aged 10–24): mortality, unintentional injury, violence, substance use and mental health, reproductive health, and the prevention of chronic diseases during adulthood.

Obj. #	Objective	Baseline (year)	2010 Target
16-03 (a,b,c)	Reduce deaths of adolescents and young adults.		
	10- to 14-year-olds	21.5 per 100,000 (1998)	16.8 per 100,000
	15- to 10-year-olds	69.5 per 100,000 (1998)	39.8 per 100,000
	20- to 24-year-olds	92.7 per 100,000 (1998)	49.0 per 100,000
Unintentional Injury			
15-15 (a)	Reduce deaths caused by motor vehicle crashes. 15- to 24-year-olds	25.6 per 100,000 (1999)	[1]
26-01 (a)	Reduce deaths and injuries caused by alcohol- and drug-related motor vehicle crashes. 15- to 24-year-olds	13.5 per 100,000 (1998)	[1]
15-19	Increase use of safety belts. 9th–12th grade students	84% (1999)	92%
26-06	Reduce the proportion of adolescents who report that they rode, during the previous 30 days, with a driver who had been drinking alcohol. 9th- to 12th-grade students	33% (1999)	30%
Violence			
18-01	Reduce the suicide rate. 10- to 14-year-olds	1.2 per 100,000 (1999)	[1]

	15- to 19-year olds	8.0 per 100,000 (1999)	[1]
18-02	Reduce the rate of suicide attempts by adolescents that required medical attention. 9th- to 12th-grade students	2.6% (1999)	1.0%
15-32	Reduce homicides. 10- 14-year-olds 15- 19-year-olds	1.2 per 100,000 (1999) 10.4 per 100,000 (1999)	[1] [1]
15-38	Reduce physical fighting among adolescents. 9th- to 12th-grade students	36% (1999)	32%
15-39	Reduce weapon carrying by adolescents on school property. 9th- to 12th-grade students	6.9% (1999)	4.9%

Substance Use and Mental Health

26-11 (d)	Reduce the proportion of persons engaging in binge drinking of alcoholic beverages. 12- to 17-year-olds	7.7% (1998)	2.0%
26-10 (b)	Reduce past-month use of illicit substances (marijuana). 12- to 17-year-olds	8.3% (1998)	0.7%
06-02	Reduce the proportion of children and adolescents with disabilities who are reported to be sad, unhappy, or depressed. 4- to 17-year-olds	[2]	[2]
18-07	(Developmental) Increase the proportion of children with mental health problems who receive treatment.	[3]	[3]

(continued)

TABLE 5.1 21 Critical Health Objectives for Adolescents and Young Adults* (*Continued*)

Obj. #	Objective	Baseline (year)	2010 Target
Reproductive Health			
09-07	Reduce pregnancies among adolescent females. 15- to 17-year-olds	68 per 1,000 (1996)	43 per 1,000
13-05	(Developmental) Reduce the number of new HIV diagnoses among adolescents and adults. 13- to 24-year-olds	16,479 (1998) [4]	[3]
25-01 (a,b,c)	Reduce the proportion of adolescents and young adults with Chlamydia trachomatis infections. 15- to 24-year olds		
	Females attending family planning clinics	5.0% (1997)	3.0%
	Females attending sexually transmitted disease clinics	12.2% (1997)	3.0%
	Males attending sexually transmitted disease clinics	15.7% (1997)	3.0%
25-11	Increase the proportion of adolescents who abstain from sexual intercourse or use condoms if currently sexually active. 9th- to 12th-grade students	85% (1999)	95%

Chronic Diseases

27-02 (a)	Reduce tobacco use by adolescents. 9th- to 12th-grade students	40% (1999)	21%
19-03 (b)	Reduce the proportion of children and adolescents who are overweight or obese. 12- to 19-year-olds	11% (1988–94)	5%
22-07	Increase the proportion of adolescents who engage in vigorous physical activity that promotes cardiorespiratory fitness 3 or more days per week for 20 or more minutes per occasion. 9th- to 12th-grade students	65% (1999)	85%

Note: Critical health outcomes are italicized, and behaviors that substantially contribute to important health outcomes are in normal font.

[1] 2010 target not provided for adolescent/young adult age group.

[2] Baseline and target inclusive of age groups outside of adolescent/young adult age parameters.

[3] Developmental objective—baseline and 2010 target to be provided by 2004.

[4] Proposed baseline is shown but has not yet been approved by the Healthy People 2010 Steering Committee.

*From U.S. Department of Health and Human Services *Healthy People 2010.* With Understanding and Improving Health and Objectives for Improving Health. 2 Vols. Washington, DC: U.S. Government Printing Office, 2000. This information can also be accessed at http://wonder/cdc/gov/data2010/

responsive clinical care is postulated to be one of several key strategies for addressing this problem (Brach & Fraser, 2000).

Drawing from the field of anthropology, early writers pointed out that culturally determined values, beliefs and preferences influence such health-related issues as problem identification, health-seeking, and adaptation to illness (Chrisman & Kleinman, 1983; Leininger, 1988); therefore, clinicians were advised to incorporate these understandings into illness care. More recently, awareness of the impact of cultural attitudes on motivation to engage in healthy behaviors has been recognized as an important aspect of health promotion interventions. As an illustration, *Be Proud! Be Responsible!*—a curriculum that was found to effectively promote healthy sexual behavior for African American adolescents—used pride and concern for protecting one's ethnic community as factors to motivate behavior change (Jemmott, Jemmott, & Fong, 1992). For adolescents, a strong ethnic identity is associated with better self-esteem and psychological adjustment (Carlson, Uppal, & Prosser, 2000; Yasui, Dorham, & Dishion, 2004) and is protective for violence (Soriano, Rivera, Williams, Daley, & Reznik, 2004). Ethnic identity, as defined by Phinney (1996), is "a commitment and sense of belonging to one's ethnic group, positive evaluation of the group interest in and knowledge about the group, and involvement in activities and traditions of the group" (p. 145). Nurses should be mindful of the role this cultural attitude plays in healthy development and offer parents guidance about the advantages of fostering ethnic identity for young children of color. Incorporating such cultural understandings into nursing interventions will enhance the quality of care.

Poor communication due to language differences between clients and providers is a culturally related aspect of care that is thought to have major consequences for health. The specific role that discordant language plays in child health disparities remains under investigation; but overall, children of parents with limited English proficiency fare worse with respect to access to care and health status than those whose primary language is English (Flores, 2004; Yu, Nyman, Kogan, Huang, & Schwalberg, 2004). Timmins' (2002) review of literature on language's influence on the health of U.S. Latinos of various ages similarly points out that language serves as a barrier to accessing care and is also associated with negative care outcomes for non-English-speakers of this ethnic group.

To meet the challenge of effectively communicating with families of limited English proficiency, providers not fluent in the family's primary language should utilize trained medical interpreters. In addition to addressing linguistic differences through enhancing spoken communication, providers should ensure that written communication is likewise understandable to families with limited English skills or with low literacy

(American Academy of Pediatrics, 2004). Two instructive resources for guiding practice with families who have limited proficiency in English are *Ensuring Linguistic Access in Health Care Settings: An Overview of Current Legal Rights and Responsibilities* (Perkins, 2003) and *Standards for Culturally and Linguistically Appropriate Services in Health Care* (OMH, 2001). The former is available electronically through the Henry J. Kaiser Foundation (www.kff.org) and the latter through the Office of Minority Health (www.omhrc.gov/CLAS/finalcultural1a.htm). An informative compendium that discusses approaches for promoting clear communication for low-literacy families is the recently published report of Nielsen-Bohlman, Panzer, and Kindig (2004), *Health Literacy: A Prescription to End Confusion.*

Last, minority families' views of societal racism and of discrimination specifically from the health care system may also play a role in their differential poor health outcomes. Williams, Neighbors, and Jackson's (2003) review of 86 studies established that ethnic minorities' perceptions of discrimination are related to a number of negative health consequences. For example, judgments about discrimination were related to the health risk behavior of smoking for urban African American adolescent girls (Guthrie, Young, Williams, Boyd, & Kintner, 2002) and for substance use for American Indian early adolescents in the upper Midwest (Whitbeck, Hoyt, McMorris, Chen, & Stubben, 2001). Stress generated by discrimination is proposed as the underlying mechanism by which such perceptions adversely affect health. For families negatively affected by discrimination, nurses can suggest stress-reducing coping strategies and recommend community programs for youth that promote ethnic identity (Cain & Kington, 2003).

Discrimination specifically related to health care experiences is also presumed to contribute to health disparities. In a large survey of adult patients on their opinions of health care quality, perceptions of bias in health care encounters were more likely to be endorsed by African Americans, Hispanics, and Asians than by Whites (Johnson, Saha, Arbelaez, Beach, & Cooper, 2004). Minority respondents in this nationally representative sample were more likely to say their providers judged them unfairly and treated them with disrespect because of their race/ethnicity or because of their poor English fluency and were more likely to believe they would receive better care if they belonged to a different race/ethnicity. Further analysis of this sample's responses revealed that such negative opinions were related to respondents' being less likely to undergo some recommended screenings, to have a routine physical exam, and to follow their physician's advice (Blanchard & Lurie, 2004). Although providers may not intentionally discriminate against clients of color, studies of physician practice have found that unconscious bias and negative stereotyping of minorities are prevalent in medical encounters (Burgess, Fu, & van Ryn, 2004). Racism and discrimination have been inadequately explored in nursing to date (Porter & Barbee, 2004); however, it follows that sensitivity to cultural values, beliefs, and preferences in the delivery of nursing care may help to mitigate such care perceptions by families of color and in turn help reduce disparities in health and health care.

NURSING CARE EXCELLENCE

H. L. Mencken once said, "For every complex question, there is a simple answer—and it's wrong." The rich diversity in cultural backgrounds of U.S. families presents both opportunities and challenges for nurses caring for children and families. The array of cultural beliefs provides opportunities to enrich our practice through incorporating different insights and perspectives into care. Practitioners can play a key role in helping to eliminate these disparities through culturally responsive care. Such an approach integrates family beliefs, values, and preferences into nursing interventions. This discussion will address one aspect of care.

The complexity of incorporating cultural perspectives into clinical care sometimes can be daunting. As with other complicated issues, practitioners are inclined to search for a single clinical guideline or prescription that results in culturally responsive care. However, the intricacies of culture preclude this solution. Just as the pathways are varied in which culture influences health status, health behavior, and health-service access and utilization, approaches for delivering culturally responsive care are likewise many and different. This section will offer several key principles to guide pediatric nurses' delivery of culturally responsive care, using prevention of overweight and obesity among adolescents of color as an exemplar.

If our nation is to make meaningful progress toward achieving the 21 Critical Health Objectives for adolescents of color specified in *Healthy People 2010*, greater attention will need to be given to promoting healthy behaviors through clinical encounters and community programs. Health behaviors are the result of complex, multifactorial processes that include individual, interpersonal, and environmental factors. Health promotion for adolescents is focused not only on identifying and reducing risks, but also on strengthening factors that are protective or that serve as resources for positive health outcomes (Rew & Horner, 2003). To be optimally effective, such interventions should be responsive to families' values, beliefs, and preferences. For purposes of illustration, principles of culturally responsive care will be discussed in the context of preventing overweight and obesity in ethnic/racial minority adolescents.

The prevalence of overweight children and adolescents is rapidly escalating, with approximately 16% of U.S. children estimated to be overweight in 1999–2002, based on body mass index measurements (Hedley et al., 2004). This figure represents a 45% increase from the 1988–1994 estimates of 11%. Because prevalence of obesity is high for African American, Native American, and Mexican American children, these subgroups have been identified to be at risk (Koplan, Liverman, & Kraak, 2005). Given that obesity is a key precursor of later adult chronic disease, current standards of clinical care call for measuring height, weight, and body mass index, and counseling adolescents and their parents on proper nutrition and physical activity, especially when excessive weight gain is noted (Krebs & Jacobson, 2003). The cultural negotiation model of nursing practice (Engebretson & Littleton, 2001) provides a useful framework for guiding the incorporation of family values beliefs and preferences into care focused on preventing overweight and obesity for adolescents of color.

The cultural negotiation model is predicated on a holistic view of the client and a recognition that health is shaped by sociocultural context as well as by biomedical factors. According to the model, each participant—the adolescent and the nurse—brings expert knowledge to the clinical encounter and interacts through a process of cultural negotiation. The five steps of the nursing process are augmented to include (a) an exchange of expert knowledge; (b) an analysis and interpretation of information; (c) joint decision-making; (d) implementation of mutually derived plans for action; and (e) an appraisal of expected outcomes. Additionally, this practice approach recognizes the health care system as an important cultural system that influences health (Engebretson & Littleton, 2001). Using the cultural negotiation model as a framework, several principles of culturally responsive care are discussed in the following sections.

Assessment: Exchange of Expert Knowledge

Integrating culturally responsive approaches into clinical care is a valued goal and begins with assessment. Although being culturally literate or knowing about the predominant cultural characteristics of a particular group is a good starting point for clinicians, quality nursing care for culturally diverse adolescents and their families must be based on an individualized assessment of each adolescent and family. There can be pitfalls to stereotyping, oversimplifying, or basing care on superficial features. Culture is dynamic and there is great diversity of beliefs within groups of similar race/ethnicity. Often this heterogeneity of beliefs is influenced by social and economic factors, such as family, school, and peer characteristics; income, immigration experiences, and geographic location. Such within-group differences mitigate against adopting a one-size-fits-all approach.

A culturally responsive assessment consists of interaction is which expert knowledge is interchanged between nurse and client. Because nurses are invariably older than the clients are, are often of different cultural backgrounds, and possess more professional knowledge than adolescents have, they must take care to ensure the assessment is conducted with a communication style that honors and respects adolescents and their families' beliefs, values, and preferences. Such a style builds trust and is based on empathy. Trust is especially important for adolescents of color who may be unaccustomed to interacting directly with the nurse or may have experienced past discrimination. Trust is posited to have an important role in enhancing care for low-income minority individuals (Sheppard, Zambrana, & O'Malley, 2004).

Another key aspect of assessment is determining the adolescent and family's explanatory model as it relates to a specific health issue or condition (Kleinman, Eisenberg, & Good, 1978). Explanatory models make up clients' understandings of the reasons, course, and treatments for health or disease; therefore, they are a significant feature of expert knowledge. Parents' explanatory models of such children's conditions such as attention deficit disorder and asthma have been found to vary by racial/ethnic group (Bussing, Schoenberg, & Perwein, 1998; Peterson, Sterling, & Stout, 2002). In considering childhood obesity prevention, it is important to note that several studies demonstrate that African American girls have less concern about weight than other ethnic groups or males do (Koplan et al., 2005), that some Hispanic and African American parents define obesity differently than professionals do (Myers & Vargas, 2000; Thompson & Story, 2003), and that obesity may not be seen as a health risk by African American parents of obese children (Young-Hyman, Herman, Scott, & Schlundt, 2000). Multiple cultural perspectives influence each adolescent and family; therefore, it is advantageous to directly elicit clients' meanings of healthy weight, physical activity, and diet to determine which ones may be salient to their understanding of this health issue. In addition to learning about explanatory perspectives, it is also useful to ascertain what adolescents may have already tried, who they may have previously consulted, what they think is needed, and how the nurse can help.

Nursing Diagnosis: Analysis and Interpretation of Information

At this step, nursing diagnoses based on the exchange of the nurse and adolescent's expert knowledge are presented. In offering diagnoses, careful consideration should be given to the adolescent's degree of understanding and acceptance of the nurse's biomedical explanatory model about overweight and its deleterious effect on health. Rationale for diagnoses should be given in clear terms that respect and match the language and literacy level of the adolescent and family. For example, rather than offering explanations about disease mechanisms, knowledge deficits about the relationships between obesity and chronic conditions like type II diabetes, hypertension, and high cholesterol could be addressed by simply pointing out that excess weight puts one at risk. To avoid stigma in communicating the diagnosis, consideration should be given to cultural attitudes toward being overweight and weight norms for the family.

Planning: Joint Decision-Making

Mutually derived goals and strategies are established in this phase. In general, the key behaviors to be targeted in preventing childhood overweight and obesity include limiting consumption of sweetened drinks, reducing television watching or computer time, and increasing physical activity or play (Whitaker, 2003). Culturally responsive plans that address healthful eating and physical activity should be based on a shared agreement with the adolescent. Plans that are congruent with existing cultural traditions involving food, music, and activities may more likely be incorporated into adolescents' lifestyles. Such an approach will also show respect and validate the adolescent's unique perspectives and expert knowledge. In addition, planning should be based on knowledge of the adolescent's distinctive sociocultural environment. For example, economic disadvantage may limit the family's purchasing power to make nutritious foods available and affect access to safe environments for physical activity. Strategies that consider such contextual factors and are mutually derived will have a greater likelihood of success.

Intervention: Implementation of Mutually Derived Plans for Action

Connecting adolescents with community-based programs that encourage healthful eating and physical activity is a useful and complementary intervention strategy to counseling and guidance. Like individually focused clinical interventions, quality health promotion programs should be customized to be compatible with values, beliefs, and preferences of the target population to optimize their effectiveness.

In examining the cultural responsiveness or sensitivity of health promotion programs, two dimensions are suggested for consideration, *surface structure* and *deep structure* (Resnicow, Soler, Braithwaite, Ahluwalia, & Butler, 2000). Adapting programs to the surface structure of cultures involves incorporating obvious characteristics of the target population into the intervention. Some examples of surface structure include using the language, music, settings (e.g., churches and schools), and staff that are familiar to and embraced by the cultural group. Attention to surface structure increases a program's face validity and is often achieved by soliciting the input of the target population in the planning process. Deep structure addresses how the differences in health behaviors are influenced by values associated with specific racial/ethnic groups. For example, because family, or *familismo,* is a central value for Hispanics, health promotion programs for this group might emphasize the health benefits of healthful eating for the adolescent's family as well. Contemporary nursing practice often includes negotiating referrals to community-based health promotion programs or actually conducting such programs. Care should be taken to insure that programs are culturally responsive.

Evaluation: Appraisal of Expected Outcomes

The evaluation of care is necessary to determine its effectiveness. Culturally responsive care is expected to enhance satisfaction and promote adherence to care plans. Evaluation strategies that incorporate a client's care perspectives can be invaluable in determining the degree to which clinical care and programs address cultural issues. One effective strategy for soliciting evaluation information from adolescents of color is the focus group (Jones & Broome, 2001). Through focus groups, clinicians not only can learn about salient cultural characteristics and values that influence particular health behaviors but also ascertain satisfaction with care and care preferences. For example, Dienes, Morrissey, and Wilson's (2004) evaluation with African American adolescent girls in the Southeast revealed that disrespectful communication with physicians was a negative aspect of care for many respondents. Likewise, Alexander (2004) used focus groups to capture effectively the various care preferences for a diverse sample of women who were receiving care from nurse practitioners at an urban facility in the Northeast. Such evaluations of care can also address other features of the care experience, such as insensitivity and bias experienced in making appointments and interacting with nonprofessional staff. Clinicians can use such evaluation data to address the cultural components of the care experience.

MULTIDISCIPLINARY INTEGRATION AND PARTNERSHIP

Providing culturally responsive care requires the commitment and cooperation of the entire health care team as well as representatives of community-based agencies who may be partners in care. Clients may interact with a number of persons when receiving care. Each member of the team needs to interact in ways that are culturally responsive. To insure culturally responsive care, it is recommended that health care organizations implement policies and practices that support its realization. Such system-focused efforts include diversifying the workforce, providing interpreter services, insuring availability of culturally and linguistically appropriate health education materials, and requiring ongoing staff development (Betancourt, Green, Carrillo, & Ananeh-Firempong, 2003; Frusti, Niesen, & Campion, 2003). These and similar measures will ensure a coordinated approach and guarantee sustainability of initiatives. The case that follows demonstrates an example of multidisciplinary integration and partnership.

Case Study

F.A. is a nurse practitioner of Asian descent and a member of a team that provides primary care to adolescents at an urban, mixed-income, neighborhood clinic. Members of the team include a physician, social worker, dietician, interpreter, and a bilingual community outreach worker. The clinic serves a culturally diverse population with approximately 50% of clients self-identifying as African American, 35% as White, and 15% as Hispanic.

Last Wednesday F.A. saw Maria, a 14-year-old Hispanic female, for her annual preventive screening visit. The results of the psychosocial and biomedical screenings revealed no health concerns except for a body mass index in the overweight range. When F.A asked Maria what she thought about her weight and shape, Maria shared that she would like to weigh less so that she could wear clothes that were more flattering. After cooperatively setting some goals for increasing Maria's physical activity, F.A. escorted her to the dietician's office for dietary counseling. Today during the daily team meeting, F.A. learns that the dietician invited Maria's mother, who prepares the family meals but is not fluent in English, to join Wednesday's session. The three of them jointly developed a diet plan with the help of the interpreter. Although Maria's mother participated in the planning, the dietician is concerned about her support of Maria's nutritional plan. She reports that the mother commented several times that Maria is a healthy weight.

F.A. engaged the team in a brief discussion of how to assist Maria further in achieving her goal of a healthy weight. Strategies suggested by the team included a home visit by the community outreach worker to learn more about the mother's views about obesity-related health risk, physical activity, and nutrition, and investigating a new physical activity program offered by a local youth development agency. The social worker offered to assess the cultural and linguistic appropriateness of the program for Maria and report back to the team. As the case of Maria demonstrates, culturally responsive care involves cultural competence and negotiation on the part of all the team members. In addition, culturally responsive community programs can be a useful adjunct to clinical care.

SUMMARY

The extensive ethnic and racial diversity found among contemporary American families is not reflected in today's nursing workforce and, as a result, family values, beliefs, and preferences in caring for minorities may go unaddressed. Such omissions can result in, among other things, dissatisfaction with care, decreased adherence to health care provider advice, and poor communication. This chapter offered an overview of the current thinking about some of the factors that contribute to health disparities and strategies for their elimination, as well as summarizing some of the major issues that arise in delivering culturally responsive nursing care. The clinical implications of the guideline were described in the context of strategies for addressing overweight and obesity with adolescents of color. Specific principles for incorporating family values, beliefs, and preferences into clinical care and community programs were explained according to a model of nursing care built on negotiation.

REFERENCES

Alexander, I. M. (2004). Characteristics of and problems with primary care interactions experienced by an ethnically diverse group of women. *Journal of the American Academy of Nurse Practitioners, 16,* 300–310.

American Academy of Pediatrics. (2004). Policy statement: Ensuring culturally effective pediatric care: Implications for education and health policy. *Pediatrics, 114,* 1677–1685.

Betancourt, J. R., Green, A. R., Carrillo, J. E., & Ananeh-Firempong, O. (2003). Defining cultural competence: A practical framework for addressing racial/ethnic disparities in health and health care. *Public Health Reports, 118,* 293–302.

Betz, C. L., Cowell, J. M., Lobo, M. L., Craft-Rosenberg, M., Bakken, S., Feetham S. L., et al. (2004). American Academy of Nursing Child and Family Expert Panel health care quality and outcomes guidelines for nursing of children and families: Phase II. *Nursing Outlook, 52,* 311–316.

Blanchard, J., & Lurie, N. (2004). R-E-S-P-E-C-T: Patient reports of disrespect in the health care setting and its impact on care. *Journal of Family Practice, 53,* 721–730.

Borders, T., Brannon-Goedeke, A., Arif, A., & Xu, K. T. (2004). Parents' reports of children's medical care access: Are there Mexican-American versus non-Hispanic white disparities? *Medical Care, 42,* 884–892.

Brach, C., & Fraser, I. (2000). Can cultural competency reduce racial and ethnic health disparities? A review and conceptual model. *Medical Care Research and Review, 57*(Suppl. 1), 181–217.

Burgess, D. J., Fu, S. S., & van Ryn, M. (2004). Why do providers contribute to disparities and what can be done about it? *Journal of General Internal Medicine, 19,* 1154–1159.

Bussing, R., Schoenberg, N. E., & Perwein, A. R. (1998). Knowledge and information about ADHD: Evidence of cultural differences among African-American and white parents. *Social Science and Medicine, 46,* 919–928.

Cain, V. S., & Kington, R. S. (2003). Investigating the role of racial/ethnic bias in health outcomes. *American Journal of Public Health, 93,* 191–192.

Campinha-Bacote, J. (2002). The process of cultural competence in the delivery of healthcare services: A model of care. *Journal of Transcultural Nursing, 13,* 181–184.

Campinha-Bacote, J. (2003). Many faces: Addressing diversity in health care. *Online Journal of Issues in Nursing, 8,* No. 1, Manuscript 2. Retrieved January 10, 2005 from http://nursingworld.org/ojin/topic20/tpc20_2.htm

Carlson, C., Uppal, S., & Prosser, E. C. (2000). Ethnic differences in processes contributing to the self-esteem of early adolescent girls. *Journal of Early Adolescence, 20,* 44–68.

Centers for Disease Control and Prevention. (2004). *21 critical health objectives for adolescents and young adults.* Retrieved March 20, 2005 from http://www.cdc.gov/HealthyYouth/NationalInitiative/pdf/21objectives.pdf

Chrisman, N. J., & Kleinman, A. (1983). Popular health care, social networks, and cultural meanings: The orientation of medical anthropology. In D. Mechanic (Ed.), *Handbook of health, health care and the health professions* (pp. 569–590). New York: Free Press.

Chu, S. Y., Barker, L. E., & Smith, P. J. (2004). Racial/ethnic disparities in pre-school immunizations: United States, 1996–2001. *American Journal of Public Health, 94,* 973–977.

Cross, T. L., Bazron, B. J., Dennis, K. W., & Issacs, M. R. (1989). *Towards a culturally competent system of care: A monograph on effective services for minority children who are severely emotionally disturbed.* Washington, DC: CASSP Technical Assistance Center, Georgetown University Child Development Center.

Day, J. C. (1996). *Population projections of the United States by age, sex, race, and Hispanic origin: 1995 to 2050, U.S. Bureau of the Census, current population reports* (P25-1130). Washington, DC: U.S. Government Printing Office.

Dienemann, J. A., & Dienemann, J. (Eds.). (1997). *Cultural diversity in nursing: Issues, strategies, and outcomes.* Washington, DC: American Academy of Nursing.

Dienes, C. L., Morrissey, S. L., & Wilson, A. V. (2004). Health care experiences of African American teen women in Eastern North Carolina. *Family Medicine, 36,* 346–351.

Engebretson, J., & Littleton, L. Y. (2001). Cultural negotiation: A constructivist-based model for nursing practice. *Nursing Outlook, 49,* 223–230.

Flores, G. (2004). Culture, ethnicity, and linguistic issues in pediatric care: Urgent priorities and unanswered questions. *Ambulatory Pediatrics, 4,* 276–282.

Frusti, D. K., Niesen, K. S., & Campion, J. K. (2003). Creating a culturally competent organization: Use of the diversity competency model. *Journal of Nursing Administration, 33,* 31–38.

Grunbaum, J. A., Kann, L., Kinchen, S., Ross, J., Hawkins, J., Lowry, R., et al. (2004). Youth risk behavior surveillance—United States, 2003. *MMWR Surveillance Summary, 53,* 1–96.

Guthrie, B. J., Young, A. M., Williams, D. R., Boyd, C. J., & Kintner, E. K. (2002). African American girls' smoking habits and day-to-day experiences with racial discrimination. *Nursing Research, 51,* 183–190.

Hedley, A. A., Ogden, C. L., Johnson, C. L., Carroll, M. D., Curtin, L. R., & Flegal, K. M. (2004). Prevalence of overweight and obesity among U.S. children, adolescents, and adults, 1999–2002. *Journal of the American Medical Association, 291,* 2847–2850.

Jemmott, J. B., Jemmott, L. S., & Fong, G. T. (1992). Reductions in HIV risk-associated sexual behaviors among black male adolescents: Effects of an AIDS prevention intervention. *American Journal of Public Health, 82,* 372–377.

Johnson, R. L., Saha, S., Arbelaez, J. J., Beach, M. C., & Cooper, L. A. (2004). Racial and ethnic differences in patient perceptions of bias and cultural competence in health care. *Journal of General Internal Medicine, 19,* 101–110.

Jones, F. C., & Broome, M. E. (2001). Focus groups with African American adolescents: Enhancing recruitment and retention in intervention studies. *Journal of Pediatric Nursing, 16,* 88–96.

Koplan, J. P., Liverman, C. T., & Kraak, V. I. (Eds.). (2005). *Preventing childhood obesity: Health in the balance.* Washington, DC: National Academies Press.

Kleinman, A., Eisenberg, L., & Good, B. (1978). Culture, illness, and care: Clinical lessons from anthropologic and cross-cultural research. *Annals of Internal Medicine, 88,* 251–258.

Krebs, N. F., & Jacobson, M. S. (2003). Policy statement: Prevention of pediatric overweight and obesity. *Pediatrics, 112,* 424–430.

Leininger, M. M. (1988). Leininger's theory of nursing: Cultural care diversity and universality. *Nursing Science Quarterly, 1,* 152–160.

Meleis, A. I. (1992). AAN expert panel report: Culturally competent health care. *Nursing Outlook, 40,* 277–283.

Myers, S., & Vargas, Z. (2000). Parental perception of the preschool obese child. *Pediatric Nursing, 26,* 23–30.

Newacheck, P.W., Hung, Y. Y., & Wright, K. K. (2002). Racial and ethnic disparities in access to care for children with special health care needs. *Ambulatory Pediatrics, 2,* 247–254.

Nielsen-Bohlman, L., Panzer, A. M., & Kindig, D. A. (2004). *Health literacy: A prescription to end confusion.* Washington, DC: National Academies Press.

Office of Minority Health. (2001). *Assuring cultural competence in health care: Recommendations for national standards and an outcomes-focused research agenda.* Retrieved March 10, 2005, from

Ortega, A. N., Gergen, P. J., Paltiel, A. D., Bauchner, H., Belanger, K. D., & Leaderer, B. P. (2002). Impact of site of care, race, and Hispanic ethnicity on medication use for childhood asthma. *Pediatrics, 109*, e1. Retrieved March 20, 2005 from http://www.pediatrics.org/cgi/content/full/109/1/e1

Perkins, J. (2003). *Ensuring linguistic access in health care settings: An overview of current legal rights and responsibilities.* Washington, DC: Kaiser Commission on Medicaid and the Uninsured.

Peterson, J. W., Sterling, Y. M., & Stout, J. W. (2002). Explanatory models of asthma from African-American caregivers of children with asthma. *Journal of Asthma, 39*, 577–590.

Phinney, J. S. (1996). Understanding ethnic diversity: The role of ethnic identity. *American Behavioral Scientist, 40*, 143–152.

Porter, C. P., & Barbee, E. (2004). Race and racism in nursing research: Past, present, and future. *Annual Review of Nursing Research, 22*, 9–37.

Resnicow, K., Soler, R., Braithwaite, R. L., Ahluwalia, J. S., & Butler, J. (2000). Cultural sensitivity in substance use prevention. *Journal of Community Psychology, 28*, 271–290.

Rew, L., & Horner, S. D. (2003). Youth resilience framework for reducing health-risk behaviors in adolescents. *Journal of Pediatric Nursing, 18*, 379–388.

Ronsaville, D. S., & Hakim, R. B. (2000). Well child care in the United States: Racial differences in compliance with guidelines. *American Journal of Public Health, 90*, 1436–1443.

Shen, Z. (2004). Cultural competence models in nursing: A selected annotated bibliography. *Journal of Transcultural Nursing, 15*, 317–322.

Sheppard, B. A., Zambrana, R. E., & O'Malley, A. S. (2004). Providing health care to low-income women: A matter of trust. *Family Practice, 21*, 484–491.

Smedley, B. D., Stith, A. Y., & Nelson, A. R. (Eds.). (2003). *Unequal treatment: Confronting racial and ethnic disparities in health care.* Washington, DC: National Academy Press.

Soriano, F. I., Rivera, L. M., Williams, K. J., Daley, S. P., & Reznik, V. M. (2004). Navigating between cultures: The role of culture in youth violence. *Journal of Adolescent Health, 34*, 169–176.

Stevens, G. D., & Shi, L. (2003). Racial and ethnic disparities in the primary care experiences of children: A review of the literature. *Medical Care Research and Review, 60*, 3–30.

Thompson, L. S., & Story, M. (2003). Perceptions of overweight and obesity in their community: Findings from focus groups with urban, African-American caretakers of preschool children. *Journal of National Black Nurses Association, 14*, 28–37.

Timmins, C. L. (2002). The impact of language barriers on the health care of Latinos in the United States: A review of the literature and guidelines for practice. *Journal of Midwifery and Women's Health, 47*, 80–96.

Whitaker, R. C. (2003). Obesity prevention in pediatric primary care: Four behaviors to target. *Archives of Pediatric and Adolescent Medicine, 157*, 725–727.

Whitbeck, L. B., Hoyt, D. R., McMorris, B. J., Chen, X., & Stubben, J. D. (2001).

Perceived discrimination and early substance abuse among American Indian children. *Journal of Health and Social Behavior, 42,* 405–424.

Williams, D. R., Neighbors, H. W., & Jackson, J. S. (2003). Racial/ethnic discrimination and health: Findings from community studies. *American Journal of Public Health, 93,* 200–208.

Yasui, M., Dorham, C. L., & Dishion, T. J. (2004). Ethnic identity and psychological adjustment: A validity analysis for European American and African American adolescents. *Journal of Adolescent Research, 19,* 807–812.

Young-Hyman, D., Herman, L. J., Scott, D. L., & Schlundt, D. G. (2000). Care giver perception of children's obesity-related health risk: A study of African American families. *Obesity Research, 8,* 241–248.

Yu, S. M., Nyman, R. M., Kogan, M. D., Huang, Z. J., & Schwalberg, R. H. (2004). Parent's language of interview and access to care for children with special health care needs. *Ambulatory Pediatrics, 4,* 181–187.

CHAPTER SIX

Enhancement of Family Support Systems

Martha K. Swartz
Kathleen Knafl

INTRODUCTION, DEFINITIONS, AND THEIR MEASUREMENT

The Nursing Intervention Classification (NIC) identifies family support as one of several interventions targeting family roles and functioning (McCloskey Dochterman & Bulechek, 2004). Family support is defined as "promotion of family values, interests, and goals" (p. 377) and includes activities such as those listed in Box 6.1. These supportive activities are aimed at improving or sustaining both family system and individual family member functioning (Johnson, Bulechek, McCloskey Dochterman, Maas, & Moorhead, 2001).

Supportive family interventions, especially those related to families in the childbearing and child-rearing phases of the family life cycle are in keeping with the philosophy of family-centered care (FCC). FCC had its origins in early studies of the negative effects on hospitalized children of being separated from their mothers, and efforts by parents to liberalize restrictive hospital visiting policies (Lewandowski & Tesler, 2003; Prugh, Staub, & Sands, 1953; Robertson, 1958). Since its beginnings in the 1950s, FCC has evolved from its initial focus on visiting policies and parental involvement in the child's care to conceptualizing parents as "the molders and shapers of care" (Lewandowski & Tesler, 2003). This expanded view of FCC is reflected in the Institute for Family-Centered Care's definition of the approach:

A family-centered approach to care empowers individuals and families and fosters independence; supports family care giving and decision making; respects patient and family choices and their values, beliefs, and cultural backgrounds; builds on individual and family strengths; and involves patients and families in planning, delivery, and evaluation of health care services. Information sharing and collaboration between patients, families, and health care staff are the cornerstones of family-centered care. (Institute for Family-Centered Care, 2005)

As reflected in the above definition, family support is an essential component of FCC.

Measurement of family support can occur at the institutional or individual level. For example, the Institute for Family-Centered Care has developed a self-assessment inventory for measuring FCC in pediatric care hospitals (Institute for Family-Centered Care, 2005). The inventory includes a section on patient and family support and rates the following aspects of supportive care on a 3-point scale: broad definition of family; determination of preferences for participation in care; efforts to assure positive experiences during hospital visits; developmental or child life specialists on staff; access to affordable temporary housing; financial support; peer or family support groups; a broad range of referrals; assistance in developing emergency care plans; support during the dying

---

BOX 6.1 Example of Family Support Activities

- Assure family that best possible care is being given to patient.
- Appraise family's emotional reaction to patient's condition.
- Determine psychological burden of prognosis for family.
- Foster realistic hope.
- Listen to family concerns, feelings, and questions.
- Facilitate communication of concerns/feelings between patient and family or between family members.
- Promote trusting relationship with family.
- Accept family's values in a nonjudgmental manner.
- Answer all questions of family members or assist them to get answers.
- Orient family to the health care setting, such as hospital or clinic.
- Identify nature of spiritual support for family.
- Respect and support adaptive coping mechanisms used by family.
- Provide feedback for family regarding their coping.
- Provide opportunities for peer group support

Adapted from *Nursing Interventions Classification (NIC)* (4th ed., p. 377) by J. McCloskey Dochterman & G. M. Bulechek (Eds.), 2004.

process; bereavement counseling; specialized staff for psychosocial and spiritual care. The intent of this self-assessment inventory is to measure the extent to which an organization has policies, programs, and practices in place that are likely to contribute to the creation of a supportive environment for families, and to track changes in the development of FCC over time. Assessment tools such as this one help to raise awareness among health care providers as to the nature of family support and FCC, and can be used to measure progress toward creating environments that will achieve these goals.

At the individual level, family support is an inherently subjective experience. Wide variation in how individuals define and experience family support makes measurement especially challenging. For example, some family members find health care providers' efforts to involve them in all aspects of treatment decision making to be highly supportive; others prefer to delegate decision making to professionals and feel overwhelmed by efforts to involve them in complex treatment decisions (Kirschbaum & Knafl, 1996). Because perceptions of support are highly subjective, it typically is measured by assessing family members' needs and preferences. In keeping with the NIC definition of family support, stated needs and preferences are interpreted and acted on in the context of the family's values, interests, and goals in specific health care situations. The assumption is that assessment of family members' needs and preferences will contribute to nursing interventions that family members experience as supportive. The activities listed in the NIC description of family support are a useful guide to assessment as well as intervention, and can be used to determine family members' needs and preferences. Structured measures such as the Family Empowerment Scale and the Family Needs Survey also may help measure family members' desires for certain kinds of support (Touliatos, Perlmutter, Straus, & Holden, 2001).

In the remainder of this chapter, we discuss more fully the implications of family support for children and families. Following a discussion of how family support influences child and family outcomes, the chapter addresses strategies for incorporating family support into nursing care.

INFLUENCES OF FAMILY SUPPORT ON CHILDREN

The influence of family support on children is best understood in the context of research on the relationship between family functioning and child outcomes. The relationship between family and child functioning when a child has a chronic condition typically is discussed in terms of the family's impact on the child's psychosocial adjustment, disease control, and treatment adherence. A large body of research has focused on children's psychosocial adjustment to chronic illness. This research consistently has shown that although children with chronic conditions are at increased risk for behavioral and psychological problems, the quality of family functioning can play a pivotal role in moderating the negative impact of chronic and acute illness experiences (Lavigne & Faier-Routman, 1992; Melnyk, Small, & Carno, 2004; Wallander & Varni, 1998). For example, a recent comprehensive review of the research on the physiological and psychological functioning of youth with type 1 diabetes identified a number of family variables affecting youth outcomes (Whittemore, Kanner, & Grey, 2004). These authors found that better metabolic control and adherence to the treatment regimen were related to decreased family stress; decreased family conflict; increased parental involvement; increased cohesion, warmth, and caring behaviors; and increased diabetes support behavior. In addition, the family variables of more cohesion, more organization, and less conflict consistently were associated with better psychosocial adjustment in youth with diabetes. Other studies have demonstrated a relationship between levels of parental stress and anxiety in acute care settings and child outcomes, with higher stress levels associated with poorer outcomes (Melnyk & Feinstein, 2001). Across a wide range of studies of diverse families and health care situations, the family variables of cohesion, expressiveness, and family conflict consistently have been associated with adjustment in children (Knafl & Gilliss, 2002). However, despite a compelling body of evidence demonstrating the importance of family variables as moderators of children's response to illness and other health-related challenges, few studies have investigated the interrelationships between interventions aimed at family support, family functioning, and child outcomes. Those that have tested interventions designed to support the family have reported positive child outcomes as well (Chernoff, Ireys, DeVet, & Kim, 2002; Melnyk, Alpert-Gillis et al., 2004; Sherman, 1995). For example, Melnyk, Alpert-Gillis and colleagues (2004) tested an intervention to increase knowledge and participation in the care of mothers of children hospitalized in a pediatric intensive care unit and found positive outcomes for both the mother and the child. Mothers in the experimental group reported less stress, better functioning, and greater participation in the child's emotional and physical care than mothers in the control group did; children in the experimental group evidenced fewer withdrawal behaviors at 6 months posthospitalization and fewer negative behaviors at 12 months than those in the control group. In a study explicitly targeting family support, Chernoff and colleagues (2002) tested a community-based intervention designed for families in which a child had a chronic illness (diabetes mellitus, sickle cell anemia, cystic fibrosis, moderate to severe asthma), and found significant improvements in the adjustment scores of children in the experimental

group. Their results are especially promising because the intervention—
which was delivered by a child life specialist and included telephone contacts, face-to-face visits, and special family events—was equally effective
across the four diagnostic groups. In discussing the significance of their
study, Chernoff and colleagues (2002) concluded as follows:

> Over the last decade family support programs have become an ac-
> cepted and important part of service systems for children with chronic
> health and mental health problems, but the empirical foundation for
> these efforts is thin. Our study documents a workable approach to
> implementing a family support program, and adds to the growing ev-
> idence that community-based family-centered care can make a differ-
> ence. (p. 539)

Studies such as these highlight the importance of family support and
the pivotal role of both researchers and health care providers in developing, testing, and implementing family support programs.

INFLUENCES OF SUPPORT SYSTEMS
FOR THE FAMILY

Other studies have addressed family functioning when a child has an acute
or chronic illness or other health-related condition. Numerous investigators have focused on the impact of childhood illness on family life or the
quality of family functioning in the context of childhood illness or disability (Cornman, 1993; Dashiff, 1993; Donnelly, 1994; Ferrell, Rhiner,
Shapiro, & Dierkes, 1994; Fleming et al., 1994; Kopp et al., 1995; Labbe,
1996; Sawyer, 1992). The results of these studies present a mixed picture
of the impact of illness on family life, with some reporting that families
continue to function well when a child has a health-related problem
(Bohachick & Anton, 1990; Donnelly, 1994; Rehm & Catanzaro, 1998;
Sawyer, 1992; Youngblut, Brennan, & Swegart, 1994), and others reporting negative outcomes (Cornman, 1993; Ferrell et al., 1994; Kopp et al.,
1995; Park & Martinson, 1998) or a variable illness impact across subsys-
tems within the family or different illness contexts (Dashiff, 1993; Fleming
et al., 1994; Gallo, 1990; Labbe, 1996; Zahr, Khoury, & Saoud, 1994).
Good family functioning has been reported in families facing diverse health
challenges, including childhood asthma (Donnelly, 1994), cystic fibrosis
(Sawyer, 1992), and medical fragility (Youngblut et al., 1994). Across studies, the variables of fewer family stressors, greater resources, social support, and hardiness have been linked with better family functioning.

In order to understand how health care providers can support families and contribute to optimal family functioning in the context of a

child's illness or health-related problem, researchers have studied the health care needs and preferences of families as well as family-health care provider interaction as a basis for developing and testing interventions aimed at supporting families. These studies provide insights into the kinds of interactions families perceive at supportive. Studies of both families' needs when a child has a health care problem (Balling & McCubbin, 2001; Feudtner, Haney, & Dimmers, 2003; Kirk & Glendinning, 2004; Kirschbaum & Knafl, 1996; Scott, 1998) and the quality of family-health care professional interactions (Knafl, Breitmayer, Gallo, & Zoeller, 1992; Robinson, 1994, 1996) point to the importance of both information and the quality of the interaction between family members and providers as key elements contributing to family support. These studies indicate that fulfillment of family expectations, supporting decision-making agency, information exchange, and trust are the critical components of a supportive working relationship between families and health care providers. In the next section, we address how these interactional qualities can be incorporated into the care of child and families.

NURSING CARE EXCELLENCE

A framework to guide clinical interventions when a family member becomes ill is suggested by the family systems-illness model (Rolland, 1999). With the family as the interactional focal point, the development of a health problem or chronic disorder in a child is viewed in a developmental context in which three evolutionary trends are intertwined: the type and progression of illness, disability, or loss; the impact on the life cycle of the child; and the psychosocial demands placed on the family within the context of their culture, ethnicity, and belief systems. According to the model, in order for families to master the challenges that they will face, they need to accomplish certain tasks. First, they will need to learn about the expected pattern of practical and emotional demands they will face over time as the child's illness or disorder and associated treatment plans unfold. These demands may change because illness patterns vary in terms of onset of the disorder, clinical course, expected outcome, level of incapacitation, and degree of uncertainty. Second, families will need to develop an understanding of themselves as a functional unit. Third, families will need to remain attuned to the changing stresses and demands of a chronic disorder and how these affect the continued development of the child and family. Finally, families should become aware of how their belief systems, cultural legacies, and multigenerational influences "guide their construction of meanings of the illness and their relationship with larger caregiving systems" (Rolland, 1999, p. 243).

The family systems-illness model is based upon a strength-oriented approach in which family relationships are viewed as resources capable of resiliency and growth. The model informs the practice of excellent nursing care by its emphasis on the goodness of fit between the psychosocial demands related to childhood illness or health problems, and the strengths and vulnerabilities of a family over time. The dynamic nature of the model also indicates that family support should be provided based on a thorough understanding of the trajectory of the illness and the family life cycle. The nature and value of support to the family will shift over time as their needs and resources also change.

According to a recent integrative review of the literature concerning families with chronically ill children, the enhancement of support was noted most often as the type of intervention that families perceived as being the most beneficial during times of transition (Meleski, 2002). Parents who formed a strong support system and who extended the system to include relatives, friends, health care providers, organizations, and religious resources were better able to deal with the demands of a child's chronic illness, cope with chronic sorrow and manage the disequilibrium in their lives. General nursing interventions to enhance support include a comprehensive family assessment, the evaluation of existing support systems, and case management services that involve the family, the primary care and specialty providers, schools, and community-based health care agencies. The remaining discussion will focus on steps to enhance family support systems within the nursing process.

Assessment

A comprehensive assessment of families is crucial to the success of a family centered-care approach and should be viewed as an ongoing, dynamic, and mutual process (Lewandowski & Tesler, 2003). As situations, stressors, and resources change over time, a family's ability to understand, function, and cope may also change. There should also be sufficient documentation and effective sharing of information across time and setting among all of the health care professionals caring for the family. Children and families should be given the opportunity to contribute actively to this documentation. In some settings, parents are offered the opportunity to contribute information directly into the medical record. At Cincinnati Children's Medical Center, adolescents with respiratory problems are also given the opportunity to document their thoughts, observations, and feelings directly into their record (Lewandowski & Tesler, 2003).

Assessing the need for family support should be based on a determination of the parents' understanding of their child's illness, and their perception of the stress. An assessment of the adequacy of the family's coping strategies, the factors that support resiliency, and emerging maladaptive coping patterns should also be discerned. Rather than using only one or two coping strategies, families will use a variety of coping strategies as they encounter different stressors over time. Burr and colleagues (1994) identified the following categories of coping strategies of families under stress: (a) cognitive strategies (gaining useful knowledge regarding the situation); (b) communication strategies (effective, open, and honest listening to one another); (c) emotional strategies (expressing feelings and affection, acknowledging negative feelings); (d) relationship strategies (increasing trust and cooperation, drawing on spiritual faith); (e) environment/community strategies (seeking support from others); and (f) individual development strategies (increasing self-sufficiency and independence).

A review by Coyne (1997) of coping mechanisms employed by parents of children with cystic fibrosis (CF) revealed that during the diagnostic phase of the illness, many parents used denial as a temporarily effective form of coping, as they sought to deal with the shock, anger, and disbelief they were experiencing. As parents moved beyond this initial phase, most parents employed more cognitive coping strategies and sought information about the nature of the illness, its early progression, and cause so that they could begin to understand and plan for the future. Similarly, a meta-synthesis of the findings of 10 qualitative studies on parenting preterm infants revealed that, for many parents, concerns about their baby's health and development were pervasive (Swartz, 2005). They, too, employed cognitive coping strategies so that they could be as informed as possible about their infant's care.

A family-centered approach during the assessment process sets the stage for including family members at future decision-making junctures. Operationally, a parent-professional partnership is defined as an association between parents and professionals that functions collaboratively, using agreed upon roles in the pursuit of common interests (Judge, 2002). Ideally, such partnerships are based on mutual trust, honesty, open communication, and respect for cultural diversity. Through this mutual process, parents are empowered to make informed decisions about the best course of action on behalf of their child and family.

Planning

As the family systems-illness model (Rolland, 1999) implies, a focus on illness or chronic disease as the key influence is inadequate because it does not acknowledge the role of other variables in family adjustment when caring for an ill child. Mutual planning among nurses and family members should acknowledge the internal resources of the family, such as adaptation and integration. Nurses should also work with family members to establish the use of family supports as an effective coping strategy. Effective planning in this regard will enable the family to make use of interpersonal supports, community resources, and social support and assist the family in adopting a future orientation.

Health care providers may find it a challenge to work with parents who are raising a child with a significant health problem. The may feel they are being tested and challenged, and may not be prepared for angry responses from parents. Thorne and Robinson (1988) described three phases of the relationship between health care providers and family caregivers. Initially, there is a phase of naïve trust, where families believe that health care professionals share their perspectives. Family members assume that all health professionals are highly skilled and knowledgeable, and that they will be honest and direct in communication. As family members engage in interactions that challenge their assumptions about the relationship with providers, they move into a second phase of disenchantment. Anger is often expressed and reflects their loss of trust in health care providers as they mobilize to protect the child. Finally, family members move to a phase of guarded alliance, where trust is shared with individual professionals, and it has to be earned. For the hospitalized child, the timing of this final phase may occur as the child approaches discharge. At this point, nurses and care coordinators may intervene to guide families through the referral process and coordinate services. If parents have confidence in the health professional at this stage of the process, they may be more likely to achieve appropriate follow-up for their child.

The opportunities and challenges for families seeking support for the care of their children will vary according to the developmental level of the child. For younger children (ages zero to 3) with chronic conditions or disabilities who are at risk for developmental delay, most communities will offer early intervention services as provided for by Public Law 99-457. The development of the Individualized Family Service Plan (IFSP) is a process that includes the family in planning services for the child that may be offered through the school system, health department, or developmental programs. Nurses and primary care providers may also be involved in the multidisciplinary meetings where the IFSP is developed. On a policy level, nurses should be familiar with community resources, and educate community leaders and legislators about the developmental needs of children with health problems.

Public Law 94-142, enacted in 1975, addresses the needs of children older than 3, and mandates that schools provide education to all children with developmental delays, including the opportunity for mainstreaming the child into the regular classroom. Special services are put into place through the multidisciplinary development of an Individualized Educational Plan (IEP).

The interface between families and schools concerning the plan to meet the developmental issues and health care needs of the child can be particularly difficult. In general, parents want their children to be placed in situations where the have the maximum opportunity to be successful. Many parents also strive to create a life for their child that is experienced as normal (Knafl, Deatrick, & Kirby, 2000). Sydnor-Greenberg and Dokken (2000) offer these five recommendations to help parents and children cope when planning experiences in school, camp and other settings: (a) communicate details about the child's needs; (b) recognize that education and knowledge about chronic illness vary among individuals; (c) be flexible concerning rules surrounding treatment; (d) advocate for parents' needs; and (e) promote self-care and self-advocacy for the children themselves.

Effective care-coordination techniques should be in place early in the planning process. Care coordination is the process of linking children and families with health care needs to special services in a coordinated manner that provides optimum care and maximizes the potential of the child. The care coordination process may be complicated by the following impeding factors: (a) there is usually no single point of entry into multiple systems of care; (b) the availability of funding and services from private and public payers is complex; and (c) sociocultural and economic barriers may impede efforts of families and professionals to maximize care (Lewandowski & Tesler, 2003). Some of these problems may be mitigated by the efforts of case managers and hospital discharge planners who can enact strategies to surmount the barriers that may exist. It is also anticipated that advances in information and communication technologies will enhance coordination efforts. The expanded use of electronic health records will ideally enable data entry, the incorporation of decision support tools into care, and the ability to measure patterns of care and outcomes across cases.

Implementation

In their study of factors associated with the adaptation of parents with a chronically ill child, Hentinen and Kyngas (1998) reported that families who experienced conflict and who felt deep sorrow and fear for their child's illness and future received little support from relatives and health care professionals. Parents who received abundant support from health care professionals reported fewer family conflicts and a better acceptance of their situation than did parents who received little or moderate support. Although there are many reasons for poor coping and adaptation in families, nurses and health care professionals should strive to identify and continually assess families who are experiencing difficulty, and should implement effective interventions that utilize support as a mediator. Because levels and type of needed support change over time, intervention needs to be based on continual assessment and attention to changes in the child's condition and family needs. For example, though the parents of children with diabetes and asthma studied by Hentinen and Kyngas (1998) reported a strong need for emotional support, Scott's (1998) study of parents of critically ill children indicated that their need for information, assurance, and proximity to their child was more important than support and comfort needs. Professionals should also be aware that differences can exist between their perceptions and the parents' perceptions of support needs. Furthermore, when support services are offered, providers should ensure that services are easily accessible, comprehensive in scope, and coordinated with other services that are provided.

Four types of support have been identified (House, 1981; Lewandowski & Tesler, 2003):

- *Informational support* involves providing factual information to help parents understand their child's illness and carry out procedures, and offering suggestions for coping and problem solving;
- *Emotional support* involves active listening, reassuring, encouraging, and conveying genuine concern for the family members;
- *Tangible support* includes providing transportation, child care, meals, financial aid;
- *Esteem support* involves conveying acceptance, respect, and value to family members.

Support may be exchanged within the family unit among parents and siblings, and may also be obtained in the contexts of relationships formed with other families with ill children. Broader sources of support emerge from the family's interface with the community (friends, clergy, employment networks) as well as health care providers and agencies.

The studies reporting the clinical implementation of family support encompass a number of sites including intensive care units, hospital units prior to discharge, and school based care settings. Dokken and Sydnor-Greenberg (1998) have recognized that the impact of technological advances and shortened hospital stays has resulted in more children with complex health needs being cared for at home. They have outlined steps that enable nurses actively to help parents mobilize their personal resources prior to discharge. They recommend that nurses encourage families to ask for help as a first step in this process, and to reassure them that asking for help does not mean relinquishing control but rather is a means to gain control over their lives. Nurses should remind families that other family and friends may want to help but are not sure what to do or whether they are qualified. Families should then take inventory of what their specific needs are, and match those needs with the interests and skills of those offering to help.

Kauffmann, Harrison, Burke, and Wong (1998) offer a research-based intervention for parents of repeatedly hospitalized children known as Stress-Point Intervention by Nurses, or SPIN. The intervention is based on a proactive approach to preparation before a child's hospitalization, and enhances family access to the nurse during and after hospitalization. With family nursing as the theoretical underpinning, SPIN utilizes some of the tools and processes associated with the Calgary family assessment and intervention model (Wright & Leahy, 1994). Overall, SPIN is a process whereby the nurse and parent sort through impending issues to discover the family's critical stress points, then design a customized family intervention that promotes continuity of care as the family moves through stressful periods.

Facilitating support groups is another intervention process that has been effectively implemented for parents of children who are coping with a wide spectrum of diseases and disorders. Such groups may be found through established supportive networks such as the American Cancer Society, the March of Dimes, the American Brain Tumor Association, Candlelighters, and so on. Nurses may assist families to access such a group. To manage support groups effectively, facilitators should have a solid understanding of group dynamics and the ability to remain objective throughout the group process. They should also be familiar with techniques that promote cohesion within a group, and create an emotional climate that is safe for parents who are coping with very personal and emotional issues. Parents have reported that support groups can be very helpful as they provide an opportunity for information gathering and sharing with other parents who have had similar experiences (Holaday, 1984). However, not all parents feel that participation in a group is beneficial. Some may choose to remain unaffiliated, especially if they feel that attendance reinforces the knowledge that their child's disease is progressive and incurable (Coyne, 1997).

Evaluation

As noted earlier, until recently relatively few studies examined the outcomes of specific nursing interventions that provide family support. With the current paradigm shift in academic nursing to derive practice implications from scholarship that is based on evidence as well as theory, more studies may be anticipated that report outcomes based on clinical findings. Nevertheless, some studies illustrate additional methods of enhancing family support systems while also reporting measurable outcomes of the intervention.

Sherman (1995) reports the results of the implementation of a home-based pediatric respite care program. This program was geared towards reducing stress and improving the quality of life for families caring for children with chronic illness through the provision of nursing services in the home. Utilization of the respite services was associated with a reduction in somatic complaints of the primary caregivers, and a decrease in the number of hospitalization days required by the children. The findings of the study were corroborated by qualitative reports of parents indicating the success of the program. Nurses involved in the provision of respite care also reported satisfaction with their work.

Sadler and colleagues (2003) present the results of a pilot study examining the effect of an intensive high-school-based parenting program (including the availability of a child-care center) for adolescent parents and their children on parental competence, parent-child interaction, and the development of the young child. The school-based program served as a mediating intervention that enhanced the contextual factors, including social support, that are associated with better outcomes in adolescent parents. Mothers in the intervention group scored higher on scales measuring maternal confidence, and also reported minimal levels of stress. These young mothers also scored significantly higher on the NCATS Teaching Scale, which measures the quality of parent-child interactions, when compared to a larger national sample. The initial founding of the parenting program and child-care center at the high school stemmed from mutual collaboration and planning among school officials, community leaders, and child-care health consultants. The results of the study indicated that educational and social supports offered at the center effectively mediated many potential adverse outcomes for this group of young parents and their children.

Although there has been some success in enhancing family support through linkages in the communities and schools, other findings indicate that the development of effective community-based services has not kept pace with the complex technological advances that allow children with intensive needs to be discharged from the hospital (Kirk & Glendinning, 2004). Often, appropriate and accessible support services are not readily available. The supply and funding of durable medical equipment and consumables may be fragmented and poorly disorganized. These problems call for a multi-agency approach with effective interprofessional collaboration at operational levels. The role of a designated case manager to coordinate the delivery of services and to be a point of contact between parents and the health care system is also important.

MULTIDISCIPLINARY INTEGRATION
AND PARTNERSHIP: CASE STUDY

A transdisciplinary team approach composed of family members and professionals who represent a variety of disciplines is crucial for the development of effective family-based support programs across settings. Such an approach overcomes the confines of individual disciplines, maximizes communication, interaction, and cooperation, and sets the stage for the ultimate success of family support initiatives. For children with assistive technology needs, variety in the team membership is particularly important because technology outcomes may be value-laden and may differ in importance according to who is evaluating them (Judge, 2002). By pooling the resources and integrating the expertise of all the team members and the strengths of the family, the chances for success in providing expert health care and improving the quality of family life is maximized. The following case study illustrates a multidisciplinary team approach and the mobilization of varied resources to improve the quality of life for a young girl with asthma.

To illustrate the multidisciplinary collaboration within a team of health professionals caring for children with moderate to severe asthma, we present the case of Lauren.

> Lauren is a 13-year-old adolescent who is obese and classified as having severe, persistent asthma. She lives in a crowded home with an older sister who smokes and who has a young child in day care who experiences frequent upper respiratory tract illnesses. Over a 12-month period, Lauren had experienced nine hospital admissions (including two admissions to the intensive care unit) for asthma exacerbations.
>
> Because of the severity of her asthma, Lauren had been referred by her primary care provider (PCP) to the Pediatric Respiratory Specialty service of a large academic health center and children's hospital. The specialty team consisted of attending pulmonologists, fellows, a pediatric nurse practitioner (PNP), and a respiratory therapist. Because Lauren was not improving despite taking an increasing number of medications, she and her family were then referred by the specialty team to the Asthma Outreach Program (AOP), a comprehensive adjunct outreach service that was affiliated with the Pediatric Respiratory Specialty and the hospital's Department of Environmental Health.
>
> The AOP is a unique multidisciplinary program that conducts home visits for children with poorly controlled moderate or severe persistent asthma. The team consists of PNPs, social workers, a psychologist, a bilingual outreach worker, and attending physicians. The program offers a comprehensive, ecologic approach to asthma case management for affected children and their families. The service is

coordinated with the care that the child also receives from the primary care provider and the pediatric pulmonology team.

As part of the AOP, the PNP intervenes for the child and family by providing case management services across settings in the home, clinical setting, and hospital. In the home setting, the nurse continually assesses the level of family functioning, their coping abilities and need for additional support, as well as the quality of the home environment. The PNP provides education regarding the disease process, medications, and equipment, and adjusts the clinical plan as appropriate. The nurse also assists in locating community resources, such as those sponsored by the American Lung Association (ALA). Case management in the hospital setting includes monitoring the child's progress, providing consultation, working with the family regarding discharge planning, and ensuring follow-up care at the specialty clinic or with the PCP.

In Lauren's case, the outreach team met with Lauren and her mother and older sister at their home to begin to assess the family's interests and goals for participating in the program. Upon environmental assessment by the AOP team, the home was found to be mostly carpeted. The mattresses were worn with no covers, and there were visible cockroaches. Because of her frequent illnesses, Lauren was not attending school on a regular basis, had repeated a grade, and had limited social contact with peers.

The following mutual goals were agreed upon: To improve the consistency of Lauren's health care; decrease hospitalizations and emergency department visits; decrease Lauren's absenteeism from school and the mother's absenteeism from work; and improve the family's overall quality of life. The family indicated that although they realized significant changes needed to be made in their home environment, they lacked the needed resources.

Frequent home visits were scheduled with the PNP and social worker to ensure the removal of asthma triggers and to provide ongoing support and education to the family. A written action-care plan for asthma, which clearly documented her medications, was provided for Lauren and her family, and also shared with her school nurse. Through active problem-solving, the family was empowered to negotiate with the landlord to remove carpeting and arrange for an exterminator. By working with the insurance providers and medical supply companies, the team was able to obtain mattress covers, an air conditioner, a purifier, and a dehumidifier for Lauren's room. Through mutual goal-setting and negotiation, the older sister agreed to smoke only outside the house, and also enrolled in a smoking cessation program.

In the 12 months following the referral to the AOP, Lauren experienced only three hospitalizations. She returned to school on a regular basis, and she attended Camp Treasure Chest (sponsored by the ALA) the following summer. The family reported much less stress in their lives, the mother was able to continue her work commitments, and the entire family experienced more opportunities for quality time together.

As this case study illustrates, the disparities in effective health care for children with asthma are often linked with the effects of poverty, problems with clean air, housing problems, and education. By adopting a team approach in the home setting, the family's interests and goals were determined, and resources needed to implement recommended changes were mobilized. The team providing ongoing care-coordination services was able to reconcile the recommendations of the specialty clinic staff with the treatment barriers faced in the home and at school. As a result, the family obtained the needed knowledge and was empowered to make changes in their physical environment and lifestyle in order to improve their child's health status and relieve some of the stress in the family's life.

SUMMARY

This chapter has reviewed the enhancement of family support systems as a key intervention targeting family roles and functions. The provision of family support should be based on mutual and ongoing comprehensive assessment, knowledge of the development of the child and family unit, and a consideration of the trajectory of the illness or disability. Effective family support and functioning have been associated with better adjustment in chronically ill children. Studies have also highlighted the pivotal role of both researchers and health care providers to develop, test, and implement family support programs.

REFERENCES

Balling, K., & McCubbin, M. (2001). Hospitalized children with chronic illness: Parental caregiving needs and valuing parental expertise. *Journal of Pediatric Nursing, 16,* 110–119.

Burr, W., Klein, S., Burr, R., Doxey, C., Harker, B., Holman, T., et al. (1994). *Re-examining family stress: New theory and research.* Thousand Oaks, CA: Sage.

Bohachick, P., & Anton, B. B. (1990). Psychosocial adjustment of patients and spouses to severe cardiomyopathy. *Research in Nursing and Health, 13,* 385–392.

Chernoff, R. G., Ireys, H. T., DeVet, K. A., & Kim, Y. J. (2002). A randomized, controlled trial of a community-based support program for families of children with chronic illness: Pediatric outcomes. *Archives of Pediatric and Adolescent Medicine, 156,* 533–539.

Cornman, B. J. (1993). Childhood cancer: Differential effects on the family members. *Oncology Nursing Forum, 20,* 1559–1566.

Coyne, I. T. (1997). Chronic illness: The importance of support for families caring for a child with cystic fibrosis. *Journal of Clinical Nursing, 6,* 121–129.

Dashiff, C. J. (1993). Parents' perceptions of diabetes in adolescent daughters and its impact on the family. *Journal of Pediatric Nursing, 8,* 361–369.

Dokken, D. L., & Sydnor-Greenberg, N., (1998) Helping families mobilize their personal resources. *Pediatric Nursing, 24,* 66–69.

Donnelly, E. (1994). Parents of children with asthma: An examination of family hardiness, family stressors, and family functioning. *Journal of Pediatric Nursing, 9,* 398–408.

Ferrell, B. R., Rhiner, M., Shapiro, B., & Dierkes, M. (1994). The experience of pediatric cancer pain, Part I: Impact of pain on the family. *Journal of Pediatric Nursing, 9,* 368–379.

Fleming, J., Challela, M., Eland, J., Hornick, R., Johnson, P., Martinson, I., et al. (1994). Impact on the family of children who are technology dependent and cared for in the home. *Pediatric Nursing, 20,* 379–388.

Feudtner, C., Haney, J., & Dimmers, M. A. (2003). Spiritual care needs of hospitalized children and their families: A national survey of pastoral care providers' perceptions. *Pediatrics, 111,* e67–72.

Gallo, A. M. (1990). Family management style in juvenile diabetes: A case illustration. *Journal of Pediatric Nursing, 5,* 23–32.

Hentinen, M. & Kyngas, H. (1998). Factors associated with the adaptation of parents with a chronically ill child. *Journal of Clinical Nursing, 7,* 316–324.

Holaday, B. (1984). Challenges of rearing a chronically ill child: Caring and coping. *Nursing Clinics of North America, 19,* 361–368.

House, J. S. (1981). *Work, stress and social support.* New York: Addison Wesley.

Institute for Family-Centered Care. (2005). *What is family centered care.* Retrieved January 14, 2005, from http://www.familycenteredcare.org/about_us/what-is-fcc.html

Johnson, M., Bulechek, G., McCloskey Dochterman, J., Maas, M., & Moorhead, S. (2001). *Nursing diagnoses, outcomes, and interventions: NANDA, NOC, and NIC linkages.* St. Louis, MO: Mosby.

Judge, S. (2002). Family-centered assistive technology assessment and intervention practices for early intervention. *Infants and Young Children, 15,* 60–68.

Kauffmann, E., Harrison, M. B., Burke, S. O., & Wong, C. (1998) Stress-point intervention for parents of children hospitalized with chronic conditions. *Pediatric Nursing, 24,* 362–366.

Kirk, S., & Glendinning, C. (2004). Developing services to support parents caring for a technology-dependent child at home. *Child: Care, Health, & Development, 30,* 209–218.

Kirschbaum, M., & Knafl, K. (1996). Major themes in parent-provider relationships: A comparison of life threatening and chronic illness experiences. *Journal of Family Nursing, 2,* 195–216.

Knafl, K., Breitmayer, B., Gallo, A., & Zoeller, L. (1992). Parents' views of health care providers: An exploration of the components of a positive working relationship. *Children's Health Care, 21*(2), 90–95.

Knafl, K., Deatrick, J., & Kirby, A. (2000). Normalization promotion. In M. Craft-Rosenberg & J. Dennehy (Eds.), *Nursing interventions for infants, children, and families* (pp. 373–387). Thousand Oaks, CA: Sage.

Knafl, K., & Gilliss, C. (2002). Families and chronic illness: A synthesis of current research. *Journal of Family Nursing, 8,* 178–198.

Kopp, M., Richter, R., Rainer, J., Kopp-Wilfing, P., Rumpold, G., & Walter, M. H. (1995). Differences in family functioning between patients with chronic headache and patients with chronic low back pain. *Pain, 63,* 219–224.

Labbe, E. E. (1996). Emotional states and perceived family functioning of caregivers of chronically ill children. *Psychological Reports, 79,* 1233–1234.

Lavigne, J. V., & Faier-Routman, J. (1992). Psychological adjustment to pediatric physical disorders: A meta-analytic review. *Journal of Pediatric Psychology, 17,* 133–157.

Lewandowski, L. A., & Tesler, M. E. (2003). *Family-centered care: Putting it into action: The SPN/ANA guide to family-centered care.* Washington, DC: American Nurses Association.

McCloskey Dochterman, J., & Bulechek, G. M. (Eds.). (2004). *Nursing interventions classification (NIC)* (4th ed.). St. Louis, MO: Mosby.

Meleski, D. D. (2002). Families with chronically ill children. *American Journal of Nursing, 102,* 47–54.

Melnyk, B. M., Alpert-Gillis, L., Feinstein, N. F., Crean, H. F., Johnson, J., Fairbanks, E., et al. (2004). Creating opportunities for parental empowerment: Program effects on the mental health/coping outcomes of critically ill young children and their mothers. *Pediatrics, 113,* e597–607.

Melnyk, B. M., & Feinstein, N. (2001). Mediating functions of maternal anxiety and participation in care of young children's post hospital adjustment. *Research in Nursing and Health, 24,* 18–26.

Melnyk, B. M., Small, L., & Carno, M. (2004). The effectiveness of parent-focused interventions in improving coping/mental health outcomes of critically ill children and their parents: An evidence-based guide to practice. In B. Melnyk & E. Fineout-Overholt (Eds.), *Evidence-based practice in nursing and healthcare: A guide to best practice* (pp. CD–22). Philadelphia: Lippincott, Williams, and Wilkins.

Park, E. S., & Martinson, I. M. (1998). Socioemotional experiences of Korean families with asthmatic children. *Journal of Family Nursing, 4,* 291–308.

Prugh, D., Staub, E., & Sands, H. (1953). Study of the emotional reactions of children and families to hospitalization and illness. *American Journal of Orthopsychiatry, 23,* 70–106.

Rehm, R. S., & Catanzaro, M. L. (1998). "It's just a fact of life": Family members' perceptions of parental chronic illness. *Journal of Family Nursing, 4,* 21–40.

Robertson, J. (1958). *Young children in hospitals.* New York: Basic Books.

Robinson, C. A. (1994). Nursing interventions with families: A demand or an invitation to change. *Journal of Advanced Nursing, 19,* 897–904.

Robinson, C. A. (1996). Health care relationships revisited. *Journal of Family Nursing, 2,* 152–173.

Rolland, J. S. (1999). Parental illness and disability: A family systems framework. *Journal of Family Therapy, 21,* 232–266.

Sadler, L. S., Swartz, M. K., & Ryan-Krause, P. (2003). Supporting adolescent mothers and their children through a high school-based child care center and parent support program. *Journal of Pediatric Health Care, 17,* 109–117.

Sawyer, E. H. (1992). Family functioning when children have cystic fibrosis. *Journal of Family Nursing, 7,* 304–311.

Scott, L. D. (1998). Perceived needs of parents of critically ill children. *Journal of the Society of Pediatric Nurses, 3,* 4–12.

Sherman, B. R. (1995). Impact of home-based respite care on families of children with chronic illness. *Children's Health Care, 24*(1), 33–45.

Sydnor-Greenberg, N., & Dokken, D. (2000). Family matters, coping and caring in different ways: Understanding and meaningful involvement. *Journal of Pediatric Nursing, 26,* 185–190.

Swartz, M. K. (2005). Parenting preterm infants: A meta-synthesis. *MCN: The American Journal of Maternal Child Nursing, 30*(2), 1–6.

Thorne, S. E., & Robinson, C. A. (1988). Health care relationships: The chronic illness perspective. *Research in Nursing and Health, 11,* 293–300.

Touliatos, J., Perlmutter, B., Straus, M. A., & Holden, G. (2001). *Handbook of family measurement techniques: Instruments and index* (Vol. 3). Thousand Oaks, CA: Sage.

Wallander, J. L., & Varni, J. N. (1998). Effects of pediatric chronic physical disorders on child and family adjustment. *Journal of Child Psychology and Psychiatry and Allied Disciplines, 39,* 29–46.

Whittemore, R., Kanner, S., & Grey, M. (2004). The influence of family on physiological and psychosocial health in youth with type 1 diabetes: A systematic review. In B. Melnyk & E. Fineout-Overholt (Eds.), *Evidence-based practice in nursing and healthcare: A guide to best practice* (p. CD 22). Philadelphia: Lippincott, Williams, and Wilkins.

Wright, L., & Leahy, M. (1994). *Nurses and families: A guide to family assessment and intervention.* Philadelphia: Davis.

Youngblut, J. M., Brennan, P. F., & Swegart, L. A. (1994). Families with medically fragile children: An exploratory study. *Pediatric Nursing, 20,* 463–468.

Zahr, L. K., Khoury, M., & Saoud, N. B. (1994). Chronic illness in Lebanese preschoolers: Impact of illness and child temperament on the family. *American Journal of Orthopsychiatry, 64,* 396–403.

CHAPTER SEVEN

Genetic Assessment and Counseling

Janet K. Williams

INTRODUCTION, DEFINITIONS, AND THEIR MEASUREMENT

The topic of genetics in child health care can seem incomprehensible to some, familiar to others, and at times full of exciting possibilities for new treatments and hoped-for cures. However, new genetic testing options also may pose a risk for individual health or societal well-being, and some genetic discoveries that guide diagnosis have not led yet to new treatment options. Some nursing practitioners and educators note that their own nursing background has not prepared them to use new genomic concepts in their professional nursing practice, whereas for many new students and graduate nurses, genetics principles are a familiar part of their basic science preparation. With emerging awareness of the importance of genetic factors in contributing to the cause of common chronic diseases (National Coalition for Health Professional Education in Genetics [NCHPEG], 2004; Skirton & Patch, 2003), children and families are now being asked to describe their genetic family histories, and genetic discoveries are employed in clinical assessment for children with rare as well as more common diseases.

The term *genetics* refers to units of heredity, that is, genes that contain instructions for production of a functional cellular product (Jorde, Carey, Bamshad, & White, 2003; Skirton & Patch, 2003). The use of the term *genetic* generally refers to this heritable information, and in clinical terms the idea of a genetic condition often refers to uncommon, medically complex disorders that are passed on in families, and are managed by teams of specialists. A newer term is *genomics*. This refers to the study and function of all the genetic information in an organism, including interactions of these genetic factors with environmental factors (Guttmacher, Collins, Drazen, & Zerhouni, 2004). The field of genomics is very new. However, when today's children become adults, the knowledge of genomic factors influencing their health is likely to be applied not only to diagnose a clinical problem, but also to help guide treatment, or help prevent, postpone, or lessen the manifestations of the disease (Zerhouni, 2004).

The genetic family history provides information on factors within the family that put a child at risk for a disease with a major genetic component. Used with data on the shared environment, common behaviors, and other disease risk factors, the genetic family history is an important component of a comprehensive health assessment (Yoon et al., 2002). The November 2004 announcement of a new national family history initiative program, by the U.S. Surgeon General (http://www.hhs.gov/familyhistory/) means that families will expect health professionals to include family history risk factors in assessments and subsequent plans of care. The view of health and disease from a genomic perspective requires that information about genetic and environmental factors be considered throughout the clinical assessment, treatment, and evaluation period, moving the inclusion of a genomics perspective closer to the holistic view of children, families, and health that is familiar to the profession of nursing. However, in order to use genetic information and a genomic perspective wisely, nurses must be prepared to understand basic elements of genomic nursing practice.

Guidelines for inclusion of genetics content into nursing practice have been issued by several national professional health care organizations (Table 7.1). These efforts are not completed and guidelines are needed for documenting competencies as evidenced by licensing and certification procedures. NCHPEG guidelines (2000) pertain to all health care professionals. Statements contained in the report from the Expert Panel on Genetics and Nursing (2000), and the report entitled *Essentials of Baccalaureate Education* (American Association of Colleges of Nursing [AACN], 1998) address the knowledge and skills that professional nurses should possess. The National Organization of Nurse Practitioner Faculties (NONPF) (2002), the International Society of Nurses in Genetics (ISONG) (1998), and the Oncology Nursing Society (ONS) (2003) delineate additional knowledge and skills for advanced practice nurses. The American Academy of Nursing has called for documentation of competencies through licensure and certification mechanisms (Lea, 2002). Core elements for baccalaureate and graduate nursing

TABLE 7.1 Standards of Practice in Genomic Health Care Statements

Organization	Topics
American Association of Colleges of Nursing	The essentials of baccalaureate nursing education for professional nursing practice
American Academy of Nursing	Statement on genetic nursing competencies
International Society of Nurses in Genetics	Statement on scope and standards of genetics
American Nurses Association	Clinical nursing practice
National Coalition for Health Professional Education in Genetics	Core competencies
Oncology Nursing Society	Guidelines for oncology nurses
Report of the Expert Panel on Genetics and Nursing	Implications for education and practice
The National Organization of Nurse Practitioner Faculties	Primary care competencies in specialty areas

education have been proposed, but not yet adopted, by licensure or credentialing bodies (Jenkins, Dimond, & Steinberg, 2001; Williams, 2002). A small expert group has discussed plans to build upon past efforts of nurse leaders and design a competence-based education framework for U.S. nurses in the genomics era. A plan has been developed to hold at least three meetings over the next 2 years with the goal of working with stakeholders to set an agenda for nursing education. Invited meeting participants will contribute to the identification of minimum common core competencies for nurses in the United States, determining learning objectives, and setting expected outcomes. Efforts are continuing to create national standards and exemplars that will be presented for consideration by representatives of education, licensing, and credentialing bodies that may be useful for redesigning curricula to include preparation of nurse competency in genomics.

There are multiple publications, including the Health Resources and Services Administration's (HRSA)–sponsored Expert Panel Report on Genetics and Nursing (2000), that encourage the integration of genomics into nursing education, certification, and licensure. The foundation is now in place, but we must move forward to create the building blocks that facilitate integration of genomics into practice to improve health outcomes.

Genomic health care is a new and a rapidly expanding field. Elements of nursing excellence in this field will continue to be identified as the knowledge base emerges and changes. Several components of excellence for professional nursing practice are shared by the current guidelines. These focus on the need for genomic knowledge, integration of this knowledge into the practitioner's skills, and ability to work within a multidisciplinary health care system in order to ensure that children and families receive genomic health care that is appropriate for their needs.

INFLUENCES OF GENETIC ASSESSMENT AND COUNSELING FOR INFANTS AND CHILDREN

Core elements are based upon knowledge of genetics and genomics in professional nursing practice. Although current documents do not specify the extent of knowledge needed, a baseline of genetics knowledge must underlie the ability to incorporate understanding of genomic concepts in professional nursing practice, regardless of clinical population or setting (Feetham & Williams, 2004). Documentation of education in clinical genetics and genetic counseling are required for nurses who seek credentialing as advanced practice genetic nurses (Cook, Kase, Middelton, & Monsen, 2003). Traditional genetic health care has focused on individuals with single-gene or chromosomal disorders that have a clear pattern of inheritance. Ability to provide comprehensive nursing care for these children, such as those with cystic fibrosis (CF), includes a comprehensive and current understanding of the role of genetic factors in the detection and management of these single-gene disorders. For example, children with CF who have specific mutations in the CFTR gene may have fewer pancreatic symptoms than children with other CFTR mutations have (Zielenski, 2000). This basic genetic knowledge is also applied during the diagnostic process when a genetic factor is suspected. For example, understanding health effects of alterations in the FMR1 gene, associated with Fragile X syndrome, is an essential component of knowledge for persons providing care to infants and children with developmental delay (Bailey, Skinner, & Sparkman, 2003).

A second core element is the ability to collect and communicate a genetic family history. Assessment of genetic components of risk for disease is based upon the drawing of a genetic family history in the form of a three-generation pedigree, using standardized symbols (NCHPEG, 2004). In order to maintain privacy of health history information, health care providers should not share with other family members the individual health data from a person's genetic family pedigree in their personal medical record without the permission of the person who provided the information. In addition to identification of single-gene disorders that may be present in a family, the genetic family history can also identify the presence of conditions for which there is a major genetic component, but for which that component is not fully understood. An example of this situation is the presence of asthma in more than one family member. Recognition of potential genetic aspects of asthma may be useful in the overall plan of care, including drug selection and future development of genetic tests that predict drug response (University of Washington Center for Genomics and Public Health, 2004).

Understanding of genetic factors that contribute to health and disease is of little use without the accompanying interpersonal skills upon which nursing communication relies. The term *genetic counseling* is used both within the provision of specialized services by persons with advanced training in genetic health care, and as a component of health care practice that reflects the scope of the health care professional's knowledge. The definition of genetic counseling, as stated by the American Society of Human Genetics (ASHG) (1975), is a communication process that deals with human problems associated with the occurrence, or the risk of occurrence, of a genetic disorder in a family. This process involves an attempt by one or more appropriately trained persons to help the individual or family to (1) comprehend the medical facts, including the diagnosis, probable course of the disorder, and the available management; (2) appreciate the way heredity contributes to the disorder, and the risk of recurrence in specified relatives; (3) understand the alternatives for dealing with the risk of recurrence; (4) choose the course of action which seems to them appropriate in view of their risk, their family goals and their ethical and religious standards, and to act in accordance with that decision; and (5) make the best possible adjustment to the disorder in an affected family member and/or the risk of recurrence of that disorder. (pp. 240–241).

When used to describe a nursing intervention, Genetic Counseling (Iowa Intervention Project, 2000) is defined as the "use of an interactive helping process focusing on assisting an individual, family, or group, manifesting or at risk for developing or transmitting a birth defect or genetic condition, to cope" (p. 357). Activities that illustrate the use of these interpersonal counseling skills for children and their families include providing privacy and confidentiality, supporting the person's coping process, and providing referral to genetic health care specialists, as necessary.

INFLUENCE OF ASSESSMENT AND COUNSELING FOR THE FAMILY

The core skills for nurses who apply knowledge of genetics and genomics to care of infants and children are also skills that form the basis for care of that child's family. As they provide genomic health care to family members, nurses must be able to elicit and use understanding of the family's perceptions about illness and disease risk. The theory of lay representation of disease includes five domains that are used by the individual to create a psychological construct of the illness. The five domains are disease identity (name, signs, and symptoms), timeline, consequences, causes, and controllability (Lau & Hartman, 1983). When one member of a family believes a condition is caused by a situation that does not include genetic factors, decisions about symptom management—as well as response to information regarding recurrence risk—may influence not only that person, but other family members as well. This situation is illustrated in a family where several young men had mental retardation, but their parents believed this situation was due to mistakes made by the physicians or nurses at the time of their sons' births rather than by a genetic factor, such as a gene mutation leading to Fragile X syndrome.

Psychosocial Typology of Genetically Influenced Illnesses (Rolland & Williams, in press) focuses on family adaptation to the potential or existence of an inherited disease in one or more family members. This typology includes the concepts of timing of disease or information within the life cycle, severity of the condition, likelihood that symptoms of the disease will occur, and extent of prevention or treatment options for the disorder. For example, Huntington's disease (HD) is a genetic disorder, but it usually isn't apparent until adulthood. Although symptomatic treatments are available, at this time there are no treatments that will prevent or alter the course of the disease. Decisions about obtaining genetic information by one person in a family can have an impact on others in the family. For example, a young adult woman whose father has HD may be reluctant to ask for any information about her own risk to have this disorder, out of a fear that this may be perceived as evidence that she does not love her father. Yet, her reluctance to ask for information may leave her with misconceptions or incomplete information about her own health status as well as potential reproductive options. The recognition of components of genetic illnesses that can influence psychosocial responses within a family can guide assessment and intervention choices by nurses and other health care providers.

Throughout the nursing care of infants, children, and their families, principles of medical ethics also underlie health care practice. Ethics principles can help guide, not necessarily what decisions must be made, but how they can be made (Lea, Williams, & Donahue, in press). The principle of autonomy is demonstrated when a person's activities in a decision, such as having a genetic test, is voluntary, and the person has had the opportunity to understand information about the test. This principle is especially important when genetic testing is considered for children. A second principle, privacy, is respected when one person's medical information is not disclosed to others, even family members, without that person's consent. The obligation to do no harm and the principle of justice also apply in the process of ensuring that people provide consent that is informed, and that all persons have an equal opportunity to receive genetic health care.

NURSING CARE EXCELLENCE IN GENETIC ASSESSMENT AND COUNSELING

Application of the major components of genomic nursing practice reflects standards of nursing practice addressed by professional nursing organizations, the Expert Nursing Panel, and the core competencies for health professionals, including nurses (Table 7.1).

Genomic Education

Education to support nursing knowledge includes basic genetic principles, clinical genetics topics, and factors that interact with genes to increase risk for disease. Although existing guidelines do not specify content for education, the following topics are suggested as foundational for baccalaureate graduates. Basic genetic principles include the principles of human genetics, that is, genes, their structure and function, their roles in cellular activities, proteins and other products produced from genetic instructions, and interactions with other factors influencing cell function. Education also should include chromosomal function and abnormalities; single gene, multifactorial, and nontraditional inheritance; and the principles of population genetics. This information is of limited use to nurses unless there is content that links these basic science principles to human health and disease. Here, the application of these principles throughout the nursing curriculum is essential. Courses such as physiology and pharmacology will increasingly use genetic principles as disease processes and new treatments are developed. Examples of application of genetics in these courses are the molecular testing of cancer cells for targeting therapies to specific pathways within the cell (Capriotti, 2004) and potential use of genotyping to predict drug response in asthma (University of Washington Center for Genomics and Public Health, 2004).

This education must continue throughout the curriculum, so that nurses can apply principles of genetics and genomics throughout the nursing process for health care of children and families. Maintaining a perspective of genomics is essential in identifying ways in which gene and environmental interactions influence the health care of persons with relatively uncommon genetic conditions, as well as those who have or are at risk to have common conditions affecting larger components of the population. For example, in an undergraduate child-health course, nursing diagnoses, outcomes, and interventions for a toddler with Down's syndrome would include an understanding of the health risks that accompany this disorder, reproductive options that may be desired by the child's parents, health promotion issues at this age in the child's life, and strategies to promote family functioning. Discussion of nursing care for the child with asthma would include genetic and environmental factors that influence symptom management.

Genetic Family History

One of the most basic genomic health-care skills for all health care providers is the ability to obtain and record a three-generation family history. Although DNA-based testing may someday become available to identify risk for common chronic diseases, DNA testing is now largely limited to analysis of highly penetrant genes with mutations that account for approximately 5% of the total population disease burden (Yoon et al., 2002). However, a genetic family history can be useful to identify familial components of risk for single-gene as well as common chronic diseases. The symbols and procedures for recording a genetic family pedigree are straightforward and resources for constructing a genetic family pedigree are available (NCHPEG, 2004). Using this skill within nursing practice relies on several other skills. One is that child health nurses should have adequate understanding of patterns of inheritance, so that evidence of a disorder that may be genetic can be recognized in the family's pedigree. For those who provide care to a specific population of children, this knowledge should be more specialized, so that during the obtaining of the family genetic history, the nurse can focus questions about health risks on specific diseases. An example would be a nurse who specializes in pediatric cardiology. The nurse should be knowledgeable about the inheritance, age of onset, range, and severity of symptoms for cardiac diseases presenting in childhood that have genetic components.

Application of genomic knowledge in assessment of children and families for genetic disease risk factors also includes knowledge of alterations in physical growth and development that are consistent with specific clinical disorders. Fragile X syndrome is an example of a clinical disorder that results from a gene mutation, and has variable severity and clinical presentation. The disorder may be recognized because of a pattern of clinical symptoms in one child, or through a careful analysis of the genetic family history. When health care providers are not knowledgeable about this condition, the diagnosis is delayed, with considerable frustration resulting for parents who report a substantive lag between the time they first became concerned about their child and confirmation of the diagnosis (Bailey et al., 2003). When a nurse obtains a family history of learning disabilities, or mental retardation, or behavioral disorders in males and females within a family, the nurse should recognize that these findings might be consistent with the presence of Fragile X syndrome in the family members. Although the family history will not reveal all the information that is needed to establish the diagnosis, an astute clinician can recognize the clinical information and inheritance patterns that would be consistent with this disorder.

Interpersonal Communication Skills

It is also necessary for the nurse to possess skills that allow for sensitive and supportive teaching and counseling regarding management of genetic health risks (Iowa Intervention Project, 2000). When developing genetic history taking skills, nurses must be able to apply their knowledge of communication principles when families or children are asked to discuss potentially sensitive topics. Such aspects as consanguinity, a pregnancy outside of marriage, mental retardation or mental illness, nonpaternity, or other events that may be regarded by the family as secret or potentially stigmatizing may not be easily revealed to the nurse.

Therapeutic communication skills are necessary when the child-health nurse discusses sensitive topics that arise throughout the trajectory of genetic conditions. One such topic is end-of-life decisions. Genetic conditions may improve, remain stable, or slowly worsen over time, and in some, life span is shortened. Little is known about the end-of-life preferences of children with life-shortening genetic disorders. However, once preferences of children and their families are known, nursing interventions can be applied to this population. One example is the opportunity that children with a fatal genetic disease may wish to have to express their wishes for end-of-life care. In a clinical study of end of life preferences, teens with Duchenne muscular dystrophy (DMD) and their mothers had differing views on end-of-life preferences, but expressed gratitude for the opportunity to express their fears and preferences (Trout, Mathews, & Williams, 2004).

Rather than reflecting the opinion of the health care professional, nondirectiveness, or the provision of genetic information in a way that keeps decisions about reproduction within the family, is considered to be a cornerstone for the practice of genetic counseling. This principle differs from the more traditional health care approach where the goal may be to reduce the incidence of disease (Jorde et al., 2003). When a family is considering health care decisions that focus on reproductive decisions, the principle of nondirectiveness focuses on supporting a family's values and beliefs, rather than on the ultimate reduction of the number of persons with a genetic disorder. Both the Code of Ethics for Nurses (American Nurses Association [ANA], 2001) and the ISONG guidelines (ISONG,

1998) reinforce support of this principle. Yet, there are circumstances where individuals and families expect that nurses, as well as other health care providers, will provide sound and knowledgeable advice, for example, regarding treatment options for a familial cancer risk or decisions regarding genetic testing for inherited disorders. The nurse should use therapeutic communication skills in a manner that supports a family's abilities to become informed and to weigh options, and assist the family in determining a course of action that is consistent with current standards of practice, yet also consistent with their own family values and goals.

Lay Beliefs and Psychosocial Adaptation

Applying genomic knowledge in nursing practice also includes assessment and integration of knowledge about family responses to illness. One's beliefs about a situation may be influential in determining which courses of action a person would consider. Comparison of new information to familiar beliefs may make it difficult for individuals or families to accept new genomic information. In one family where several people had a diagnosis of HD, the belief within the family was that only males could develop the disorder, because that had been the pattern in the family. When one of the daughters of a man with HD learned that this was an autosomal dominant disorder, in which males and females both could inherit the disease, she had difficulty accepting the new and potentially frightening information. Likewise, in families in which a woman has learned, through genetic testing, that she has a mutation in a gene for familial breast or ovarian cancer, it may be difficult for her sons to understand that they too have the potential to have inherited the gene mutation, and thus the potential to pass it on to their sons and daughters.

Adaptation to the possibility of an inherited disease also challenges a family's ability to cope with the stresses of the onset of an inherited disease. Adaptation to a genetic condition may occur in phases that begin prior to the onset of a disorder and extend beyond the life span of the person with the disease (Rolland & Williams, in press). The period prior to the onset of classic motor symptoms in HD is an example of a phase of the disorder in which family members have difficulty adapting to changes in the person with HD as well as within the family system. HD typically appears in the middle adult years, creating caregiving challenges for family members, including children of persons with this disorder. Psychosocial issues for teens in families in which there is a parent with HD include the possibility that the teen may also develop the disease; how to have a normal life when one's parent is beginning to demonstrate loss of neurologic and cognitive function; and attempts to decrease the stress within the family (Williams, 2002).

Ethics

The profession of nursing is guided by the Code of Ethics (ANA, 2001). Ethics principles used to resolve dilemmas in nursing practice regarding genetics issues include autonomy, privacy, beneficence, and fairness. When mutation(s) in a gene associated with an inherited disorder have been identified, individuals with a positive family history may request genetic testing. The purposes of the testing include predicting the likelihood that the person will develop the condition in the future, or identifying if the person is a carrier of the mutation in an autosomal recessive or x-linked gene. Ethical issues arise when parents request that predictive or carrier testing be conducted on their minor age children.

Guidelines for use of genetic testing recommend that unless the results may have medical benefit for the child, genetic testing of minor age children not be performed (ASHG and American College of Medical Genetics [ACMG], 1995). Reasons include the potential for misunderstanding of the purpose of the test by the child, and potential risk to the child's insurability when he or she is no longer included in the parents' health insurance plan. In this situation, the nurse applies knowledge of guidelines regarding genetic testing of minor-age children, plus knowledge of the developmental level of the child and the ability of the child to understand the purposes and limitations of the test. The request for genetic testing of minor-age children provides the nurse with the opportunity to help parents determine why they want the test, what information they would like to have regarding their child's genetic status, and what the potential consequences for their child could be. In some instances, parents request this information soon after a diagnosis is made in one of their children and parents want to be reassured that their other children will not be at risk to have or pass on a gene mutation for the disorder. For some parents, discussing the potential benefits of delaying genetic testing until their minor-age children can give their own consent may be beneficial, and nurses share in the responsibility to assist parents to examine all options.

MULTIDISCIPLINARY INTEGRATION AND PARTNERSHIPS: CASE STUDY

Genetic health care involves many health care disciplines. Interdisciplinary approaches to education will enhance the ability of health care providers to work together in applying new genomic knowledge (Expert Panel on Genetics and Nursing, 2000). One example of interdisciplinary health care is in expanded newborn screening. Several U.S. states are adding newborn screening for CF to the newborn screening programs. CF is an autosomal recessive condition, meaning that each parent of a child with CF is a carrier.

> Jodie and Mark are the parents of a newborn son, Austin. He is their second child, and his older sister, Molly, is healthy. Jodi and Mark are notified that Austin's newborn screening test was positive for CF. When they spoke with Todd, their child-health nurse, they asked how the test could be positive, because no one in their family has this illness. Discussing the family history is an opportunity for Todd to use health-teaching skills to promote understanding of why a family history may be negative for CF, even though CF is a genetic disorder. In Jodie and Mark's family histories, no one has CF. This is a common situation, as the condition is present only when both parents (who do not have signs of CF) pass on the gene mutation to their child. Children of that couple could inherit both copies of the CF gene, and would be expected to have CF; or could inherit one copy of the gene with the mutation and become a carrier; or inherit neither copy of the gene with the mutation. Todd would also use this opportunity to help Jodie and Mark understand that Austin's test only indicates that he may have CF, as the test was a screening rather than a diagnostic test. In his teaching, Todd also notes that the screening test has the purpose of identifying children who may have CF but that a more definitive test will be needed to actually determine if that is true. He recognizes that Mark and Jodie are frightened by the results of the screening test and he assists them in identifying what questions they want to ask the team that will perform the diagnostic tests on Austin. He writes down the questions that Mark and Jodie mention, and suggests information they also may want to ask about. Examples of questions on Mark and Jodie's list are, If Austin doesn't have CF, why would the screening test be positive? Is CF always a fatal disease? If Austin has CF why does he appear so normal now? What will happen when Austin has more tests, and is it possible that Molly could also be sick?
>
> Todd's interventions reflect his educational preparation on principles of human genetics, Mendelian inheritance patterns, the purposes and policies governing newborn screening, and mechanisms for referral to genetics and CF specialists. He does not have current information regarding the specific mutations that can be present in a person who has CF, and he explains that if Austin is found to have CF, the team at the CF testing and management program can help Mark and Jodie understand the specific test findings. Further health teaching by genetics nursing or genetic counseling specialists regarding the genetic components of CF would include more technical information regarding the specific mutation present in Austin; genotype/phenotype relationships, if known, from Austin's

test results; and implications for Austin's future health. In this situation, Todd will collaborate with genetics and CF specialists during the time that Austin is being evaluated for CF.

After Austin's evaluation by the CF diagnosis and management team, it is found that he has this diagnosis. Todd continues to communicate with Jodie and Mark about Austin's care, and notes that their understanding of the disorder and its inheritance may need further clarification. Mark's mother has mentioned that she is not convinced the diagnosis is correct, as she has read about a baby who had a newborn test but actually did not have anything wrong. In these conversations, Todd applies his knowledge of genetics, newborn screening, and family dynamics as he identifies lay beliefs that extended family members may have about CF or newborn screening. In addition to exploring the source of the information (that is, Todd and Jodie's concerns), Todd reviewed the differences between diagnosis and screening, noting that not all babies with a positive screening test will be found to have a disease. He also recognizes that coping with the diagnosis can be difficult, and he explores how Mark and Jodie feel their family members, including Mark's mother, are handling the news.

Child-health nurses apply understanding of the psychosocial adjustment of family members throughout the trajectory of the disease, and the changing roles for family members. Collaboration and partnerships may extend into the community and can be especially challenging for children with CF, with the knowledge that their disease may lead to death in childhood or early adult years. Throughout Austin's life, many child-health and family nurses will participate in his health care. When he enters school, the school nurse can communicate with Mark and Jodie and also provide information to Austin's teachers to ensure that his health care needs will be met throughout the school day. Despite the hope for more effective treatments for CF and other genetic disorders, health care may also involve coordination among family, CF specialists, and community health care providers when end-of-life issues are to be addressed. Achieving excellence in applying genetic and genomic principles to child- and family-health nursing includes the ability to share knowledge with members across health care disciplines.

SUMMARY

Knowledge of genetic and genomic aspects of health and disease in children and their families is a foundational component of child-health nursing. This knowledge is an essential component of child and family assessment, and appropriate use of nursing interventions including health teaching, coping enhancement, and participation in interdisciplinary child-health services. Identification of minimum common core competencies for nurses creates the basis for integration of genomics into nursing education, certification, and licensure, leading to improved health care outcomes for children and their families.

ACKNOWLEDGMENT

The author would like to acknowledge support for this chapter provided by the National Institute for Nursing Research Award R01 NR07970, "Family Health After Predictive HD Testing."

REFERENCES

American Association of Colleges of Nursing. (1998). *The essentials of baccalaureate education for professional nursing practice.* Washington, DC: American Association of Colleges of Nursing.

American Nurses Association. (2001). *Code of ethics.* Retrieved August 20, 2004, from http://www.nursingworld.org

American Society of Human Genetics Ad Hoc Committee on Genetic Counseling. (1975). Genetic counseling. *American Journal of Human Genetics, 27,* 240–242.

American Society of Human Genetics and American College of Medicine Genetics. (1995). Points to consider: Ethical, legal, and psychosocial implications of genetic testing in children and adolescents. *American Journal of Human Genetics, 57,* 1233–1241.

Bailey, D. B., Jr., Skinner, D., & Sparkman, K. L. (2003). Discovering Fragile X syndrome: Family experiences and perceptions. *Pediatrics, 111,* 407–416.

Capriotti, T. (2004). New oncology strategy: Molecular targeting of cancer cells. *MEDSURG Nursing, 13,* 191–195.

Cook, S. S., Kase, R., Middelton, L., & Monsen, R. B. (2003). Portfolio evaluation for professional competence: Credentialing in genetics for nurses. *Journal of Professional Nursing, 19,* 85–90.

Expert Panel on Genetics and Nursing. (2000). Implications for education and practice. In Health Resources and Services Administration and the National Institutes of Health, *Report of the expert panel on genetics and nursing: Implications for education and practice* (BHP 00177). Washington, DC: U.S. Department of Health and Human Services.

Feetham, S., & Williams, J. (2004). Introduction. In *Nursing and 21st century genetics: Leadership for global health.* Geneva, Switzerland: International Council of Nurses.

Guttmacher, A. E., Collins, F. S., Drazen, J. M., & Zerhouni, E. (2004). *Genomic medicine: Articles from the New England Journal of Medicine.* Baltimore: Johns Hopkins University Press.

Iowa Intervention Project. J. C. McCloskey & G. M. Bulechek (Eds.). (2000). *Nursing interventions classification (NIC)* (3rd ed.). St. Louis: Mosby

International Society of Nurses in Genetics. (1998). *Statement on the scope and standards of genetics clinical nursing practice.* Silver Springs, MD: American Nurses Association.

Jenkins, J. F., Dimond, E., & Steinberg, S. (2001). Preparing for the future through genetics nursing education. *Journal of Nursing Scholarship, 33,* 191–195.

Jorde, L., Carey, J., Bamshad, M., & White, R. (2003). *Medical genetics* (3rd ed.). St. Louis, MO: Mosby

Lau, R. R., & Hartman, K. A. (1983). Common sense representations of common illnesses. *Health Psychology, 2,* 167–185.

Lea, D. H. (2002). Position statement: Integrating genetics competencies into baccalaureate and advanced nursing education. *Nursing Outlook, 50,* 167–168.

Lea, D. H., Williams, J. K., & Donahue, M. P. (in press). Ethical, legal, and social issues in genetic testing. *Journal of Midwifery and Women's Health.*

National Coalition for Health Professional Education in Genetics. (2000). *Core competencies in genetics essential for health-care professionals.* Retrieved August 20, 2004, from http://www.nchpeg.org

National Coalition for Health Professional Education in Genetics. (2004). *Genetics family history resources.* Retrieved August 20, 2004, from http://www.nchpeg.org

National Organization of Nurse Practitioner Faculties. (2002). *Nurse practitioner primary care competencies in specialty areas: Adult, family, gerontological, pediatric, and women's health.* Rockville, MD: American Association of Colleges of Nursing, Department of Health and Human Services, Health Resources and Services Administration, Bureau of Health Professions, Division of Nursing.

Oncology Nursing Society. (2003). *Genetics and cancer care: A guide for oncology nurses.* Retrieved November 26, 2003, from http://www.ons.org/clinical/PreventionDetection.shtml

Rolland, J. S., & Williams, J. K. (in press). Psychosocial typology of 21st century genetics. In S. Miller, S. McDaniel, J. Rolland, & S. Feetham (Eds.), *Individuals, families, and the new era of genetics: Biopsychosocial perspectives.* New York: Norton.

Skirton, H., & Patch, C. (2003). *Genetics for healthcare professionals: A lifestage approach.* New York: Routledge.

Trout, C., Mathews, K., & Williams J. (2004). *Knowledge and concerns about respiratory illness in males with Duchenne muscular dystrophy and their parents.* Unpublished data.

University of Washington Center for Genomics and Public Health. (2004). *Asthma genomics: Implications for public health.* Seattle, WA: Center for Genomics and Public Health.

Williams, J. K. (2002). Education for genetics and nursing practice. *AACN Clinical Issues, 13,* 492–500.

Yoon, P. W., Scheuner, M. T., Peterson-Oehlke, K. L., Gwinn, M., Faucett, A., &

Khoury, M. (2002). Can family history be used as a tool for public health and preventive medicine? *Genetics in Medicine, 4,* 304–310.

Zerhouni, E. (2004). Forward. In A. E. Guttmacher, F. S. Collins, J. M. Drazen, & E. Zerhouni (Eds.), *Genomic medicine: Articles from the New England Journal of Medicine* (pp. ix–xi). Baltimore: Johns Hopkins University Press.

Zielenski, J. (2000). Genotype and phenotype in cystic fibrosis. *Respiration, 67,* 117–133.

CHAPTER EIGHT

Supporting Emotional Health

Ann Marie McCarthy
Shelly Eisbach

INTRODUCTION, DEFINITIONS, AND THEIR MEASUREMENT

In the past two decades, the recognition and treatment of children and adolescents with emotional and behavioral problems has increased dramatically (Zito et al., 2003). Between 12% and 25% of school-aged children have a behavioral or emotional problem, or both (Albrecht, Dore, & Naugle, 2003), with the Surgeon General estimating that one in four children will have mental health difficulties sometime during their child and adolescent years. In addition, children are currently prescribed psychiatric medications at unprecedented rates (Zito et al., 2003). However, it is still estimated that two thirds of children with mental health problems do not receive care (Melnyk, Brown, Jones, Kreipe, & Novak, 2003). In response to this significant child health concern, the U.S. Surgeon General initiated a task force, the 2001 Surgeon General's National Action Agenda for Children's Mental Health, to prevent mental health problems in children and adolescents (report available at www.surgeongeneral.gov/topics/cmh/childreport.htm).

The concept of mental health is complex and encompasses more than just the absence of mental illness. The core features of mental health involve an ability to maintain meaningful relationships, to respond effectively to stress and adversity, to have an accurate perception of reality, and to maintain mental function in work, love, and play (Vaillant, 2003). Emotional difficulties in children include a wide range of concerns. Some children experience transitory emotional problems, often related to developmental or situational factors. For example, a 3-year old child may have difficulty with the birth of a new sibling and display regressive behaviors; a school-age child may be upset about his or her parent's divorce and become noncompliant with parent and school requests; and an adolescent may seek peer approval by participating in risk-taking behaviors. These situations are often resolved within the family, with time, or with the assistance of health care professionals such as pediatric nurses and physicians. However, other children display ongoing emotional difficulties that need more intensive intervention. For example, a preschooler may display autistic symptoms, a 12-year-old may experience a mood disorder, or an adolescent may have symptoms of an eating disorder. Each of these problems will require in-depth assessment and management by a multidisciplinary team.

Emotional problems in children are commonly divided into two major groups, externalizing and internalizing problems (Achenbach & Ruffle, 2000; Shapiro & Kratochwill, 2000). Children with externalizing problems typically display behaviors that are externally directed and disruptive to those around them, such as noncompliant, oppositional, inattentive, hyperactive, or aggressive behaviors (MacDonald, 2003). Children with internalizing problems such as anxiety, depression, or social withdrawal typically direct their feelings inwardly, and may not display overt problem behaviors. Because children with internalizing problems may not be disruptive to the adults in their environment, their problems may not be recognized (Albano, Chorpita, & Barlow, 2003). The *Diagnostic and Statistical Manual of Mental Disorders (DSM-IV-TR)*, published by the American Psychiatric Association (APA), is a classification of mental disorders into more specific diagnostic categories that is commonly used in clinical, research, and education settings (APA, 2000).

Emotional health in children ranges from children who are well-adjusted, to those experiencing situational difficulties, to children with significant mental health problems. A complex combination of factors impacts a child's emotional adjustment, such as child characteristics, family interactions, and social context. This chapter reviews some of the factors impacting children's emotional health, provides guidelines for identifying children with mental health problems, and discusses interventions that support the development of positive mental/emotional health in children.

CHILD AND FAMILY INFLUENCES
ON CHILD MENTAL HEALTH

Until recently, much of the research on children's mental health has focused on factors that have a potential negative impact on the child's well-being. However, one postmodern paradigm shift within the scientific research community is the concept of resilience. In studying strengths and adaptation, the focus becomes less problem-oriented and more connected with identifying and nurturing strengths.

Resilience as a concept denotes overcoming adversity and involves two critical conditions: the exposure to a significant threat or adverse situation, and the achievement of positive outcomes in the face of challenges to the child's development (Heller, Larrieu, D'Imperio, & Boris, 1999; Luthar, Cicchetti, & Becker, 2000). Many children face difficult situations in their lives, such as parental divorce, bullying, and poverty. Although these situations create adversity, every child has some ability to handle stress and to cope with difficulties in his or her environment (Masten, 2001). Resilience is no longer viewed as an extraordinary phenomenon that only a few invulnerable individuals possess. It is now recognized that resilience occurs when the risks or difficulties an individual faces are outweighed by the protective factors they possess.

In the following sections, variables impacting a child's emotional adjustment are presented. These variables include vulnerability or risk factors that negatively impact mental health, and protective factors that have been identified as contributing to a child's resilience. Protective factors contributing to resilience fall into three categories: individual attributes, family qualities, and supportive systems in and outside the family (Masten & Powell, 2003).

Child Influences

Individual attributes that may be protective factors contributing to a child's resilience include intelligence, which can enhance problem solving abilities; easy temperament, which may decrease irritability and therefore assist a child in being sociable and engaging with peers; and positive self-concept that increases self efficacy and is related to the development of an internal sense of control, which can enhance coping. Development and temperament are two characteristics that contribute to children's overall emotional health (Christophersen & Mortweet, 2002).

A developmental perspective is important in addressing the concept of mental health because what may be seen as developmentally appropriate at one age will be unhealthy and indicative of a problem at another age. For example, a 2–year-old child having a temper tantrum in a store may be viewed as developmentally appropriate, whereas a 9-year-old having a similar outburst in the same setting would be viewed as displaying inappropriate behavior. For older children, puberty is a milestone of physical development that may impact emotional adjustment. Girls who experience early onset of puberty have an increase in both internalizing and externalizing difficulties, and boys with early pubertal onset have an increase in externalizing symptoms (Kaltiala-Heino, Marttunen, Rantanen, & Rimpela, 2003). Adolescence is a time often associated with an increase in the prevalence of mental health disorders such as eating disorders, anxiety disorders, depression, and substance abuse (Kaltiala-Heino et al., 2003).

In addition to development, a child's personality traits can influence overall mental health. Temperament is the innate behavioral style of the individual. Each person's temperament is distinct and varies in characteristics such as activity, rhythmicity, approach, adaptability, intensity, mood, persistence, distractibility, and threshold (Thomas & Chess, 1977). Based on these characteristics, children are identified as being difficult, easy, or slow to warm up. Children with temperaments that are difficult or slow to warm up have more emotional difficulties than easy-tempered children have. For example, caregivers are thought to respond differently to children with different temperaments. Children who have difficult temperaments are more likely to be the objects of parental irritability, which increases the risk for verbal or physical abuse (Corcoran & Nichols-Casebolt, 2004).

Family Influences

Family factors can influence a child's mental health, either positively or negatively. Family qualities that support resilience in children include a warm and caring structured environment, positive parenting, and close parental relationships. Negative parenting styles, inappropriate developmental expectations, marital discord, and parents' experiencing psychosocial problems may negatively impact a child's mental health (Campbell, 2002). In addition to these nurturing or environmental factors, the role of nature or genetics in mental health is increasingly recognized. The relationships between phenotypic characteristics such as depression and genetic variations are being identified using molecular genetic analysis.

Positive parenting styles are described as warm, nurturing, responsive, stimulating, supportive, engaging, and stable, whereas negative parenting styles are described as inconsistent, punitive, harsh, and disapproving (Boyle et al., 2004). Positive parenting and stable parent-child relationships create the warm and nurturing environment necessary to bolster the child's emotional health and cognitive functioning, and results in better behavioral outcomes for children and adolescents (Boyle et al., 2004). Negative styles tend to increase the possibility of internalizing and externalizing behavioral difficulties.

Marital separation or the dissolution of a marriage can create stress for all family members as everyone transitions from an intact family system to one that is divided. Although many parents expect that the conflicting relationships between them will end once the separation begins, studies have shown that this early stage of separation is a time of great conflict and vulnerability within the family (Cohen, 2002; Melnyk & Alpert-Gillis, 1997). During this period, children often witness arguing and the emotional lability of their parents due to the parents' dissolved relationship. Parents are also more likely to experience feelings of worthlessness, anxiety, anger, and guilt, which may translate into the use of poor coping skills such as smoking, overcompensating in dating relationships, and substance abuse. Children's immediate responses to separation and divorce are mediated developmentally. Younger children display more regressive and aggressive behaviors, irritability, separation anxiety, heightened fears of abandonment, gastrointestinal difficulties, and problems sleeping (Cohen, 2002). School-age children will tend to show depressed feelings, poor academic performance, difficulties in peer relationships, anger, and low self-esteem (Cohen, 2002; Melnyk & Alpert-Gillis, 1997). During adolescence, children will become angry or depressed, attempt to gain control, have loyalty conflicts, and may engage in risky peer behavior such as drug, sexual activity, and alcohol use (Cohen, 2002; Melynk & Alpert-Gillis, 1997).

Although not all children and adolescents experience long-term mental health problems, divorce and separation can have lasting effects on emotional health (Cohen, 2002; Melnyk & Alpert-Gillis, 1997; Richardson & McCabe, 2001). Individuals who experienced a parental divorce in childhood may have long-term emotional difficulties such as difficulties with intimacy and long-term relationships (Cohen, 2002; Richardson & McCabe, 2001). These effects can be buffered by ensuring positive relationships between parent and child. Psychosocial adaptation outcomes improve when the child is able to maintain positive child-to-adult relationships with both parents (Richardson & McCabe, 2001).

SOCIAL INFLUENCES ON CHILD EMOTIONAL HEALTH

Although family provides a strong influence on a child's emotional health, other social factors play a direct and indirect role in a child's adjustment. For example, a child's role models, close peer relationships, and supportive community networks provide an emotionally safe environment and are associated with positive adaptation (Corcoran & Nichols-Casebolt, 2004). Three powerful influences on a child's emotional adjustment are school, peers, and poverty.

School

Children spend a significant amount of their time in school, an environment that typically expects all children to learn and behave in a similar manner. Although many children are able to navigate the school environment successfully, for other children the demands of school may contribute to or exacerbate emotional or behavioral problems. For example, a child with undiagnosed learning problems may display disruptive behaviors to try to escape from academic demands. Another child diagnosed with remediate learning problems may display depressed and anxious symptoms as a result of academic stress encountered in the school environment (Grier, Morris, & Taylor, 2001). Children with learning problems often have a comorbid mental health problem, such as the child with attention deficit hyperactivity disorder (ADHD) who is also depressed.

Most children display emotional or behavioral problems across multiple settings. The child with oppositional behavior is typically defiant both at home and at school. It is important to recognize the possibility that a child who is displaying negative behavior or emotional problems only in the school setting may have a learning problem, difficulty with other children, or a conflict with a specific teacher (Pianta, 1999).

Peers

Peer relationships are an important part of the social development of children and adolescents, both in and out of the school environment. As children develop socially, their interactions with their peers become more complex and important (Fopma-Loy, 2000). Children as young as 7 begin to value the opinions of their peers and recognize the importance of looking at another's point of view. These children are moving away from egocentric play towards a cooperative partnership that creates an atmosphere where social comparisons with others become possible (Fopma-Loy, 2000).

During adolescence, cooperative relationships become more emotionally connected as adolescents form close friendships and romantic relationships with their peers (Stiles & Raney, 2004). Social competence becomes critical during adolescence. Difficulties in peer relationships have been linked with aggressive behavior, poor academic performance, and psychopathology (Riley, Ensminger, Green, & Kang, 1998). Addressing feelings of love, intimacy, and sexuality can pose challenges to the social and emotional development of adolescents (Russell & Consolacion, 2003). Teens are uncovering their sexual identities during this period and at the same time are given norms and expectations from society as to how these relationships should develop and with whom.

Although visibility and acceptance of alternative lifestyles is increasing for lesbian, gay, and bisexual youths, there continues to be pressure by heterosexual peers and society to engage in "normative" dating patterns during the high-school experience. These adolescents may delay acting on sexual feelings due to fears of rejection or due to sexual prejudice by others. Lesbian, gay, and bisexual youths are at an increased risk for mental health difficulties due to increased feelings of isolation, depression, anxiety, and suicidal ideation (Russell & Consolacion, 2003).

Positive peer relationships provide a medium for the development of emotional health, and negative peer relationships such as bullying may contribute to detrimental mental health effects. Being bullied is a form of peer abuse that affects approximately 5% to 15% of school-age children and 3% to 10% of adolescents each week (Kaltiala-Heino, Rimpela, Rantanen, & Rimpela, 2000). The act of bullying creates a situation in which victims become isolated and singled out by select peers. This negative attention has been shown to increase the likelihood of alienation, loneliness, and further rebuffing by the bully and other peers (Fekkes, Pijpers, & Verloove-Vanhorick, 2004; Kumpulainen & Rasanen, 2000). Victims of bullying commonly experience an increased incidence of psychosomatic complaints such as fatigue, difficulty sleeping, school refusal, and nausea in response to the increased stress of being isolated from social support networks. Long-term mental health difficulties have also been described in children and adolescents who were victims of bullying. These children are more likely to display internalizing difficulties such as depression, suicidal ideation, anxiety, and eating disorders (Fekkes et al., 2004; Kaltiala-Heino et al., 2000; Kumpulainen & Rasanen, 2000).

The act of bullying may actually be a reaction to the bully's own environmental stress and can indicate underlying mental health concerns (Kaltiala-Heino et al., 2000). Children who bully participate more in risky behaviors such as substance abuse and antisocial or criminal behavior during adolescence (Kumpulainen & Rasanen, 2000). Survey research also shows that children who bully may also have been bullied themselves. These children and adolescents have an increased incidence of internalizing difficulties similar to any child who has been bullied (Kaltiala-Heino et al., 2000; Kumpulainen & Rasanen, 2000).

Poverty

A variety of social factors such as unemployment, limited financial resources, inadequate child-care services, limited education, and disadvantaged neighborhoods influence a family's economic stability, thus impacting the development of children's behavior problems (Campbell, 2002). Poverty also can impact maternal health, which in turn can strongly influence child adjustment (Garmezy, 1993). The basic needs of children who live in poverty may not be met, with some children experiencing hunger, overcrowded conditions, and homelessness.

Children living in poverty have difficulty gaining access to health care and may not have resources at their disposal to receive the early intervention necessary for prevention of detrimental health outcomes (Evans & Kantrowitz, 2002). Living in impoverished neighborhoods also places children and adolescents at increased risk for problems with internalizing and externalizing behavior. Exposure to violence, lack of social structure, and negative peer influences are associated with substance abuse and delinquency for adolescents (Leventhal & Brooks-Gunn, 2000). Research has demonstrated a link between neighborhood violence and anxiety, depression, oppositional defiant disorder, and conduct disorder in children and adolescents (Corcoran & Nichols-Casebolt, 2004).

Children and adolescents living in poverty have home environments that may not facilitate learning. These children are less likely to have access to books in the home, or to have parents that read to them (Evans & Kantrowitz, 2002). According to the National Center for Education Statistics (2004), children from public schools with a high percentage of low-income families experience overcrowding in the schools and more teachers not adequately prepared for teaching their assigned class content. In addition, overcrowded schools are at risk for concerns with safety. Children from these schools report more exposure to violence (weapons and fighting) in the school than children from wealthier neighborhoods do.

NURSING CARE EXCELLENCE

Pediatric nurses play a central role in the emotional health of children. They are in ideal positions to recognize that the children they care for have mental health needs. School nurses in the community, nurse practitioners in primary care, and pediatric nurses in acute care settings all have opportunities to promote mental health and identify children in need of mental health services. Four standards of nursing care excellence that all pediatric nurses should provide are (1) developing safe environments that promote emotional health, (2) screening children for emotional health concerns, (3) providing families with primary management interventions, and (4) referring families to mental health providers when needed.

Promoting Mental Health

Pediatric nurses should be advocates for children and families who are coping with mental health problems. They need to assist families by identifying available services, negotiating funding sources, and explaining the child's unique needs to others in the child's environment. The stigma associated with a mental health diagnosis, and concerns with labeling their child, may interfere with a families willingness to seek appropriate care (Corrigan, 2004). However, the support of a nurse may facilitate a family's seeking the services needed.

In addition to advocating for individual children with mental health problems, pediatric nurses must be active in developing programs and supporting environments that promote mental health for all children. Programs typically involve providing direct services to children in order to prevent psychosocial difficulties. Two examples are parenting and school-based programs. Many parents benefit from structured parenting programs. Although one child in a family may have an easy temperament and respond readily to parent requests, another child may have a more difficult temperament and may require different approaches. Parents may need to be taught alternative parenting skills. Most parenting programs incorporate basic behavior theory and interventions. One example of a parenting program developed for parents of aggressive children and written by a nurse is the Incredible Years Parent Program developed by Webster-Stratton (Webster-Stratton, 1998). This program, which incorporates videotaped modeling, is developed for parents, teachers, and other adults who live and work with children 2 to 8 years old (Christophersen & Mortweet, 2002).

School personnel, including school nurses, often develop positive behavior support (PBS) programs that focus on prevention and early intervention for children who display chronic problem behaviors at school. These programs typically involve establishing a code of conduct for students to follow, developing plans for teaching students appropriate behaviors, and incorporating strategies to support students who practice these desired behaviors (Lewis, Powers, Kelk, & Newcomer, 2002; Scott, 2001; Taylor-Greene & Kartub, 2000).

In addition to providing direct services to children, pediatric nurses must recognize the need for public health policies that support mental health services for children. Unfortunately, obtaining mental health services for children may be difficult. Families often discover that their health insurance provides limited coverage for mental health services (Melnyk et al., 2003). Studies have shown that private and public insurance programs frequently do not pay for specific treatments and services that would benefit children with mental health problems (Fox, McManus, & Reichman, 2003; Fristad, Gavazzii, & Mackinaw-Koons, 2003). Nurses need to work with legislators to advocate for coverage of mental health problems equal to that provided for physical health problems (mental health parity).

Professional nursing organizations can also play an important role in promoting positive mental health in children. The National Association of Pediatric Nurse Practitioners (NAPNAP) developed a plan of action, titled "Keep Your Children/Yourself Safe and Secure (KySS)," to improve the mental health needs of children across the country and to decrease risk-taking behaviors. Strategies were implemented to identify the knowledge, worries, and needs of parents and children, to assess health professionals' practices, and to improve the skills of primary care providers to screen children for mental health concerns and provide preventive interventions (Melynk et al., 2003).

Screening

Screening children for mental health problems is an integral part of all pediatric nurses' practices. When a nurse is asked to assess a child with a potential emotional problem, the nurse needs to obtain information from multiple sources, including parents, the child, and possibly teachers or other adults in the child's life. Information may be obtained through interviews, structured questionnaires, and direct observation of the child's behavior.

Interviews

The nurse will want to obtain a description of the problem by talking with the child, the parent(s), and other adults such as teachers, if needed. It is helpful to find out if the child's problem occurs across multiple settings. For children displaying disruptive behaviors, the interview should include questions that clarify what precedes or precipitates the occurrence of the disruptive behavior and what follows the behavior that might be encouraging the child to continue the disruptive behavior. Interventions that have been tried to address the child's problem and the results of these interventions should be identified.

Children, regardless of age, should be interviewed to assess their perceptions of themselves and their understanding of the problem. The nurse may be able to obtain information from the child that the child has not shared with others, particularly if the nurse has built a trusting relationship with the child. In all interviews, confidentiality must be addressed. The nurse needs to be honest about what will happen with the information discussed in the interview. It is important that children and adolescents understand that if they indicate they may harm themselves or others, this information must be shared with others and appropriate action taken. When talking with a child, it may be easier to begin talking about general, nonthreatening topics, before discussing the problem. Allow the child to talk by using open-ended questions and active listening. Obtain information from the child about daily activities such as sleep and eating patterns, school performance and activities, family interactions, and outside activities. Some physical complaints such as encopresis, urinary incontinence, frequent stomachaches, or other somatic complaints may be associated with the child's emotional problems (van Zanten, 2003).

Children may be encouraged to share their feelings by normalizing their experience. Many children are encouraged to discuss their feelings or experiences by statements such as "Other children have told me . . ." or "It's common for children your age to . . . ." When interviewing an adolescent, an effective interview approach is the HEADSS(W) Interview (Deering & Cody, 2002). In this approach, questions are asked about Home, Education/employment, Activities, Drugs, Sexuality, Suicide/depression, and Weight, in that order, from less threatening topics to more difficult ones. At the end of the interview with a child or adolescent, review what was discussed, clarify what information will be shared with others in accordance with the new Health Insurance Portability and Accountability Act (HIPAA) regulations, and end with a plan that includes what you will do with the information (School Mental Health Project, 2002).

Parents should also be interviewed to review the child's medical history, obtain the parent's description of the child's problem, and assess parenting skills and the home environment (Shapiro & Kratochwill, 2000). Ask if other family members have experienced similar problems or behaviors. See if there have been any recent changes in the family, such as a separation, that may contribute to the child's current problem. Remember to consider cultural differences, because behaviors accepted as normal in one culture may not be acceptable in another.

If a child's teacher is interviewed, information on the child's overall academic and social performance and relationships of the child with teachers and classmates should be discussed. Ask about school-avoidance behavior, which may occur in general or in response to specific classes or teachers. A teacher-student mismatch, unrealistic expectations of the child by a teacher, and academic demands that exceed a child's abilities may all contribute to a child's having problems with school adjustment. Ask the teacher if bullying or teasing from other students might be contributing to the child's difficulties, although unfortunately teachers are not always aware if this type of behavior is occurring in the school.

Structured Questionnaires

Checklists and questionnaires are helpful in assessing a child's emotional adjustment and overall behavior (Achenbach & Ruffle, 2000; Glascoe, 2000; Perrin & Stancin, 2002). It is important to remember that structured questionnaires reflect the perceptions of the person completing the form, either the child or an adult in the child's life, such as a parent or teacher, and may not be an accurate interpretation of what is actually happening. The purpose of using standardized checklists or questionnaires is that in the development of these instruments, data were collected on a large number of children to document the typical responses of children of various ages. Using normative checklists or questionnaires allows comparisons of a child with other children. These instruments often are available in several versions that allow the child, a parent, or a teacher to complete similar versions of the instrument and for responses to be compared.

Examples of checklists and rating scales include general behavior checklists such as the Child Behavior Checklist (CBCL), and checklists that are more specific, such as the Child Depression Inventory (Achenbach & Ruffle, 2000). Some instruments are copyrighted and require fees for use, and some need a psychologist or mental health professional to score and interpret the results.

An example of a screening instrument that may be appropriate for pediatric nurses to use in multiple settings to identify children with adjustment is the Pediatric Symptom Checklist (PSC) (Jellinek et al., 1988). The PSC has both parent and child versions available. The tool is a one-page, 35 item screening questionnaire that is completed by parents and is designed to help clinicians in outpatient practice settings identify children ages 4 to 16 years old with difficulties in psychosocial functioning. The Web site provides information on the reliability and validity of the PSC. An overall score is obtained and compared with the cutoff score for referral. This instrument is free and available at www.massgeneral.org/allpsych/PediatricSymptomChecklist/psc_home.htm.

Observations

A child's behavior can provide valuable information about the child's overall mental health. Change in a child's behavior may be the first indicator of emotional difficulties. Unstructured observations of behavior during a child interview or from parent or teacher reports may provide valuable insight into the child's emotional health. Children with externalizing problems may display hyperactive or impulsive behaviors, distractibility, noncompliance to requests, and difficulties communicating feelings (Shapiro & Kratochwill, 2000). Children with internalizing problems also may display overt, concerning behaviors such as the child with obsessive compulsive disorder (OCD) engaging in ritualistic behaviors, a depressed children having increased somatic complaints and irritability, and a child with an eating disorder preferring to eat alone or eating a large amount of food at one sitting.

For some children, structured observation of the problem behavior may be helpful in understanding factors that trigger the behavior and in developing possible interventions. The specific behavior may be observed and the frequency of occurrence in a designated time period may be documented (Alberto & Troutman, 2003). An example of observing a specific behavior in which school nurses often participate is the on-task behavior of children with ADHD (Shapiro & Kratochwill, 2000).

In addition, children without diagnosable disorders may display risk behaviors that indicate potential emotional difficulties. These children may not have problems that meet diagnostic criteria for a mental health diagnosis, but they may require intervention from a primary care provider to decrease progression to a more serious problem. For example, at the birth of a new sibling, a preschool child may show regressive behaviors such as bed-wetting or a school-age child may refuse to do homework.

Management

Pediatric nurses should be knowledgeable about the wide range of evidence-based, effective interventions available for assisting children with emotional and behavioral problems (Barrett & Ollendick, 2004; Christophersen & Mortweet, 2002). These interventions incorporate approaches based on multiple theories, such as behavioral, cognitive-behavioral, and social learning theory. In addition, medications, which are not discussed here, increasingly are used to assist effectively in the management of mental health problems in children. Some behavioral and cognitive-behavioral interventions that might be incorporated into primary care practice or school setting are discussed in the following section.

Behavioral Interventions

The goals of behavioral interventions for children are to teach appropriate behaviors and discourage inappropriate behaviors. Behavioral interventions may be used as part of a treatment plan for an individual child or incorporated into programs for encouraging appropriate behaviors in group settings such as classrooms. To understand behavioral interventions it is important to understand the underlying behavior theory. Often referred to as the ABC model, behavior is viewed in relationship to *antecedent* factors in the environment that trigger a *behavior* to occur and the results or *consequences* in the environment that occur after the behavior and influence the likelihood that the behavior will occur again

(Alberto & Troutman, 2003; Shapiro & Kratochwill, 2000). Antecedent stimuli include a word, a situation, a person, or a request that triggers a specific behavioral response in a child. Behavior includes whatever the individual's response is to the antecedent stimuli. Consequences include events or behaviors that occur in the environment in response to the child's behavior. Consequences may be reinforcing, which increase the chance that the behavior will be repeated, or punishing, which decrease the chance that the behavior will be repeated.

Behavioral interventions focus on changing antecedents that trigger problem behaviors and altering the consequences that maintain behaviors. Multiple stimuli can trigger problem behaviors in children and, if identified, may be altered (Conroy & Stichter, 2003; Grier et al., 2001). For example, chaotic, unstructured environments may confuse and overstimulate some children, particularly children with decreased impulse control. Providing a more structured environment can decrease disruptive behaviors in these children.

A number of behavioral interventions change what children experience as a consequence of their behavior. For inappropriate behaviors, the consequences may be to ignore the behavior, thus decreasing the likelihood the behavior will occur again. When an acceptable behavior occurs, the consequence may be positive reinforcement that encourages the child to repeat the behavior. Positive reinforcement, or a reward, occurs when something is provided following a behavior, such as praise or stickers, and as a result the occurrence of the behavior increases (MacDonald, 2003). Two examples of positive reinforcement that are frequently used are token systems and contracts. A token economy is a system in which a child can earn rewards contingent on engaging in specified behaviors. Typically, the child earns something other than the actual reward, like points, stars on a chart, or poker chips, which can be exchanged for the desired reward (Christophersen & Mortweet, 2002). For some children, particularly older children, a formal, written contract is helpful in encouraging the appropriate behavior in the child. A contract describes the desired behavior of the child and the rewards the child will receive when the desired behavior occurs (Carns & Carns, 1994; Garrick-Duhaney, 2003).

Two examples of punishing consequences, which tell a child which behaviors are not acceptable, are time-out and natural consequences. Time-out is actually time out from positive reinforcement and is more commonly used for younger children. Time-out is often used to decrease the occurrence of a behavior that cannot be ignored, such as hitting or acting out (Turner & Watson, 1999). With time-out, the child is removed from a situation that is reinforcing the problem behavior to one that is not reinforcing for the child (MacDonald, 2003). Time-out is usually brief, from 1 to 10 minutes; the younger the child, the shorter the time-out (Coucouvanis & McCarthy, 2001). Natural consequences are the events that follow a behavior unless someone does something to prevent them. For example, a child who does not turn in homework will get a failing grade on that assignment. Children who experience the naturally occurring negative consequences that follow an inappropriate behavior are less likely to repeat that behavior in the future.

Cognitive-Behavioral Interventions

Cognitive-behavioral interventions build on the behavior model of treatment, but in addition incorporate the role of cognitive processes that individuals use as they think about the antecedents and consequences that occur in relationship to their behaviors. The basic assumption of cognitive behavioral therapy is that cognitive schemata, our attitudes and beliefs about something, will influence how we perceive and process incoming stimuli, which in turn will affect our behavior (Grave & Blissett, 2004).

The overall goal of cognitive-behavioral therapy is to identify and restructure our thinking patterns to correct cognitive distortions (Grave & Blissett, 2004). Cognitive distortions are common to individuals experiencing self-doubt, depressed thoughts, and anxiety (Grave & Blissett, 2004; Prochaska & Norcross, 2003). These distortions are a cognitive process in which individuals view the world through a negative lens; they have a negative self-view, view the surrounding environment as demanding and hostile, and see their future as lacking value (the cognitive triad) (Prochaska & Norcross, 2003).

Cognitive behavioral interventions are used with children to foster coping, to encourage self-control, and to enhance self-efficacy. When tailoring cognitive interventions for use with children and adolescents, it is necessary to address the child's level of growth and development (Grave & Blissett, 2004; Hudson, Hughes, & Kendall, 2004). Young children have difficulty in separating themselves from the environment; they also have difficulty in self-observation and self-evaluation (Grave & Blissett, 2004). Because of these difficulties, children under the age of 9 may not receive the full benefit of cognitive-behavioral interventions. Using cognitive behavioral interventions with children and adolescents can be as simple as helping an anxious child to become aware of when he or she feels frightened, and to recognize the negative self-talk surrounding these anxious feelings. In helping the child gain awareness of the fear, the nurse can then work through problem-solving activities to help the child cope with the anxiety-producing situation. For example, a child with a health problem might be anxious about leaving her mother and attending school. A teacher might approach the school nurse and ask for help with the situation. In talking with the child and the child's mother, the school nurse might be able to understand their concerns (fear of the child's becoming sick in school). The nurse can assist the mother and child in identifying their assumptions regarding the anxiety (cognitive restructuring), and develop a reward system for attending school (behavioral reinforcement).

Due to their close proximity to their patients in providing daily and around-the-clock care, nurses are in a good position to listen empathetically and to foster cognitive behavioral techniques. The expectation is not that nurses become therapists, but that they use their communication and listening skills to help the child develop positive coping skills.

Referrals

Pediatric nurses need to assess continuously a child's need for referral to a mental health specialist. Use of an accurate history and normative screening instruments, coupled with a professional relationship with children and their families, will guide the nurse in making the decision to refer a child for more in-depth mental health assessment and treatment. Although the nurse may refer a child for mental health services, the family's insurance coverage may have limited mental health benefits resulting in the child not receiving the care needed. When a child is referred to a mental health specialist, the nurse should follow up with the family to ascertain if the child and family are comfortable with the provider. Families may need to see more than one mental health provider before they are able to establish a comfortable, effective, therapeutic relationship.

MULTIDISCIPLINARY INTEGRATION
AND PARTNERSHIP: CASE STUDY

Children at risk for mental health problems, as well as children with an established diagnosis, present complex management situations requiring the collaborative services of multiple providers. Often the pediatric nurse is the health professional who identifies the need for services and initiates the referral process for appropriate care. In addition to referral, the nurse may be involved in monitoring adherence to treatment, assessing medication effectiveness and side effects, and advocating for the child across multiple settings.

Comprehensive care of a child with a mental health problem often requires involvement of individuals from a wide range of disciplines and services outside of classic health care settings. In addition to health care providers, personnel from schools, social services, juvenile services, and volunteer agencies may all be involved with these children. The following case study provides an example of a child with emotional health difficulties and the multiple health care providers involved in his care.

As a school nurse, Ms. R is concerned with the emotional health of all the children in her school. She was a key participant in developing the school's positive-behavior support program, and as a result is recognized by the staff as a resource for children with emotional and behavioral difficulties. Joshua M. is a 9-year-old fourth grader who is new to the school. His teacher, Mr. B, notes that Joshua is impulsive, frequently out of his seat without permission, fights with classmates, and is having academic difficulties. Mr. B asks the school nurse for assistance with Joshua. Ms. R talks with Joshua about his behavior and meets with his mother, Mrs. M, to obtain family information, past health history, and school history. She discovers that Mrs. M had recently divorced Joshua's father, an abusive husband, and that Joshua has had difficulty in school since first grade. The school nurse and teacher meet with Mrs. M and with her permission and support from the principal, initiate evaluations that include assessments of Joshua by the school psychologist and reading specialist. The school counselor and social worker meet with both Joshua and Mrs. M. The school nurse also arranges an assessment of Joshua by a local behavioral pediatrician who, in consultation with the school psychologist, diagnoses attention deficit hyperactivity disorder (ADHD) and recommends a trial of medication. After all the evaluations have been completed, the school's Child Study Team, which includes the child's principal, teacher, school nurse, school counselor, school psychologist, and reading specialist, meet with Mrs. M. The school nurse presents her information as well as the reports from the local doctor and the social worker. As a result of this multidisciplinary team meeting, an Individualized Educational Plan (IEP) is proposed for Joshua, which includes involvement in a remedial reading program and educational support. The school nurse works with the pediatrician to monitor the effectiveness of the medication prescribed for Joshua's ADHD. She also collaborates with the teacher and school counselor to develop a behavior management plan to improve Joshua's behavior in the classroom, and meets with Mrs. M to assist her in carrying out similar behavior management approach at home. Over the next few moths, each member of the team works closely and in collaboration with Joshua and his mother. At the end of the school year, Joshua's behavior has improved, his reading skills have advanced almost 2 academic years, and he is beginning to make friends.

SUMMARY

Maintaining the emotional health of children is central to their overall health and well-being. This chapter summarizes the wide range of factors that influence the emotional health of today's children. Pediatric nurses must recognize the importance of emotional health for children and understand the potential emotional problems children may experience. In the wide range of settings that pediatric nurses practice, they are in ideal positions to develop safe and emotionally healthy environments, screen children for emotional health concerns, provide families with primary interventions, and refer families to mental health providers when needed.

REFERENCES

American Psychiatric Association. (2000). *Diagnostic and statistical manual of mental disorders* (text revision). Washington, DC: Author.

Albano, A. M., Chorpita, B. F., & Barlow, D. H. (2003). Childhood anxiety disorders. In E. J. Mash, & R. A. Barkley (Eds.), *Child psychopathology* (2nd ed., pp. 279–329). New York: Guilford

Alberto, P. A., & Troutman, A. C. (2003). *Applied behavior analysis for teachers* (6th ed.). Upper Saddle River, NJ: Prentice-Hall.

Albrecht, S. J., Dore, D. J., & Naugle, A. E. (2003). Common behavioral dilemmas of the school-aged child. *Pediatric Clinics of North America, 50,* 841–857.

Achenbach, T. M., & Ruffle, T. M. (2000). The Child Behavior Checklist and related forms of assessing behavioral/emotional problems and competencies. *Pediatrics in Review, 21,* 265–271.

Barrett, P. M., & Ollendick, T. H. (2004). *Handbook of interventions that work with children and adolescents: Prevention and treatment.* West Sussex, England: Wiley.

Boyle, M. H., Jenkins, J. M., Georgiades, K., Cairney, J., Duku, E., & Racine, Y. (2004). Differential-maternal parenting behavior: Estimating within- and between-family effects on children. *Child Development, 75,* 1457–1476.

Campbell, S. B. (2002). *Behavior problems in preschool children: Clinical and developmental issues* (2nd ed.). New York: Guilford.

Carns, A. W., & Carns, M. R. (1994). On the scene: Making behavioral contracts successful. *The School Counselor, 42,* 155–160.

Christophersen, E. R., & Mortweet, S. L. (2002). *Treatments that work with children: Empirically supported strategies for managing childhood problems.* Washington DC: American Psychological Association.

Cohen , G. J. (2002). Helping children and families deal with divorce and separation. *Pediatrics, 110,* 1019–1023.

Conroy, M. A., & Stichter, J. P. (2003). The application of antecedents in the functional assessment process: Existing research, issues, and recommendations. *Journal of Special Education, 37,* 15–25.

Corcoran, J., & Nichols-Casebolt, A. (2004). Risk and resilience ecological framework for assessment and goal formulation. *Child and Adolescent Social Work Journal, 21,* 211–235.

Corrigan, P. (2004). How stigma interferes with mental health care. *American Psychologist, 59,* 614–625.

Coucouvanis, J. A., & McCarthy, A. M. (2001). Behavior modification. In M. J. Craft-Rosenberg & J. A. Denehy (Eds.), *Nursing interventions for infants, children, and families* (pp. 427–460). Thousand Oaks, CA: Sage.

Deering, C. G., & Cody, D. J. (2002). Communicating with children and adolescents. *American Journal of Nursing, 102,* 34–41.

Evans, G. W., & Kantrowitz, E. (2002). Socioeconomic status and health: The potential role of environmental risk exposure. *Annual Review of Public Health, 23,* 303–331.

Fekkes, M., Pijpers, F. I., & Verloove-Vanhorick, S. P. (2004). Bullying behavior and associations with psychosomatic complaints and depression in victims. *Journal of Pediatrics, 144,* 17–22.

Fopma-Loy, J. (2000). Peer rejection and neglect of latency-age children: Pathways and a group psychotherapy model. *Journal of Child and Adolescent Psychiatric Nursing, 13,* 29–38.

Fox, H. B., McManus, M. A., & Reichman, M. B. (2003). Private health insurance for adolescents: Is it adequate? *Journal of Adolescent Health, 32*(Suppl. 6), 12–24.

Fristad, M. A., Gavazzi, S. M., & Mackinaw-Koons, B. (2003). Family psychoeducation: An adjunctive intervention for children with bipolar disorder. *Biological Psychiatry, 53,* 1000–1008.

Garmezy, N. (1993). Resiliency and vulnerability to adverse developmental outcomes associated with poverty. *American Behavioral Scientist, 34,* 416–430.

Garrick-Duhaney, L. M. (2003). A practical approach to managing the behavior of students with ADD. *Interventions in School and Clinic, 38,* 267–280.

Glascoe, F. P. (2000). Early detection of developmental and behavioral problems. *Pediatrics in Review, 21,* 272–279.

Grave, J., & Blissett, J. (2004). Is cognitive behavior therapy developmentally appropriate for young children? A critical review of the evidence. *Clinical Psychology Review, 24,* 399–420.

Grier, R., Morris, L., & Taylor, L. (2001). Assessment strategies for school-based mental health counseling. *Journal of School Health, 71,* 467–469.

Heller, S. S., Larrieu, J. A., D'Imperio, R., & Boris, N. W. (1999). Research on resilience to child maltreatment: Empirical considerations. *Child Abuse and Neglect, 23,* 321–338.

Hudson, J. L., Hughes, A. A., & Kendall, P. C. (2004). Treatment of generalized anxiety disorder in children and adolescents. In P. M. Barrett & T. Ollendick (Eds.), *Handbook of interventions that work with children and adolescents: Prevention and treatment* (pp. 115–144). West Sussex, England: Wiley.

Jellinek, M. S., Murphy, J. M., Robinson, J., Feins, A., Lamb, S., & Fenton, T. (1988). Pediatric symptom checklist: Screening school-age children for psychosocial dysfunction. *Journal of Pediatrics, 112,* 201–209.

Kaltiala-Heino, R., Marttunen, M., Rantanen, P., & Rimpela, M. (2003). Early puberty is associated with mental health problems in middle adolescence. *Social Science and Medicine, 57,* 1055–1064.

Kaltiala-Heino, R., Rimpela, M., Rantanen, P., & Rimpela, A. (2000). Bullying at school—An indicator of adolescents at risk for mental disorders. *Journal of Adolescence, 23,* 661–674.

Kumpulainen, K., & Rasanen, E. (2000). Children involved in bullying at elementary school age: Their psychiatric symptoms and deviance in adolescence. *Child Abuse & Neglect, 24,* 1567–1577.

Leventhal, T., & Brooks-Gunn, J. (2000). The neighborhoods they live in: The effects of neighborhood residence on child and adolescent outcomes. *Psychological Bulletin, 126,* 309–337.

Lewis, T. J., Powers, L. J., Kelk, M. J., & Newcomer, L. L. (2002). Reducing problem behaviors on the playground: An investigation of the application of schoolwide positive behavior supports. *Psychology in the Schools, 39,* 181–190.

Luthar, S. S., Cicchetti, D., & Becker, B. (2000). The construct of resilience: A critical evaluation and guidelines for future work. *Child Development, 71,* 543–562.

MacDonald, E. K. (2003). Principles of behavioral assessment and management. *Pediatric Clinics of North America, 50,* 801–816.

Masten, A. (2001). Ordinary magic. *American Psychologist, 56,* 227–238.

Masten, A., & Powell, J. (2003). A resilience framework for research policy and practice. In S. Luthar (Ed.), *Resilience and vulnerability: Adaptation in the context of childhood adversities* (pp. 1–25). United Kingdom: Cambridge University Press.

Melnyk, B. M., Brown, H. E., Jones, D. C., Kreipe, R., & Novak, J. (2003). Improving the mental/psychosocial health of US children and adolescents: Outcomes and implementation strategies from the National KySS Summit. *Journal of Pediatric Health Care, 17*(Suppl. 6), S1–S24.

Melnyk, B. M., & Alpert-Gillis, L. J. (1997). Coping with marital separation: Smoothing the transition for parents and children. *Journal of Pediatric Health Care, 11,* 165–174.

National Center for Education Statistics. (2004). *The condition of education.* Retrieved February 28, 2005, from http://nces.ed.gov/pubs2004/2004077.pdf

Pianta, R. C. (1999). *Enhancing relationships between children and teachers.* Washington, DC: American Psychological Association.

Perrin, E. C., & Stancin, T. (2002). A continuing dilemma: Whether and how to screen for concerns about children's behaviors. *Pediatrics in Review, 23,* 264–275.

Prochaska, J. O., & Norcross, J. C. (2003). *Systems of psychotherapy: A transtheoretical analysis* (5th ed.). Pacific Grove, CA: Wadsworth.

Riley, A. W., Ensminger, M. E., Green, B., & Kang, M. (1998). Social role functioning by adolescents with psychiatric disorders. *Journal of the American Academy of Child and Adolescent Psychiatry, 37,* 620–628.

Richardson, S., & McCabe, M. P. (2001). Parental divorce during adolescence and adjustment in early adulthood. *Adolescence, 36,* 467–489.

Russell, S. T., & Consolacion, T. B. (2003). Adolescent romance and emotional health in the United States: Beyond binaries. *Journal of Clinical Child and Adolescent Psychology, 32,* 499–508.

Scott, T. M. (2001). A school-wide example of positive behavioral support. *Journal of Positive Behavioral Interventions, 3,* 88–94.

Shapiro, E. S., & Kratochwill, T. K. (Eds.). (2000). *Conducting school-based assessments of child and adolescent behavior.* New York: Guilford.

Stiles, A. S., & Raney, T. J. (2004). Relationships among personal space boundaries, peer acceptance, and peer reputation in adolescents. *Journal of Child and Adolescent Psychiatric Nursing, 17,* 29–40.

School Mental Health Project. (2002). *Talking with kids. Center quick training aid: Re-engaging students in learning.* Center for Mental Health in Schools at UCLA. Retrieved June 6, 2003, from http://smhp.psych.ucla.edu

Taylor-Green, S. J., & Kartub, D. T. (2000). Durable implementation of school-wide behavior support: The high five program. *Journal of Positive Behavioral Interventions, 2,* 233–235.

Thomas, A., & Chess, S. (1977). *Temperament and development.* New York: Brunner/Mazel.

Turner, H. S., & Watson, T. S. (1999). Consultant's guide for the use of time-out in the preschool and elementary classroom. *Psychology in the Schools, 36,* 135–148.

Vaillant, G. E. (2003). Mental health. *American Journal of Psychiatry, 160,* 1373–1384.

van Zanten, S. V. (2003). Diagnosing irritable bowel syndrome. *Reviews of Gastroenterological Disorders, 3*(Suppl. 2), S12–S17.

Webster-Stratton, C. (1998). Preventing conduct problems in Head Start children: Strengthening parenting competencies. *Journal of Consulting and Clinical Psychology, 66,* 715–730.

Zito, J. M., Safer, D. J., DosReis, S., Gardner, J. F., Magder, L., Soeken, K., et al. (2003). Psychotropic practice patterns for youth: A 10-year perspective. *Archives of Pediatric and Adolescent Medicine, 157*(1), 17–25.

CHAPTER NINE

Providing for
Physical Safety

Marilyn J. Krajicek
Barbara U. Hamilton

INTRODUCTION, DEFINITIONS,
AND THEIR MEASUREMENT

Safety has been defined as a state in which hazards and conditions leading to physical, psychological, or material harm are controlled in order to
preserve the health and well-being of individuals and the community
(Maurice et al., 2001). Types of physical safety issues that affect children
in early education and child care include abuse and violence, burns, chok-
ing, drowning, falls, fire, improper infant sleep positioning, lead poisoning, medication error, playground injury, poisoning, toxic exposure, and
motor vehicle accidents. Injuries related to these safety issues happen to
children in a variety of settings such as child care and early education
(preschool) programs, community and public areas, homes, and schools.
Studies show that the risk of serious injury to children in child care settings is no greater than that of children in home care (Kotch et al., 1997).
One of four children in the United States (14 million) is injured every year
(National Center for Injury Prevention and Control [NCIPC], 2001). It is
clear that nurses are being called upon to fill an important role in health
promotion and injury risk prevention for children as child-care health
consultants in addition to their traditional provision of nursing care for
children with injuries in health clinics, hospitals, and schools (Alkon,
Sokal-Gutierrez, & Wolff, 2002; Evers, 2002; Ulione, 1997; Ulione &
Dooling, 1997).

Nurse child-care health consultants utilize a wide range of tools to support their activities in health promotion and injury risk prevention. These tools include a number of nationally recognized guidelines developed within a multidisciplinary theoretical framework, such as (a) *Caring for Our Children: National Health and Safety Performance Standards— Guidelines for Out-of-Home Child Care Programs,* (American Academy of Pediatrics, American Public Health Association, National Resource Center for Health and Safety in Child Care [AAP/APHA/NRCHSCC], 2002); (b) *Head Start Program Performance Standards and Other Regulations* (Head Start Bureau, 1997); (c) *Accreditation Criteria and Procedures of the National Association for the Education of Young Children* (National Association for the Education of Young Children, 1998); and (d) *Quality Standards for NAFCC Accreditation* (National Association for Family Child Care, 2003). Nurse child-care health consultants also may use nationally established evaluation tools to measure risk levels, such as the Infant/Toddler Environmental Rating Scale (Harms, Cryer, & Clifford, 2002) and the Early Childhood Environment Rating Scale (Harms, Clifford, & Cryer, 2004). *Stepping Stones to Using Caring for Our Children* checklist (AAP/APHA/NRCHSCC, 2003) is used by nurse child-care health consultants to compare health and safety practices used in specific child-care programs. The standards cover broad areas such as program development, health promotion/protection, nutrition, facilities, infectious disease prevention, children with special needs, and administrative health and safety policies.

INFLUENCES OF PHYSICAL SAFETY PROVISIONS FOR CARE OF INFANTS AND CHILDREN AND THEIR IMPACT ON THE FAMILY

In the past decade, nurse child-care health consultants have increased their knowledge and use of child-care quality indicators empirically identified in research literature and based on the *Stepping Stones* standards (Fiene, 1988, 1994; Fiene & Nixon, 1981, 1983). These standards are key predictors of children's positive outcomes while in child care and are statistical indicators of overall compliance with child care regulations by child care providers (Fiene, 2002). The predictor/indicator system combines the two licensing measurement methodologies (Fiene & Kroh, 2000) of licensing weighting and indicator systems. Licensing weighting and indicator systems are two licensing measurement tools that have been utilized in the licensing literature for the past 20 years. These two methodologies are part of the licensing curriculum developed by the National Association for Regulatory Administration.

These methodologies constitute the most researched tools for conducting inferential inspections by licensing agencies (Fiene, 2002). Historically, these indicators have helped state child-care agencies implement standards in their regulations that are most protective of children's health and safety in child care. When determining the health and safety of young children in child care and the overall quality of a child care program, research clearly documents the importance of the 13 indicators, which are as follows: child abuse reporting and clearances, proper immunizations, staff child ratio and group size, director qualifications, teacher qualifications, staff training, supervision/discipline, fire drills, administration of medication, emergency plan/contact, outdoor playground safety, inaccessibility of toxic substances, and proper handwashing/diapering. The related standards of *Stepping Stones* are those most likely to prevent frequent or severe disease, disability, and death (morbidity and mortality) in child care settings. In addition to child-care health consultants, many parents and family advocacy groups, public and private organizations such as state child care, health, and resource and referral agencies, as well as a variety of professionals who work in child care settings use *Stepping Stones* to target limited resources to these priority standards.

Nurses using the 13 indicators when consulting and educating on the prevention of physical injury to children in child care can focus on several topics of current national significance. The topics chosen for discussing in this chapter are child abuse, medication administration, playground safety, and sudden infant death syndrome (SIDS) risk reduction training. These four topics are selected for discussion because of their vital importance in view of the national statistics presented by the Centers for Disease Control and Prevention (CDC) National Center for Injury Prevention and Control (NCIPC, 2001).

During 2001, 903,000 children in the United States experienced or were at risk for child abuse or neglect or both. Thirteen hundred children died from maltreatment, with 35% of these deaths caused by neglect and 26% from physical abuse. In most cases, the abuser is someone known to the child, including a parent, family member, teacher, or regular caregiver (U.S. Department of Health and Human Services, Administration for Children and Families, 2003).

Medication administration is required by 15% to 18% of children in the United States who have a chronic health condition (Perrin, Lewkowicz, & Young, 2000), such as asthma, allergies, and diabetes. These children may require the administration of medications during the day while attending a child care program. In a review of state child-care regulations conducted in March 2004, data showed that 26 states require providers to have training on the administration of medications (NRCH-SCC, 2004). Nurse child-care health consultants are being asked to fulfill that training need and help develop policies regarding medication administration for child care programs (Healthy Child Care America, 2004).

Playground safety is the third topic to be discussed. About 45% of playground-related injuries are severe, such as fractures, internal injuries, concussions, dislocations, and amputations (Tinsworth & McDonald, 2001). About 75% of nonfatal injuries related to playground equipment occur on public playgrounds (Tinsworth & McDonald, 2001). Most occur at schools and care centers (Phelan, Khoury, Kalkwarf, & Lanphear, 2001). Between 1990 and 2000, 147 U.S. children ages 14 and younger died from playground-related injuries (Tinsworth & McDonald, 2001).

SIDS risk reduction will be the last topic to be presented. Between 1983 and 1992, SIDS deaths ranged from 5,000 to 6,000 per year. Deaths have declined significantly since the Back-to-Sleep campaign began in 1992. This campaign is sponsored by the National Institute of Child Health and Human Development, the Maternal and Child Health Bureau, AAP, the SIDS Alliance, and the Association of SIDS and Infant Mortality Programs. It has been successful in promoting infant back-sleeping to parents, family members, child care providers, health professionals, and all other caregivers of infants.

In 2003, the Health Resources and Services Administration launched an effort to unite child care, health, and SIDS-prevention partners across the United States to reduce the incidence of SIDS in family child-care homes and center-based child care programs. In 2001, 2,236 SIDS deaths were reported. Even though SIDS rates have declined for all babies since the introduction of Back-to-Sleep campaigns, the need for training of nurse child-care health consultants is evident in statistics showing that the SIDS rate for African American babies is more than two times greater than it is for White babies (CDC, Office of Minority Health, 2004). Also, a disproportionate number of all SIDS deaths, 20%, occur in child care settings (Moon, Patel, & Shaefer, 2000).

Working with families and child care providers, nurse child-care health consultants utilize focused questions in a tool called *A Parent's Guide to Choosing Safe and Healthy Child Care* (NRCHSCC, 2003) and culturally sensitive information to evaluate risk and to educate families and providers on best practice for each of the four topics selected for discussion (see Table 9.1).

NURSING CARE EXCELLENCE

The role of child-care health consultants is to promote health and safety practices and to prevent harm to children and child care workers in child care and early education settings. Working with child care providers,

TABLE 9.1 Questions Parents and Nurse Child Care Health Consultants Should Use to Make Decisions About Child Care

Safety Concerns	Questions
Child Abuse	Can caregivers be seen by others at all times, so a child is never alone with one caregiver?
	Have all caregivers gone through a background check (such as employment history, criminal history)?
	Have the caregivers been trained in how to prevent child abuse and how to report suspected child abuse?
Medications	Does the child care program keep medication out of reach of children?
	Are the caregivers trained and the medications labeled to make sure the right child gets the right amount of the right medication at the right time?
Playgrounds	Is the playground inspected for safety often?
	Is the playground surrounded by a fence?
	If there is a sandbox, and is it clean?
	Is the playground equipment safe, with no sharp edges, and kept in good shape?
	Are the soil and playground surfaces checked often for dangerous substances and hazards?
	Is the equipment the right size and type for the age of children who use it?
SIDS Risk Reductions	Are all child care staff, volunteers, and substitutes trained in, and do they implement infant back-sleeping and safe sleep policies to reduce the risk of SIDS (sudden infant death syndrome, or crib death)?
	When infants are sleeping, are they on their backs with no pillows, quilts, stuffed toys, or other soft bedding in the crib with them?

families, and other health professionals, the consultants are prepared to address four interventions, including assessment/monitoring, program development and implementation, evaluation, and policy development. Nurse child-care health consultants identify the child care health needs within the setting and the community. They develop and offer information regarding resources available for children and families, particularly for children with special needs, such as medical home, assistance with developing Individual Education Programs (IEP), Individualized Family Service Programs (IFSP); produce staff and parent education material about health- and safety-related issues; and facilitate clinical experiences in child care programs for nursing students. They provide direct health services for children and staff, provide ongoing health and safety information, and offer educational programs for child care providers and parents. In order to make a difference in the community, nurse child-care health consultants also work as advocates on task forces and commissions to influence policy decisions in order to improve health and safety for the pediatric population (Crowley, 1988).

Assessment/Monitoring

Within the child care settings, the nurse consultants have a large role in assessing the quality of the health and safety practices. Their observation must include the environment, such as playgrounds, sanitation, and storage of toxic substances; staff qualifications and training; child-to-staff ratio, and the identification of needs of individual children and staff members, including occupational health risk.

An example of excellence in nursing care in assessment in the child care setting would be examination of the playground area to include the safety of the equipment, its condition (state of repair), and the play surfaces. Nurses can use an array of resources including standards from *Caring for Our Children* (AAP/APHA/NRCHSCC, 2002), *Handbook for Public Playground Safety* (U.S. Consumer Product Safety Commission, 1997), and the ASTM International standards (ASTM International, 2003a, 2003b, 2003c). Other areas of playground assessment include age-appropriateness of equipment, requirements for children with special needs, and hazards, such as standing bodies of water or hanging ropes. Nurses link child care providers with local playground safety consultants for more in-depth guidance and act as a liaison with community pediatricians to distribute safety information to providers and parents.

Nurse child-care health consultants rely on the standards in *Caring for Our Children* (AAP/APHA/NRCHSCC, 2002) for appraisal of a number of other areas of concern for health and safety. Assessment of the environment also includes the consultants' examination of practices for storage of toxic substances, such as cleaning agents or pesticides. Nurse child-care health consultants also support providers with information on *Caring for Our Children* standards for cleaning and sanitation of areas and toys used by children, diaper changing areas, food service areas and equipment, toilets and bathrooms, as well as safe treatment of spills of blood and body fluid. Throughout the assessment process, nurses build a partnership with the child care providers and staff, through problem-solving issues that are identified (Dooling & Ulione, 2000; Evers, 2002).

Interaction with staff includes the nurse child-care health consultant's assessment of individual staff members' health status and needs, qualifications and participation in appropriate training, as well as collaboration in developing written guidelines and health plans for the children in care, and maintaining the level of quality by instituting quick health check procedures for use in the child care setting (Colter & Perreault, 1999).

Program Development

The partnerships between nurse child-care health consultants' and child care directors and staff progresses in the program development process as the consultant introduces model safety policies, procedures, and maintenance plans for health records. They utilize model child health policies (Aronson, 2002) as a prototype, shaping the policies to meet the existing needs of the individual program. Examples of areas of critical need for policy implementation are medication administration and emergency preparedness. Basing their recommendations about medication administration policy on applicable state nursing and medical practice acts, nurses give particular consideration to the needs of children with special health care needs to support inclusion in child care. To illustrate, nurse child-care health consultants in Colorado worked with a statewide multidisciplinary team to create a course on medication administration that is currently required for staff of child care centers throughout the state (Colorado Office of Resource and Referral Agencies, n.d.). This course work continues to be used as a training model by other states. The consultants have also collaborated with state licensing agencies to write statewide policies, as exemplified by the development of a manual for emergency preparedness produced by the Healthy Child Care Vermont and Vermont Department of Licensing (Vermont Child Development Division and Healthy Child Care Vermont, 2002).

Implementation

The nurse child-care health consultant plays an active role in ensuring that quality health and safety practices are actually implemented and adhered to in child care on a regular basis. Opportunities abound for the sharing of the expertise in the ongoing partnership between consultants and child care providers. In the area of child maltreatment, the consultation on staff selection, staff supervision, staff training, and operational policies—such as always having providers within sight of other providers when caring for children—can serve to minimize risk (AAP/APHA/NRCHSCC, 2002).

To ensure safe standards of medication administration, the nurse child-care health consultant trains staff on proper medication procedures, such as use of the EpiPen within the parameters of a state's nurse practice act. Follow-up observation and retraining are another component of the nurse child-care health consultant's responsibility. They advise on up-to-date health and safety practices based on new scientific knowledge, such as discontinuance of use of syrup of ipecac (Bull et al., 2003).

There are many facets of consultation related to safety issues, such as observing sleeping practices, including checking compliance with Back-to-Sleep policies and training, performing on-site inspection of playground surfacing, and monitoring immunization record-keeping. As educators, nurse child-care health consultants conduct educational sessions for families and staff regarding health and mental health information and services across settings to promote continuity of care (Crowley, 2001; Gaines, World, Spencer, & Leary, 2005). This consultation also includes linking staff, families, and children with community health resources, such as medical home and health insurance. They also offer practical training such as teaching hand-washing technique in various situations, food handling, diapering, toileting, and age-appropriate nutrition, often reviewing menus to suggest substitutes that are more nutritious.

Evaluation

The evaluation role of the child care health consultant encompasses review and revision of policies, plans, and procedures based upon state and local regulations and what is considered nationally best health and safety practices included in documents such as *Caring for Our Children* (APA/APHA/NRCHSCC, 2002) and *Stepping Stones to Using Caring for Our Children* (APA/APHA/NRCHSCC, 2003). Using the *Stepping Stones* compliance/comparison checklist as a framework for evaluation, consultants can analyze collected data to identify opportunities for improvement in a number of areas including the following:

- Reviewing child and staff immunization records for completeness and timeliness in comparison with state health department requirements;
- Reviewing records of scheduled fire and evacuation drills;
- Reviewing emergency preparedness plan;
- Examining child and staff health records for completeness of required content, for example, history of hearing, oral health, and vision screenings;

- Reviewing staff training records with regard to health and safety continuing-education requirements;
- Inspecting child care program records of outbreaks of infectious disease, number of children affected, and analysis trends.

Statewide child-care health networks are contributing data on service areas through the Quality Enhancement Project funded by the Division of Child Development of North Carolina's Department of Health and Human Services (Kotch, 2004). Technical assistance by national consultants Health Systems Research and John Snow, Inc. has also supported evaluation efforts. These consultants are contacted by the National Child Health Bureau.

In a study of the impact of child health consultants in 20 California counties, preliminary data released by Kern County reveals the following impact that child care health consultants have made:

- 403 children received a health or developmental assessment for a particular concern; 267 children were linked to a health care provider.
- 260 children were assessed for a behavioral health concern; 69 children were linked to mental health services.
- 242 children were assessed for special needs; 152 children have been referred to special education for further evaluation and intervention (Healthy Child Care America, 2004).

Nurse child-care health consultants engage in ongoing data collection in order to establish the effectiveness of their practice. Five centers that received health consultation services showed marked improvement in child care center's staff health knowledge, the acknowledgement of an increased need for more health information, and an increased center compliance with national health standards (Alkon et al., 2002).

MULTIDISCIPLINARY INTEGRATION AND PARTNERSHIP: CASE STUDY

In working to support health and safety in child care, nurse child-care health consultants work with multiple levels of partnerships. Within health these include state health department contacts (such as infectious disease control experts and the state Title V programs); a particular child's health provider or established medical home; other specialized consultants (such as mental health consultants) and providers; child and adult food-care program experts; and other intervention service representatives, as needed. In the area of safety, nurse child-care health consultants work with state licensing inspectors, local fire officials, playground safety inspectors, building and zoning inspectors, and local homeland security specialists. The following case study illustrates their role.

D.M. is the nurse child-care health consultant for Happy Crayons Child Care Center, which is an inclusive program serving children with and without disabilities and chronic health conditions. As the nurse child-care health consultant, she is responsible for making weekly health visits to the center, training staff teachers and aides about several health topics. These topics include proper sanitation and hygiene, such as preventing the spread of disease, maintaining personal health and hygiene, recognizing illness in children, procedures for infectious disease, and first-aid training. D.M. also provides general and specific training to the staff about the disabilities and chronic health conditions, which may affect young children. In addition, she is available to the center's director, Susan, by pager for consultation on urgent health questions. Today, Susan called D.M. in a panic. One of the children, Luis, had fallen from the merry-go-round in the city park, where the preschoolers had been taken for an outing. An older child, who was not from the child care center, was pushing the merry-go-round so it would go faster, and Luis accidentally let go. He fell on his outstretched right arm, and immediately started crying inconsolably. One of the aides who accompanied the children to the park returned with Luis right away and applied a plastic splint and ice to the arm, which had a visible swelling just above the right wrist. When the aide returned to the Happy Crayons center with Luis, Susan administered Motrin syrup to Luis, which was allowed as a PRN medication by his doctor. Child care providers are allowed to administer medications to children while they are at the center, as long as the provider has passed a medication administration course and as long as there is an up-to-date prescription on the child's chart and a permission form signed by the parents. When D.M. called back, Susan asked her if they should call an ambulance to take Luis to the emergency room. D.M. asked if the parents had been notified, and Susan replied that she had a call into Luis's mother. Susan further stated that Luis had settled down now, and was quietly sucking his thumb and fingering his old quilted security blanket. She said that he wasn't crying as long as he wasn't being moved. The splint and ice were still in place.

D.M. advised that Susan should page the mother once again, letting her know it was an urgent call, and ask if the mother wished them to call an ambulance or wait until she could get there. At that moment, Luis's mother called back, and said she would be there right away and take him to the local children's hospital emergency room, as it was only a few blocks away. She thanked Susan for calling her promptly and for applying the appropriate first aid. The next day, during the weekly health consultation visit, D.M. and Susan discussed the event. Luis's mother had called that morning, and informed them that the ER doctor had taken x-rays and diagnosed a nondisplaced fracture of the wrist, which was then put in a cast. She thanked them for their quick and accurate treatment of the injury.

D.M. and Susan were very concerned about the problem of unsafe playground equipment. The equipment at the park was old, but it was close to the center and convenient for outings and picnics when the weather was favorable. The playground equipment and the park environs were maintained by the city Department of Recreation. Susan and D.M. decided to contact the department and inform them of the unsafe merry-go-round. Other children from the child care center had fallen and skinned knees while playing on it, but this was the first time a child had acquired a serious injury. Additionally, the surface of the playground was gravel, which can contribute to injuries. They prepared their case for the city, using information on playground safety found on the Web site of the National Resource Center for Health and Safety in Child Care and other consumer protection Web sites.

D.M. contacted the Department of Recreation and informed them of the injury and other potential risks, providing them with the resources they had found. The director of the Department of Recreation was very impressed by the statistics and recommendations and invited D.M. and Susan to make their presentation to the city council, to urge them to release funds to make the playground safer, and to consider making the playground accessible for all children. D.M. suggested that they enlist the parents of children with disabilities and chronic conditions at the child care center, to help to design the new playground so that it would be safe for all children.

Eight months later, D.M., the president of the local parent support group for parents of children with disabilities, and the city council attended the ribbon-cutting ceremony for the new, safer, fully accessible playground. The merry-go-round had been removed, and the new equipment met the guidelines of the U.S. Consumer Product Safety Commission. The gravel had been removed and replaced with double shredded bark mulch, an approved surface. Now, Susan and the teachers and aides at Happy Crayons Child Care Center could take the children to play in the park without any worry about unsafe equipment.

SUMMARY

This chapter examines the role of the nurse child-care health consultant in ensuring the physical safety provision of care for children in out-of-home child care. Nurse child-care health consultants provide expertise and consultation on health education, policy and procedure development, and health promotion in the areas of physical safety. In addition, they may provide assistance in resources for provider health, physical examinations, and health care resources. The consultant can serve a critical role in providing information and skills related to proper medication administration and safe delivery of invasive health-care procedures for the increasing number of children with special health care needs in child care. Ensuring the physical safety and health of children in child care is of paramount importance as more children spend increasing time in out-of-home child care settings.

REFERENCES

Alkon, A., Sokal-Gutierrez, K., & Wolff, M. (2002). Child care health consultation improves health knowledge and compliance. *Pediatric Nursing, 28,* 61–65.

American Academy of Pediatrics, American Public Health Association, and National Resource Center for Health and Safety in Child Care. (2002). *Caring for our children. National health and safety performance standards: Guidelines for out-of-home child care programs* (2nd ed.). Elk Grove Village, IL: American Academy of Pediatrics.

American Academy of Pediatrics, American Public Health Association, and National Resource Center for Health and Safety in Child Care. (2003). Stepping stones to using caring for our children. In *National health and safety performance standards: Guidelines for out-of-home child care programs* (2nd ed.). Elk Grove Village, IL: American Academy of Pediatrics.

Aronson, S. S. (2002). *Model child care health policies* (4th ed.). Elk Grove Village, IL: American Academy of Pediatrics.

ASTM International. (2003a). *F1292-04 Standard specification for impact attenuation of surfacing materials within the use zone of playground equipment.* West Conshohocken, PA: ASTM International.

ASTM International. (2003b). *F1487-01e1 Standard consumer safety performance specification for playground equipment for public use.* West Conshohocken, PA: ASTM International.

ASTM International. (2003c). *F2223-04 Standard guide for ASTM standards on playground surfacing.* West Conshohocken, PA: ASTM International.

Bull, M. J., Agran, P., Dowd, M. D., Garcia, V., Gardner, H. G., Smith, G. A., et al. (2003). Policy statement: Poison treatment in the home. *Pediatrics, 112,* 1182–1185.

Centers for Disease Control and Prevention, Office of Minority Health. (2004, February). *Highlights in minority Health.* Retrieved December 15, 2004, from http://www.cdc.gov/omh/Highlights/2004/HFeb04IF.htm

Colorado Office of Resource and Referral Agencies. (n.d.). *Medication administration training.* Retrieved December 15, 2004, from http://www.corra.org/CORRAPrograms/MAT.asp

Colter, J., & Perreault, C. (1999). *Child care health and safety assessment and suggested child health and public health consultative activities in out of home child care settings.* Denver, CO: Department of Public Health and Environment.

Crowley, A. A. (1988). The child care dilemma: Expanding nurse practitioner involvement. *Journal of Pediatric Health Care, 2,* 128–134.

Crowley, A. A. (2001). Child care health consultation: An ecological model. *Journal of the Society of Pediatric Nurses, 6,* 170–181.

Dooling, M. V., & Ulione, M. S. (2000). Health consultation in child care: A partnership that works. *Young Children, 55,* 23–26.

Evers, D. B. (2002). The pediatric nurse's role as health consultant to a child care center. *Pediatric Nursing, 28,* 231–235.

Fiene, R. (1988). Human services instrument based program monitoring and indicator systems. In B. Glastonbury, W. LaMendola, & S. Toole (Eds.), *Information technology and the human services* (pp. 147–159). Chichester, England: Wiley.

Fiene, R. (1994, Summer). The case for national early care and education standards: Key indicator/predictor state childcare regulations. *NARA Licensing Newsletter,* 6-8.

Fiene, R. (2002). *13 Indicators of quality child care; Research update.* Retrieved October 1, 2004, from http://aspe.hhs.gov/hsp/ccquality-ind02/

Fiene, R., & Kroh, K. (2000). Measurement tools and systems. In *The NARA licensing curriculum* (pp. 1–38). Minneapolis, MN: National Association for Regulatory Administration.

Fiene, R., & Nixon, M. (1981). *An instrument-based program monitoring information system: A new tool for day care monitoring.* Washington, DC: National Children's Services Monitoring Transfer Consortium.

Fiene, R., & Nixon, M. (1983). *Indicator checklist system for day care monitoring.* Washington, DC: National Children's Services Monitoring Transfer Consortium.

Gaines, S. K., World, J. L., Spencer, L., & Leary, J. M. (2005). Assessing the need for child-care health consultants. *Public Health Nursing, 22*(1), 8–16.

Harms, T., Clifford, R. M., & Cryer, D. (2004). *Early childhood environment rating scale* (Rev. ed.). New York: Teachers College Press.

Harms, T., Cryer, D., & Clifford, R. M. (2002). *Infant/toddler environment rating scale* (Rev. ed.). New York: Teachers College Press.

Head Start Bureau. (1997). *Head Start program performance standards and other regulations.* Washington, DC: Head Start Bureau.

Healthy Child Care America. (2004, Summer). *Telling the healthy child care America story: Making a positive difference in the health of children in child care.* Elk Grove Village, IL: American Academy of Pediatrics.

Kotch, J. B. (2004). *Health and safety in child care: Relation to rating scales.* Presentation at the North Carolina Rated License Assessment Project Conference, Greensboro, NC, August 31.

Kotch, J. B., Dufort, V. M., Stewart, P., Fieberg, J., McMurray, M., O'Brien, S., et al. (1997). Injuries among children in home and out-of-home care. *Injury Prevention, 3,* 267–271.

Maurice, P., Lavoie, M., Laflamme, L., Svanstrom, L., Romer, C., & Anderson, R. (2001). Safety and safety promotion: Definitions for operational developments. *Injury Control and Safety Promotion, 8,* 237–240.

Moon, R. Y., Patel, K. M., & Shaefer, S. J. (2000). Sudden infant death syndrome in child care settings. *Pediatrics, 106,* 295–300.

National Association for the Education of Young Children. (1998). *Accreditation criteria and procedures of the National Association for the Education of Young Children—1998 edition.* Washington, DC: National Association for the Education of Young Children.

National Association for Family Child Care. (2003). *Quality standards for NAFCC accreditation* (3rd ed.). Salt Lake City, UT: National Association of Family Child Care.

National Center for Injury Prevention and Control. (2001). *Injury fact book 2001–2002.* Atlanta, GA: Centers for Disease Control and Prevention, National Center for Injury Prevention and Control.

National Resource Center for Health and Safety in Child Care. (2003). *A parent's guide to choosing safe and healthy child care.* Retrieved October 1, 2004, from http://nrc.uchsc.edu/RESOURCES/ParentsGuide.pdf

National Resource Center for Health and Safety in Child Care. (2004). *Medication administration language in state licensing regulations.* Aurora, CO: National Resource Center for Health and Safety in Child Care.

Perrin, E. C., Lewkowicz, C., & Young, M. H. (2000). Shared vision: Concordance among fathers, mothers, and pediatricians about unmet needs of children with chronic health conditions. *Pediatrics, 105,* 277–285.

Phelan, K. J., Khoury, J., Kalkwarf, H. J., & Lanphear, B. P. (2001). Trends and patterns of playground injuries in United States children and adolescents. *Ambulatory Pediatrics, 1,* 227–233.

Tinsworth, D., & McDonald, J. (2001). *Special study: Injuries and deaths associated with children's playground equipment.* Washington, DC: U.S. Consumer Product Safety Commission.

U.S. Consumer Product Safety Commission. (1997). *Handbook of public playground safety.* Washington, DC: U.S. Consumer Product Safety Commission.

U.S. Department of Health and Human Services, Administration for Children and Families. (2003). *Child maltreatment, 2001.* Washington, DC: U.S. Government Printing Office.

Ulione, M. S. (1997). Health promotion and injury prevention in a child development center. *Journal of Pediatric Nursing, 12,* 148–154.

Ulione, M. S., & Dooling, M. (1997). Preschool injuries in child care centers: Nursing strategies for prevention. *Journal of Pediatric Health Care, 11,* 111–116.

Vermont Child Development Division and Healthy Child Care Vermont. (2002). *Emergency response planning guide for child care.* Retrieved December 15, 2004, from http://www.state.vt.us/srs/childcare/erp.htm

CHAPTER TEN

Protecting the Right to Privacy and Confidentiality of Information

Ann M. Rhodes

INTRODUCTION AND DEFINITIONS

The protection of a client's right to confidentiality needs to be discussed in the context within which legal rights and obligations are defined. The United States Constitution enumerates a set of basic rights and establishes a system of government with three branches: legislative, executive, and judicial. Each branch of government produces "law" or rules that create enforceable rights or obligations.

The legislative branch of the government passes statutes. The executive branch, through agencies and departments, promulgates rules and regulations. The judicial branch decides cases. The written decisions in these cases establish case law or common law that interprets or defines the Constitution, statutes, or rules.

Statutes are laws that are written by an elected legislative body, such as Congress or a state legislature. An example of a federal statute is HIPAA (Health Insurance Portability and Accountability Act),[1] and an example of a state statute is a nurse practice act[2] (professional practice as defined, supervised, and regulated by the states).

Regulations are rules that are issued by an executive agency and have the force of law. Agencies are entities of government responsible for administering programs. They also develop the rules to implement statutes, among other duties. There are federal agencies and departments (such as the Department of Health and Human Services) and state agencies (such as state Departments of Health). An example of a federal rule is the

149

Privacy Rule promulgated under HIPAA,[3] which will be discussed in detail. Another example is the Medicare Conditions of Participation,[4] which define and regulate the requirements for reimbursement through Medicare. Both sets of rules are detailed and prescriptive,[5] compliance is mandatory,[6] and there are sanctions for noncompliance.[7] Examples of state-level regulations include state nursing licensure regulations and state board of health regulations.

The final source of law is case law or common law. This is based on judicial decisions that are made by interpreting previous court decisions, applying statutes or constitutional principles to specific cases. The applicable case law can vary with location—a court in one jurisdiction may not make the same decision as a court in another jurisdiction. Because courts are different and state laws are different, similar cases in different states can have contrary results. Consequently, practitioners must know the law and legal doctrines in the state in which they practice.

Requirements pertaining to health information and confidentiality are contained in many places: federal statutes, federal rules, funding bills, state statutes, licensing requirements, and professional codes of ethics. In addition, some areas are controversial and evolving. For example, the law regarding the right to privacy is an area of great interest and it is changing rapidly.

The Right to Privacy

The right to privacy is not stated specifically in the Constitution, but as long ago as 1890, Supreme Court Justice Louis Brandeis described "a right to be left alone."[8] Over time, this right has developed into the right to make decisions without unwarranted government intrusions and the right to privacy in personal information. Although there have been a number of cases affirming the right to privacy, the extent of the right and the basis in constitutional law remain controversial.

The modern doctrine of privacy, which is still applicable, was described by Justice William O. Douglas in *Griswold v. Connecticut.*[9] In that case, the court invalidated a state statute that prevented the use of contraceptives. Douglas asserted that marriage existed with a "zone of privacy"[10] and that the specific guarantees have "penumbras formed by emanations" that create zones of privacy.[11]

There have been a number of subsequent cases that rely on this definition of a right to privacy, particularly to protect the rights of individuals to make decisions about reproduction[12] and end-of-life decisions.[13] What is critical, however, is the recognition and acceptance of a right to privacy.

The U.S. Supreme Court has specifically upheld the constitutional protection of personal health information. In *Whalen v. Roe*,[14] the Court analyzed a New York statute that created a database of persons who obtained drugs for which there was both a lawful and unlawful market. The Court, in its analysis, recognized two different types of interests within the zone of privacy. The first is the interest in making certain kinds of decisions (reproductive) independently. The other is the individual interest in avoiding disclosure of personal matters. This interest, discussed in the context of medical information, was viewed as distinct and constitutionally protected.

In addition to a constitutional right of privacy, many state statutes provide a legal right to privacy with a basis for a lawsuit in tort if there is public disclosure of private information. There are statutes that provide for protection of financial and other personal information, but the highest standard of protection is reserved for health information. The highest expectations for protecting information are of health professionals whose relationships and discussions with patients are protected by "confidentiality."

Privacy and Confidentiality

"Privacy" and "confidentiality" are different things. In the health care setting, privacy is not only a legal right to freedom from unwanted intrusion, but it encompasses psychological, social, and physical elements as well as confidentiality. "Confidentiality" in the health care setting is the agreement between a patient and a provider that information discussed in the process of a health care transaction will not be shared with other parties without the permission of the patient.

As a general rule, confidentiality refers to the privileged and private nature of information provided during the health care transaction. It is important for patients to expect that information will be held in confidence—this encourages candor and full disclosure of health history, and it forms the basis of a relationship between the nurse and the patient.

The duty to maintain patient confidentiality arises from many sources, including state licensing regulations, ethical standards of the profession, state statutes, and state and federal funding statutes (such as Title X of the Public Health Service Act).[15] Operationally, confidentiality means that there is an understanding between the child (or parent) and the nurse that information discussed or discovered in the course of treatment will not be shared with others unless there is explicit permission to share the information.

There are circumstances, however, that override the right to privacy and the duty to maintain confidentiality. For example, nurses are obligated to report child abuse and neglect and infectious diseases.[16] These compulsory disclosures to protect child welfare and the public health out-weigh individual privacy rights.

As a rule, confidentiality follows consent. This means that the nurse's duty to maintain confidentiality is tied to whoever gives consent to treat-ment. In almost all states, 18 is the age of majority (the age at which a person is considered an adult and able to consent to treatment). When the patient is under 18, the consent of a parent is required for medical care (with numerous exceptions noted below). When a parent gives consent, the nurse owes a duty of confidentiality to the child and the parent to pro-tect the information from being disclosed to other parties.

Disclosure of Information

When the issue is the appropriate use of information, the role of the nurse is twofold: protecting confidential information from being shared with people who have no right to it (unauthorized or impermissible disclo-sure), and assuring that patients have enough of the right information to make health care decisions. The legal concept of informed consent de-scribes the process through which the patient and, in the case of children, parent learn the options for treatment, the risks, benefits, and alterna-tives. Based on knowledge and understanding, the patient then makes a decision to authorize a particular type of treatment. For consent to be in-formed, the patient needs to know (and the person obtaining consent must disclose) diagnosis, the nature and purpose of the proposed treat-ment; risks and consequences of proposed treatment; adverse effects of the proposed treatment; likelihood of success; prognosis with and with-out treatment; and alternative treatments. Consent to treatment must be given after disclosure or it is not "informed."

This is a lengthy list, but courts have indicated that the disclosure of risks can be limited to those that are material or significant. The definition of a material risk is one that is significant enough that it would affect the de-cision-making process of a reasonable patient. This can be further defined to include risks that are minor but common, and risks that are rare but se-vere. There should be documentation of disclosure for consent to treatment, including the name of the person who made the disclosure and content.

CONFIDENTIALITY FOR ADOLESCENTS: RULES, EXCEPTIONS, AND ISSUES

As noted, in most states 18 is the age at which a child becomes an adult. Prior to that, the child is a minor, and an adult (a person over the age of 18 who is legally responsible for the child, usually a parent) is required to give consent to medical care. This requirement has exceptions, however, based on two broad areas: the *status* of the minor and the *type* of care being provided.

The developmental stage of adolescence has no specific legal significance; statutes generally define only the age at which a child becomes an adult. There has been, however, a line of court cases that recognizes that children are entitled to constitutional protection to the same degree as adults.[17] In *Wisconsin v. Yoder*,[18] the U.S. Supreme Court examined the historical status of children in society and the role of parents and the state. Justice Douglas, in his dissent, cited developmental theorists and asserted that the decisional capacity of adolescents was comparable to that of adults. He stated, "the moral and intellectual maturity of the fourteen-year-old approaches that of the adult."[19]

Consequently, although 18 is the age at which a child becomes an adult and prior to that the nurse's duty of confidentiality and disclosure is owed to the child and the parent, there are numerous exceptions. These exceptions limit parental decision-making authority and shift decisional authority to the minor. This means that the nurse's duty to protect and to disclose information lies exclusively with the minor child. The shifting of rights recognizes that many minors have the cognitive and decisional skills to determine their health care needs, and there are sometimes divergent interests between parents and children because families do not always function as integrated and harmonious units.

The first status-based exception to the requirement that a person be 18 before giving consent is the *emancipated minor*. Under the common law of emancipation, a person under the age of 18 who is self-supporting, is not living at home, and whose parents have surrendered parental rights and responsibilities will be considered an emancipated minor. Some states require a case-by-case determination of the facts and circumstances[20] to declare emancipation, while other states have enacted statutes defining it.[21]

Generally, marriage, military service, or financial independence suggests emancipation. Attendance at college or giving birth to a child does not automatically confer emancipation, although minor parents can consent to their child's care. If a minor presents for treatment and is not accompanied by an adult (other than the treatment-based exceptions described below), the nurse should make an effort to determine that the minor can give consent to treatment.

The other status-based exception is the *mature minor rule,* which allows children who are mature enough to understand the risks and benefits of proposed treatment to give consent. The notion of emancipation is based on an objective analysis of the minor's independence from parents, whereas the mature minor rule is based on the cognitive maturity of adolescents. The rule was developed through judicial decisions and recognizes that minors, beginning at age 14, can make thoughtful and informed decisions about their care, given the information upon which to make a determination about treatment. Some states have written the mature minor rule into statute. Arkansas, for example, states that "any unemancipated minor of sufficient intelligence to understand and appreciate the consequences of the proposed medical or surgical treatment" is authorized to give consent to his or her own care.[22]

The second major area of exception to the requirement of parental authorization of treatment and disclosure of information is based on the nature of the treatment being provided. There are several "minor treatment" statutes that allow minors to give consent to treatment. In these circumstances, the nurse's duty to maintain confidentiality is only to the patient. Reporting any information about the patient will be prescribed and limited by the law.

The minor treatment statutes give minors the authority to consent to care that is consequent to sexual activity and drug and alcohol use. The rationale is that the requirement of parental involvement might delay some minors in seeking medical treatment or cause them to avoid treatment altogether. These statutes create a privilege between the minor and the health care provider that values the needs of the minor over the authority of the parent.

As a general rule, minors can give consent to and receive treatment for pregnancy, prenatal care, delivery; family planning services, including contraception; screening for and treatment of sexually transmitted diseases; and counseling and treatment for drug and alcohol dependency. Some states permit minors to consent to mental health services.

Abortion is excluded from this list because the status of minor consent to abortion is controversial and varies from state to state. Following *Roe v. Wade,*[23] which characterized abortion as a medical decision to be made by a woman and her physician, several states passed laws that required parental consent.[24] These laws were challenged, overturned, revised, and challenged again. The result is that, at any point in time, a state might have a state law enacted by its legislature, challenged on constitutional grounds but not overturned, that imposes one or more of the following on adolescents seeking an abortion:

- parental notification requirement or, alternatively, a judicial procedure to bypass the parents
- waiting period between consent and procedure
- required counseling
- compulsory, prescribed education program

Nurses who work with adolescents should always have the following two pieces of information: the current status of state law on minor consent to abortion and a resource person from whom to seek advice in specific cases.

SURROGATE DECISION MAKING
AND DISCLOSURE TO PARENTS

The nurse owes a legal duty to the patient. This duty encompasses a variety of elements including providing quality care. This chapter addresses only the duty of the nurse to protect confidential information when bound to do so and to disclose information when necessary for treatment purposes or for other legally permissible reasons.

Nurses who care for children frequently have a dual responsibility. Their patient is a child, to whom the legal duty is owed, but decisions about care are made by surrogates: adults who have the legal authority to act on behalf of the child. In almost all cases, this will be one or both parents. In some situations, there will be a legal guardian. A guardian must be an adult (over the age of 18) designated by the court after a legal procedure. It is typical for children in foster care to have a legal guardian who is not the foster parent. This is relevant to who has the authority to authorize disclosure of information and to protection of confidential information.

For pediatric nurses, the fact that parents serve as surrogate decision makers for children means that they have a right to receive all the information necessary to make informed decisions about care. They also have the authority to release information to third parties. Under the Privacy Rule, parents are "personal representatives" of their children, and they have the rights to authorize information release and exercise other rights,[25] with exceptions discussed below.[26]

In general, when children are very young, disclosure of information should be made only to the parents as they have the right to consent to treatment. The right of the parents to determine the course of treatment for their children has been accepted as both legally and ethically appropriate, although a recent case in Texas has raised interesting challenges to this doctrine.

When children grow mature enough to understand and participate in their own care, they should be included in discussions about treatment, although there is no legal requirement that this be done. When a child is at the developmental age of 14, the child should be considered a mature minor and consent for treatment should be obtained from both the child and the parents. The child should be included in discussions about treatment options and should be present for disclosure of information.

At this point, the nurse's duty is to both the child and the parents. Conflict will arise when the duty to the child—the patient—is in conflict with the duty to the parents. The most common situation is when the child confides in the nurse and requests that the information not be shared with parents. Unless there is a legal obligation to report (such as abuse), the nurse is obliged to keep the information confidential.

In fact, with adolescent patients, the role of the nurse may no longer be that of a caregiver of a family unit with similar concerns and interests. When the patient is a teenager, the patient can give consent to certain kinds of treatment independently and have assurances of confidentiality. This means that the nurse's duty is to the adolescent, with an obligation to maintain confidentiality and to put the patient's interests first.

As noted, the principle that parents give consent to treatment, or can refuse treatment in some cases, on behalf of their children was addressed recently by the Texas Supreme Court. *Miller ex. rel. Miller*[27] is among the most recent cases to make clear that the authority of parents, acting as surrogate decision makers for their children, is not absolute. This is especially clear when the issue is refusal of treatment. The Miller case involved the parents' wish to forego resuscitation after delivery of a severely premature infant at 23 weeks' gestation. The hospital policy was to resuscitate any infant with a birth weight over 500 grams. The Miller infant weighed 615 grams, so resuscitation measures were employed.

The parents sued the hospital corporation and after extensive litigation, the Texas Supreme Court determined that parents do not have the right to refuse "urgently needed life-sustaining medical treatment for their child unless the child's condition is 'certifiably terminal' under the [Texas] Natural Death Act."[28]

The court applied the "emergency" exception—generally used only if required to provide care when parental consent cannot be obtained—to the case of a severely premature infant. This is an unusual application of this doctrine.

There is a history of government intervention to ensure treatment of newborns. It is clear in the examination of the cases, regulations and, ultimately, the statute (the Child Abuse Prevention and Treatment Act of 1984)[29] that treatment cannot be withheld from handicapped newborns (regardless of parental wishes) and that prematurity is not covered by the federal act or considered a "terminal condition" for purposes of state statutes.

THE NURSE AS ADVOCATE FOR IMPLEMENTING THE HEALTH INSURANCE PORTABILITY AND ACCOUNTABILITY ACT

HIPAA is the title of a federal statute that includes several complex health care provisions. It was originally intended to address job-lock: the problem of employees who have health conditions and change jobs to find that they are locked out of the employee health insurance due to the preexisting condition clause. HIPAA takes its name from the idea that employees can carry insurance from one job to another (thus, health insurance portability).

During congressional committee hearings, there was testimony about problems of health information being shared outside the health system and resulting discrimination. There was particular concern about electronic transmission of health information and the use of fax, cell phone, Internet communications, and database management. This led to an effort to prevent avoidable, improper disclosure of health information and access to information.

The statute authorized the Department of Health and Human Services to enact rules to create detailed standards, the Privacy Rule, which went into effect on April 14, 2003.[30] This created a national minimal threshold of privacy standards aimed at avoiding improper dissemination of "individually identifiable information."[31] Objectives of the privacy standards include streamlining and promoting efficiency in the electronic information—sharing processes, reducing costs in health care and billing functions, and establishing parameters and limitations on health information sharing.[32]

The privacy rule is intended to assure a national minimum standard of privacy protection. If there is a state standard that is more restrictive or more protective, that standard will apply.[33] Under the privacy rule, "protected health information" must remain private unless disclosure is acceptable under the rules. There are three types of disclosures described in the privacy rules: authorized, permitted, and compulsory. *Authorized* disclosures are those made pursuant to a consent to disclose given by the patient or the patient's personal representative (parent or guardian if it is a child; spouse or next of kin; person with the power of attorney).

There are a significant number of *permitted* disclosures. Those necessary for treatment, payment, and operations are specifically identified. It should be noted that "educating future health practitioners" is included in operations. This means that disclosure of information necessary to treat the patient and teach students is permissible. All disclosures are subject to a "minimum necessary" standard: only the amount of information necessary to do the job should be disclosed to the people who need to know it.[34] Other permitted disclosures are described in the rule as disclosures that do not require authorization. These disclosures are listed more fully below.

Compulsory disclosures are those required by law. Examples include reporting child abuse and neglect, reporting infectious diseases, and providing information in response to a subpoena presented by a law enforcement agency.

Note that the terms *use* and *disclosure* are not the same, although they are frequently used together in the privacy rule (sometimes conjunctively and sometimes not). The best interpretation is to apply "use" to sharing of information within an entity (between departments or units) and "disclosure" to revealing information outside the institution.

What follows is a brief summary of the Privacy Rule with guidelines for nurses:

The Privacy Rule applies to three types of entities:[35] health plans (such as insurance carriers), health care clearinghouses (such as a billing service), and health care providers who transmit any health information in electronic form. "Health care provider" is further defined in one code section by place of service, such as a hospital, skilled nursing facility, outpatient rehabilitation facility, home health agency, or hospice.[36] In another code section, "health care provider" is defined by the services provided and the nature of the provider. This specifically includes nurse practitioners and nurse midwives.[37]

Institutions must comply with the Privacy Rule, and nurses, as employees, must meet the requirements of the rules. Nurse practitioners who are in private practice will be subject to the rule, and nurse practitioners who work as independent contractors to hospitals or other agencies will probably enter into a business-associate agreement with the agency. Nurses should assume that they need to comply, in all circumstances, with the provisions of the Privacy Rule.

Several concepts are key to understanding the Privacy Rule. First, the "designated record set" means the medical records, billing records, enrollment, and case management or claims records of an individual.[38] This includes any record, in any format or medium (paper or electronic), that is used to make decisions. Second, "psychotherapy notes" are given separate recognition and protection and include documentation of the contents of counseling sessions by a mental health professional.[39]

"Protected health information" is any information that relates to the past, present, or future physical or mental health or condition of an individual, the provision of health care to the individual, or the payment for health care provided to the individual that either identifies the individual or could be combined to identify the individual. Read in conjunction with other provisions of the rule, it is clear that what constitutes protected health information (PHI) is broad.

Institutions (or NPs in practice) have several responsibilities. Institutions must designate a HIPAA Privacy Official who oversees compliance. This person can be a valuable resource person for assistance in interpreting and applying the rules. Institutions must also train all staff in the provisions of the rule, provide a notice of privacy practice to all clients, and have policies and procedures in place to implement the requirements of the rule. These are listed below. There is a specific requirement that individuals who violate the Privacy Rule and institutional policies be disciplined. There must be documentation of staff training and policies and procedures as well as compliance procedures. All consent forms and information materials must be reviewed to assure that they are HIPAA compliant, which means, simply, that the materials contain the required notices to advise patients of their rights and that the materials do not disclose, inadvertently, PHI.

Individuals, similarly, have several responsibilities. The Privacy Rule requires training in the specific provisions of its standards. At this time, there is no retraining requirement so training that was completed prior to the April 2003 effective date of the rule meets this requirement. Maintaining the confidentiality of patient information is a duty that nurses have recognized for as long as nursing care has been provided—the Privacy Rule just codifies this requirement. Nurses were required to protect patient information prior to the Privacy Rule by other legal and ethical standards, as were other professionals.

The Privacy Rule requires institutional notices and policies and procedures that may be unfamiliar and confusing to patients. Nurses need to be knowledgeable about the rights afforded to patients in the rule so that they can explain them to patients, assist patients in exercising their rights, and ensure that the institution's approach is as clear as possible.

The protection of patient privacy is an element of excellent nursing care. This means that each transaction must involve only the use and transmission of the information necessary for care, and that a respect for patient privacy and confidentiality must be built into the culture. Nurses are in a position to be role models in this regard because nurses care for families when they are at their most vulnerable and nurses occupy a position of trust and confidence among patients and the public.

As noted, the Privacy Rule is specific and prescriptive. It requires that each patient receive a Notice of Privacy Practices, the content of which is dictated by rule. There needs to be documentation that this notice was received.[40] Patients receive this on a first encounter with a health institution or clinic. Although a great deal of useful information is contained in this notice, it is reasonable to assume that patients and families are unable to comprehend much of it, due to the stress of being in the health care system and the complexity of the information. Also, patients from diverse backgrounds find the Privacy Notices difficult to interpret. Concern about the effectiveness of communication with diverse groups has been raised by a variety of consumer groups and was summarized in a report by the General Accountability Office (GAO) of the first year's experience with HIPAA.[41] This report suggested that the privacy notice be developed to meet the needs of families with a variety of reading levels and families whose native language is not English.

Under the Privacy Rule, every patient has a number of rights, which can be exercised by the patient or, on the patient's behalf, by a "personal representative." These include the following rights:

• To be assured that personal health information will be treated in a respectful manner and disclosed only when necessary.

• To request restriction of uses and disclosures.[42] Patients can request that information be restricted to use in treatment, payment, and operations; and to disclosures to family members or under emergency conditions. Nurses should discuss this with patients to make sure the patient's wishes are clear, the directions are documented, and the restriction is permissible. There should be an institutional policy to direct how this is handled and documented.

• To request confidential communications.[43] This means that patients can request that information (such as appointment letters) be sent to a selected alternate address or communicated through a selected method not generally used. The institution should have a policy and procedure for how a patient makes a request and how and to what extent it is accommodated. The obligation of the institution is "reasonable accommodation."[44]

• To access protected health information.[45] There are detailed rules that affect this right. Briefly, this right to inspect and copy the record is subject to review and approval by the health care provider and may be denied. There are various records that the patient does not have a right to access, including psychotherapy notes and information prepared in anticipation of litigation. Patients must file a request to review the record, and the institution must advise the patient of the decision and provide a system for review if the request is denied. This is a very detailed and technical section of the rules.

• To amend the record.[46] A patient can request that a change be made in part of the designated record set. Again, the rules have detailed requirements for the form of the request, institutional review, and the method for action, informing the patient, and documenting the process. The request can be denied, in which case the patient can file a statement of disagreement that will be included in the record.[47] This is an important section for pediatric nurses to note. Parents occasionally object to characterizations of parent-child interaction or other observations contained in the record. Any indication that patients or parents feel the information in the record is wrong should be taken seriously.

- To an accounting of disclosures of protected health information. If requested, a patient can receive a list of who has received PHI from the covered entity in the 6 years prior to the date the accounting was requested.[48] Note that the earliest this can be effective is the day the rules went into effect: April 14, 2003, and there are extensive exceptions to the accounting requirement. Specifically, the accounting *excludes* authorized disclosures; those made for treatment, payment, and operations for the institution's directory or to persons involved in care; disclosures made for national security or intelligence purposes; and disclosures for law enforcement purposes (subject to various technical requirements). The GAO report recommended that disclosures made for public health purposes be excluded as well, but there has been no rule change implementing this recommendation.[49]

At this time, disclosures for research purposes and for public health reporting purposes are subject to the accounting requirement.

EXCEPTIONS

There are some uses of PHI to which patients have the opportunity to object: inclusion in the institution's directory and release of information for marketing purposes.[50] In these instances, patient requests to be excluded must be respected.

Some uses and disclosures of information can occur without patient authorization. These include the following:

- Uses and disclosures required by law.[51] Examples include providing information pursuant to a subpoena, or for an administrative proceeding (including an action being taken by a professional licensing board) or for a grand jury proceeding.
- Uses and disclosures for public health activities.[52] This section specifically includes several provisions of interest to nurses: information about public health surveillance, infectious disease reporting, child abuse and neglect, adverse events of food and drugs, and to enable product recalls.
- Uses and disclosures to monitor communicable diseases.
- Uses and disclosures to monitor workplace injuries.

- Disclosures about victims of abuse, neglect, or domestic violence.[53]
- Uses and disclosures for health oversight activities;[54] examples include audits, inspections, licensure or disciplinary actions, or actions necessary to oversee benefit or other programs.
- Disclosures for judicial and administrative proceedings,[55] which is subject to a variety of procedures and protections but, in general, disclosure must be made if the request is in the proper form.
- Disclosures for law enforcement purposes.[56] This is very broad and, in summary, if a legitimate request is made by a law enforcement agency, PHI must be disclosed. The disclosure may be about a victim of a crime or to aid in the location of a suspect. If PHI is requested under this exception, the best advice is to contact the privacy officer for consultation and to determine what documentation is appropriate.
- Uses and disclosures about decedents to coroners for the purpose of identification or determining cause of death.[57]
- Uses and disclosures for organ, eye, or tissue donation purposes.[58]
- Uses and disclosures to avert a serious threat to public safety.[59]
- Uses and disclosures for specialized government functions, which includes military, national security, and intelligence activities.[60]
- Uses and disclosures for research purposes.[61]

Research

Protected health information may be used or disclosed for research purposes regardless of the source of funding, provided that there is either authorization for the use of the PHI or there is a waiver of the authorization requirement from an institutional review board (IRB) or privacy board.

The definition of research contained in the Privacy Rule[62] is identical to that in the Common Rule: "a systematic investigation, including research development, testing, and evaluation, designed to develop or contribute to generalizable knowledge."[63] There are several types of reviews of records containing PHI that can be conducted without authorization but they must be approved, meet several criteria, and be documented appropriately. These include reviews preparatory to research, such as developing a research protocol and research on decedent records.

Other Provisions

There are consequences to violating the Privacy Rule. An institution can receive civil and criminal penalties for a documented breach of a patient's privacy rights. The rules require institutions to set up complaint procedures, and the Office of Civil Rights (OCR) of the Department of Justice is the enforcement agency. The OCR can receive complaints directly and can conduct an investigation and impose penalties. The penalties, most likely fines, will be assessed against institutions.

Of course, nurses can be subject to discipline brought by licensing boards for violating patient confidentiality, and this predates the privacy rule and the penalty attaches to the individual nurse.

To summarize, there are multiple, complex provisions to the privacy rule. The principle is that PHI can only be disclosed when authorized, permitted, or compelled. There are many exceptions. There are institutional responsibilities and individual responsibilities associated with assuring compliance with the privacy rule, and there are consequences to noncompliances.

The main role of the nurse is to continue to respect the privacy of patient information, to work with patients and families to help them understand what their rights are and how they can be exercised, and to work within their institutions to create a culture in which privacy is valued, confidentiality is respected, and appropriate disclosure is managed and documented.

MULTIDISCIPLINARY INTEGRATION AND PARTNERSHIP: CASE STUDY

You are a school nurse. A ninth grader in a public school has tested positive for pertussis. You are advised by the advanced practice nurse at a pediatric health clinic of the positive result. What are the implications regarding disclosure of this information?

First, information about the child's history and symptoms must be shared with the lab that performs the test. Once the case of pertussis is confirmed, treatment of the child must be started, the family will usually be started on prophylaxis, and a variety of additional information must be obtained from and about the child.

As a general rule, you can obtain whatever relevant information is necessary to contain an outbreak of a highly infectious disease. The authority for this will be found in state public health statutes and rules, and the Privacy Rule permits public health activities to proceed without specific patient authorization for release of information.

A positive pertussis result in one child requires an immediate multidisciplinary response that includes information gathering, information sharing, treatment, and dissemination of information to the public. The result will be reported by the primary care provider to the school and the health department. The school nurse, care provider, school administrator, and health department will need to collaborate on the next steps. Legal counsel should also be included.

Both the school and the public health agency will have legal counsel available. To ensure that the privacy rights of the ill child are protected while information is collected to minimize the threat to the public, the attorney for both should be consulted. As a rule, the attorney for the public health agency (often a county attorney or specialist from a state attorney general's office) will be the most knowledgeable and can help craft the questions that will elicit the identities of people at risk and draft informational pieces that advise people of the occurrence of illness without disclosing the source.

The child must be contacted to determine whom she has had close contact with. This means the child must identify (1) immediate family and those sharing living space; (2) recent visitors, especially children under 1 year of age; (3) close friends and others (lunch partners, locker neighbors, others on the school bus); and (4) contact groups, such as sport teams. This may require that the school provide a team roster or list of students involved in an activity if exposure is possible. Obtaining all this information, and sharing it in order to identify those at risk of contracting pertussis, is legally permissible.

The second step is that the school or the public health department contacts the persons identified so that they can be aware of symptoms and can be tested if they have symptoms. In addition, the school may want to notify the entire student body about a pertussis outbreak. In these communications, the identity of the person who has the illness is *not* disclosed.

The third step is to educate the community about pertussis, signs and symptoms, and treatment and actions to be taken if symptoms develop. This requires the collaboration of nursing, school personnel, public health department staff and others to develop materials that can be distributed to children, families, practitioners, and the public.

The key principles in this case study are these: To avert threats to the public health, there is a broad authority to collect and share information. However, the identity of an individual with an infectious disease should be protected in the case-finding and education efforts. The relevant law is the state statute and regulations on public health, and the Privacy Rule provision for activities conducted by a public health authority. As always, the most effective way to achieve the goal of excellent care is through the use of a coordinated multidisciplinary team which, because of the privacy and disclosure issues, includes an attorney.

SUMMARY

Privacy and the protection of information is an element of excellent nursing care. Similarly, the disclosure of information to parents and children so that they can make informed decisions about treatment is equally important. The role of the nurse as patient advocate also requires an understanding of the patient's rights under the Privacy Rule so that the nurse can explain, clarify, and assist the patient's exercise of rights to information access and protection. To assure that the nursing care standard—*Protection of Rights for Information and Confidentiality*—is met, the following recommendations should be considered:

- Every nurse, regardless of practice setting, should be educated in the principles of privacy, confidentiality, and disclosure. In particular, nurses need to know institutional policies enacted pursuant to the Privacy Rule.
- The concepts of privacy, confidentiality, disclosure, and the management of information to promote excellence in nursing care should be emphasized in basic nursing education programs and in continuing education.
- Confidentiality and privacy must be evaluated periodically in practice settings, with particular attention paid to electronic records and electronic transmission of information.
- Expanded educational initiatives are necessary to increase nurses' knowledge of the laws and regulations in their jurisdiction that affect confidentiality and disclosure.
- Specific educational efforts should be undertaken to inform practitioners about the law affecting protection of rights for information and confidentiality of adolescents.
- When dealing with adolescents, nurses must know what care can be provided confidentially.
- When state law requires disclosure, and when disclosure is compelled, develop a disclosure plan for adolescents who do not have the capacity to consent. When possible, involve the adolescent in decisions about how the information is shared.
- Nurses should discuss with patients the general issues of privacy, confidentiality, their rights under the Privacy Rule, and the conditions under which information can be disclosed or confidentiality breached.
- Nurses should pay particular attention to assisting groups with diverse backgrounds to understand their rights under the Privacy Rule. This is not limited to individuals with language differences, but includes adolescents, parents under stress, and families from impoverished backgrounds.
- Nurses should review all institutional policies and procedures regarding confidentiality and disclosure every 2 to 3 years.

Finally, when faced with a decision about disclosing information about a child, to ensure that the privacy and information receive the highest possible level of protection, the nurse should ask two questions before making the disclosure. First, is this disclosure legally permissible? And second, but more important, Does this disclosure promote the best interests of this child, my patient? All nursing care standards are met by applying knowledge, analysis, skill, and compassion to the task of doing what is best for the children in our care.

REFERENCES

1. 29 U.S.C. § 1162 (2) (A) (V) (2000).
2. See, e.g., Iowa Code §152.
3. 45 C.F.R. 160, 164.
4. 42 C.F.R. 482.
5. See, e.g., 45 C.F.R., § 160.103; 42 C.F.R. § 482.13.
6. 45 C.F.R. § 164.530.
7. 42 U.S.C. § 1320d-5 (a) (2000); 42 C.F.R. § 160 (2003).
8. L. Brandeis, S. Warren, The Right to Privacy, *4 Harv. L. Rev.* 193 (1890).
9. 381 U.S. 479 (1965).
10. Id. at 482.
11. Id. at 484.
12. Roe v. Wade. 410 U.S. 113 (1972).
13. Cruzan v. Director, Missouri Dept. of Health, 497 U.S. 261 (1990).
14. 429 U.S. 589 (1977).
15. Pub. L. No. 91-572, 84 Stat. 1506 (codified at 42 U.S.C. 300-300 (a) (6) (1970)).
16. 45 C.F.R. §164.512 (b) (1).
17. See, e.g., Haley v. Ohio, 332 U.S. 596 (1948); In re Gault, 387 U.S. 1 (1967): Tinker v. Des Moines School District, 393 U.S. 503 (1969).
18. 406 U.S. 205 (1972)
19. Id. at 244–46.
20. See, e.g., Iowa Code Ann. § 232.
21. See, e.g., Minn. Stat.
22. Ark. Code. Ann. 20-9-602 (2000).
23. See note 12, *supra.*
24. Planned Parenthood v. Danforth, 428 U.S. 52 (1976); Bellotti v. Baird, 428 U.S. 132 (1976).
25. 45 C.F.R. § 164.502 (g) (3).
26. 45 C.F.R. § 164.502 (g) (3) (i), (ii), (iii).
27. Miller ex. rel. Miller, 47 Tex. Sup. Ct. J. 12 (September 30, 2003).
28. Id. at 12.
29. Pub. L. No. 98-457, codified at title 1 § 101; currently 42 U.S.C. Chapter 67, subchapter 1, § 5101.
30. 45 C.F.R. §§ 160 and 164.
31. 42 U.S.C. § 1320 d-2 (2000); 45 C.F.R. § 160.101–160.312, § 164.102–164.534 (2003).

32. 42 U.S.C. § 1320 d-7 (2000).
33. 45 C.F.R. § 160.202.
34. 45 C.F.R. § 164.502 (b).
35. 45 C.F.R. § 160.102.
36. 42 U.S.C. § 1395x (u).
37. 42 U.S.C. § 1395x (S) (2) (K) and (L).
38. 45 C.F.R. § 164.501.
39. Id.
40. 45 C.F.R. § 164.520.
41. GAO-04-965: Health Information First-Year Experiences Under the Federal Privacy Rule (September 2004), at 19.
42. 45 C.F.R. § 164.522 (a) (1).
43. 45 C.F.R. § 164.522 (a) (2).
44. Id. At (ii) (A).
45. 45 C.F.R. § 164.524.
46. 45 C.F.R. § 164.526.
47. Id.
48. 45 C.F.R. § 164.528.
49. GAO report, *supra,* note 41, at 24.
50. 45 C.F.R. § 510.
51. 45 C.F.R. § 512 (a).
52. 45 C.F.R. § 512 (b).
53. 45 C.F.R. § 512 (c).
54. 45 C.F.R. § 512 (d).
55. 45 C.F.R. § 512 (e).
56. 45 C.F.R. § 512 (f).
57. 45 C.F.R. § 512 (g).
58. 45 C.F.R. § 512 (h).
59. 45 C.F.R. § 512 (j).
60. 45 C.F.R. § 512 (k).
61. 45 C.F.R. § 512 (i).
62. 45 C.F.R. § 164.501.
63. 45 C.F.R. § 46.102 (d).

CHAPTER ELEVEN

Health Promotion, Maintenance, and Disease Prevention

Judith B. Igoe

INTRODUCTION, DEFINITIONS, AND THEIR MEASUREMENT

Health promotion, health maintenance, and disease prevention are integral to the practice of pediatric nursing and community-oriented maternal and child health services. Consequently, disease prevention, health maintenance, and promotion are an important component of the Health Care Quality and Outcome (HCQO) Guidelines for Nursing of Children and Families (Guideline #9), which is the topic of this chapter. In addition three other HCQO guidelines are closely related to Guideline #9 and also likely to influence efforts to enhance the health and well-being of children, youth, and their families (Betz, Cowell, Lobo, & Craft-Rosenberg, 2004; Craft-Rosenberg, Krajicek, & Shin, 2002).

> HCQO Guideline #2: The families of children and youth are partners in decisions, planning, and delivery of care.
>
> HCQO Guideline #9: Children, youth, and families receive care that promotes and maintains health and prevents disease.
>
> HCQO Guideline #16: Children's, youth's, and families' health and risky behaviors and problems are identified and addressed.
>
> HCQO Guideline #17: Children, youth, and families receive care that supports development.

Historical Overview

Beginning in the late nineteenth century, social and public health endeavors were instituted to promote the welfare of America's children. These efforts included the movement to abolish child labor, the establishment of milk stations, laws for compulsory school attendance and the resultant concern over the spread of communicable disease in schools, and the opening of settlement houses. Lillian Wald, a pioneer in public health nursing and opponent of child labor, first advocated for the creation of a federal Children's Bureau, believing it was in the best interest of the country to highlight the health, social, educational needs of children. A bill to create such a bureau was first introduced to Congress in 1906 with the support of President Theodore Roosevelt (Hutchins, 1994).

After much opposition from states that did not want the federal government usurping their responsibilities and from individuals who feared erosion of their privacy, the importance of maintaining the health of children was officially recognized in the United States on April 9, 1912. President William Howard Taft signed into law the congressional act that created the Children's Bureau. The Children's Bureau was granted broad powers to enlist specialists to investigate all the interrelated aspects of child health, dependency, delinquency, and child labor, and to help state and local groups organize and take action for child welfare (Hutchins, 1994).

The Children's Bureau's studies on mortality, morbidity, and the needs of particular groups of children strengthened and shaped the direction of maternal and child health services in this country; eventually federal grants to address these needs were established in each state and were matched with state funds. Subsequently, President Herbert Hoover, in 1930, convened the White House Conference on Child Health and Protection, which created the Children's Charter. The charter consisted of 19 statements addressing the health, education, welfare, and protection needs of children that would ensure optimal growth and development.

In 1934 Katherine Lenroot, a special agent to the Children's Bureau, suggested a new plan for poor mothers and children. The plan contained three proposals: aid to dependent children, welfare services for children with special needs, and maternal and child health services. The proposals for child welfare services and maternal and child health programs combined with services to children with disabilities (known in those days as "crippled children") were enacted as Title V of the Social Security Act (SSA) by President Franklin D. Roosevelt on August 14, 1935. Funding for this legislation came in the form of federal grants-in-aid to states. According to Hutchins (1994), "the inclusion of Title V in the SSA rather than in health legislation recognizes a critical distinction, that it is the dependence of mothers and children rather than diseases or conditions that merits societal attention" (p. 696). In the years to come, the many provisions of the SSA, including old age pensions and unemployment compensation, further protected children indirectly by shifting economic burdens away from their parents.

Between 1943 and 1949, the Emergency Maternity and Infant Care (EMIC) program, provided health supervision and medical care for infants of military men in the four lowest pay grades. EMIC was responsible for the care of 1,500,000 mothers and infants, and became the largest single public health/prevention program in the United States (Brodie, 1982).

In 1968, the programs for Maternal and Child Health and Crippled Children were transferred together, as the Maternal and Child Health Service (MCH), to the Health Services and Mental Health Administration of the U.S. Public Health Service. States were required to submit plans for their use of federal funds, which went toward wellness-oriented activities such as school health services, immunizations, population screening, and establishing standards for day care and hospital care for mothers and children (Hutchins, 1994).

The 1970s and 1980s brought more streamlining and simplification to state processes, and federal oversight was reduced. MCH collaborated with other federal agencies to promote programs dealing with prevention of lower-birth weights, improved nutrition, and enhanced mental health services, dental consultation, HIV/AIDS prevention, and breastfeeding (Olds et al., 2004; Rosenbaum, Hughes, & Johnson, 1988; Thompson, 1986).

In 1989, amendments to Title V expanded the goal of improving the health of poor mothers and children to all mothers and children. From then until the present, the pivotal role of the family and the importance of family participation have been emphasized. Most important, states are now expected to provide and promote family-centered, community-based, coordinated care for children, especially those boys and girls with special health care needs (Brodie, 1982). At present the Maternal and Child Health Bureau (MCHB) is located within the U.S. Department of Health and Human Services, Health Resources and Services Administration (HRSA).

Throughout the history of pediatrics, there has also been a focus on child safety, normal growth and development, proper nutrition, and disease prevention. Anticipatory guidance about child care practices has frequently been the strategy that pediatric nurses and physicians have utilized to reach parents and other caretakers (Palfrey, 1997). By the nineteenth century, for example, hospitals devoted entirely to the care of children were established and here parents were encouraged initially to help care for their children. At the same time, they learned improved parenting practices related to sleep, rest, feeding, and injury prevention in order to reduce the spread of disease and increase the likelihood of safer environments at home.

During the late part of the century however, with the discovery of the germ theory, dramatic changes occurred. Concern about contagion resulted in the closing of hospital wards to visitors, including parents. Hospitals began to require personnel to wear uniforms, toys were restricted, and social contact among the children became limited in order to avoid the spread of disease; these new policies lasted well into the twentieth century. According to Thompson (1986), although hospital care focused on curing physical disease and preventing its spread to others, the emotional health of hospitalized children and their families received little attention.

Throughout the twentieth and twenty-first centuries, pediatric nurses have supported and contributed to the now common belief in the importance of well-child care, adequate nutrition, immunization, and prompt attention to illness and injury. Indeed pediatric and public health nurses today are actively involved in the delivery and follow-up of much of the disease prevention, health maintenance, and health promotion care provided to children and youths in hospitals and communities.

The American Academy of Pediatrics, the Society for Pediatric Nurses, and the American Public Health Association have actively participated in many efforts to promote the health and well-being of infants, children, and youths over the years. These three initiatives in particular have contributed to primary care improvements in private practice as well as through public health programs:

1. the historic partnership with the Centers for Disease Control (CDC), other federal and state health agencies, private organizations, and professional health associations to (a) establish immunization schedules for infants, children, and youths; (b) facilitate the development and distribution of vaccines; and (c) foster the advocacy efforts undertaken to gain the public's support and willingness to adhere to the recommended schedules for immunizations;

2. the introduction of periodicity schedules for well-child exams, which advanced significantly in the 1990s when the National Clinical Prevention Task Force recommended that these services had to be evidence-based;

3. the publication of *Bright Futures: Guidelines for Health Supervision of Infants, Children and Adolescents* by the American Academy of Pediatrics (Green & Palfrey, 2002).

These interdisciplinary guidelines (with several pediatric nursing leaders contributing to all the editions) emphasize a multidiscipline and community-oriented approach to disease prevention and health maintenance and promotion for children and youth of all ages (Green & Palfrey, 2002).

Definitions

A nationwide disease prevention and health promotion initiative called Healthy People has guided the nation's health promotion and disease prevention agenda since 1976. A series of state-of-the-art papers on the major strategies, issues, and prospects of disease prevention and health promotion programs provided the original justification for Healthy People. These papers appeared first in *Healthy People: The Surgeon General's Report on Health Promotion and Disease Prevention /Background Papers* (U.S. Department of Health, Education and Welfare [HEW], 1979).

The Healthy People agenda at that time (and today) has been a combination of public and private efforts, national in scope but not federal. Initially, the Healthy People plan was divided into five life stages, with two major health problems and risks delineated for each life stage. Goals to be achieved were presented for each life stage: infancy, children (ages 1–14), adolescents and young adults (ages 15–24), adults (ages 25–64), and older adults (ages 65 plus).

For infants, the goal in 1978 was to reduce death by 25% (less than 9 per 1,000 births). Special emphasis was given to low-birth-weight infants and infants with birth defects. For children, the goal was 20% fewer deaths (less than 34 per 100,000); the targeted two problems were growth and development, and accidents and injuries. For adolescents, again the goal was 20% fewer deaths (less than 93 per 100,000) with the emphasis on fatal motor vehicle accidents and alcohol and drug misuse (USDHHS Public Health Service [PHS], 1991, p. 4).

From the outset of the Healthy People program, the terms *disease prevention, health promotion,* and *health protection* appear frequently to describe (both conceptually and operationally) the three types of services and measures included in this national initiative. Today disease prevention, health promotion, and health protection are widely accepted and commonly recognized types of health services and activities by the National Center for Health Statistics at the CDC; the National Institutes of Health Center for Scientific Review Nursing Science: Children and Families Study Section; and the Health Promotion and Evaluation section of the National Institute of Nursing Research. In addition, the use of these same definitions are reflected in reports and publications in academic and health policy journals from nursing, medicine, and a variety of other disciplines; their professional organizations; national, federal, and state funding agencies, and the public. Although it is beyond the scope of this chapter and not included in these Health Care Quality and Outcome Guidelines, the definition of health protection is included here because it is closely aligned with overall disease prevention and health promotion efforts for children and their families and is an increasingly important category within the Healthy People 2010 program.

1. Disease prevention services are risk reduction activities that have as their goal the protection of people of all ages from becoming ill because of actual or potential health threats (Stanhope & Lancaster, 2004). Usually these efforts are targeted at the specific population (Betz, Hunsberger, & Wright, 1994). According to the Surgeon General's 1979 *Healthy People* report, these services also are "usually delivered to individuals by health care providers in various clinical settings" (Iverson & Kolbe, 1983, p. 296). The five services targeted for attention were family planning, pregnancy and infant care, immunizations, sexually transmissible disease, and high blood pressure control (HEW, 1978).

2. Health promotion efforts are defined as "activities individuals and communities can undertake to promote healthy lifestyles (Iverson & Kolbe, 1983, p. 296). Health promotion activities are concerned not only with strengthening the skills and capabilities of individuals, but are also directed at actions intended to change social norms, environmental conditions, and economic conditions in order to improve population and individual health, using a broad range of political, legislative, fiscal, and administrative means (Stachtchenko & Jenicek, 1990). Furthermore, according to Pender (1994), "basic to any health promotion program is the philosophy that children can be powerful, life-long learners and that they can be empowered to care for themselves" (p. 385). Finally, Pender (1994) differentiates health promotion from disease prevention with this explanation: "To prevent is to keep something from occurring, whereas 'to promote' is to help or encourage something to be or to develop" (p. 385). The three health promotion strategies targeted for attention in *Healthy People 2000* were smoking cessation, enhancement of exercise and fitness, and management of stress (Iverson & Kolbe, 1983, p. 296).

3. Health protection measures are steps taken for which control is substantially dependent upon manipulation of the environment (Iverson & Kolbe, 1983, p. 296). Industry, government, and other agencies are in a position to take these measures. The five areas targeted for attention were toxic agent control, occupational safety and health, accident/injury control, fluoridation of community water supplies, and infectious agent control (HEW, 1978).

Health maintenance is a term that appears frequently in the nursing literature. Consequently, it is a component of HCQO Guideline #9 and deserving of a definition as well. Health maintenance has been defined by Laffrey (1990) as "activities that are directed toward keeping a current state of health and is based on the individual's reason for performing a given behavior, such as to maintain or to promote an enhanced state of health" (p. 444). Although this definition reflects the meaning of a number of the references to this term in nursing literature, the term *health maintenance* has not been formally identified and defined in the same sense as the terms *disease prevention, health promotion,* and *health protection* have been for the Healthy People initiative. Therefore, there is likely to be more variation in the interpretation of the term *health maintenance.*

Over the last three decades, the current Healthy People 2010 program has made progress in achieving goals set back in 1990 and 2000, including reducing infant mortality rates, with the latest mortality figures being up for the first time in decades. With time Healthy People initiative has evolved and at present has two overriding goals for all stages of life: to increase the quality and years of healthy life, and to eliminate health disparities. To reach these goals, Healthy People 2010 is supported by specific objectives and 28 focus areas. Additional information about the Healthy People program can be accessed through the Web site www.healthypeople.gov. Although there is less emphasis now on distinguishing disease prevention, health promotion, and health protection services from one another than was true in previous years, all three are still considered essential to include when addressing the Healthy People goals and focus areas.

Improvement of health literacy or the Health Literacy Component (HLC) is a new Healthy People focus area with numerous opportunities for nurses working with children and their families. HLC addresses the public's need for three types of health information and services related to their clinical health problems, disease prevention measures, and navigation of the health care system. Health literacy has been the subject of an Institute of Medicine report, *Health Literacy: A Prescription to End Confusion* (Nielsen-Bohlman, 2004).

Finally, Steps to a HealthierUS is a prevention-oriented by-product of Healthy People, which is aimed at reducing the risks created by obesity, diabetes, asthma, cancer, heart disease, and stroke. Given the present trend in pediatrics to return to "early in life" interventions, the Steps to HealthierUS campaign encourages the development of healthy lifestyles during infancy and early childhood (USDHHS, 2004).

Multiple Measures of the Health Status of Children

Healthy People 2010 measures the health of the nation (all age segments) according to these ten leading health indicators:

physical activity
overweight and obesity
tobacco use
substance abuse
responsible sexual behavior
mental health
injury and violence
environmental quality
immunization
access to health care

Generally, the majority of American children and youth today are free of acute diseases. The numbers with chronic disease is increasing, including asthma and the concern for the increased number with type 1 and type 2 diabetes. However, as of 2000, there were 86 million children under age 21 in the United States representing 31.2% of the total population. Of these, 11 million (15.6%) live below the poverty level; and with poverty come certain health risks, as reflected in Table 11.1. Thus, it is clear that infants, toddlers, children, and youths who are poor are the segment of the population most likely to miss out on the benefits of disease prevention, health maintenance, and health promotion services (Smith, Orleans, & Jenkins, 2004).

Childhood poverty exceeds adult poverty by 71%. Poor children who live in families headed by a single mother are 56%, compared to

TABLE 11.1 Relative Frequency of Health Problems in Low-Income Children Compared with Other Children

Health Problem	Relative Frequency in Low-Income Children
Delayed immunization	Triple
Asthma	Higher
Child deaths due to accidents	Double-triple
Child deaths due to disease	Triple-quadruple
Percent with conditions limiting school activity	Double-triple
Lost school days	40% more
Severely impaired vision	Double-triple

Note: From "Population and Selective (High-Risk) Approaches to Prevention in Well-Child Care," by B. Starfield & P. M. Vivier. In M. R. Solloway & P. P. Budetti (Eds.), *Child health supervision: Analytical Studies in the Financing, Delivery and Cost-Effectiveness of Preventive and Health Promotion Services for Infants, Children, and Adolescents* (pp. 205–226), 1995. Washington, DC: George Washington University Center for Health Policy Research. Used with permission.

38% who live with both parents (MCHB, 2002, p. 12). About 4.8% of youth drop out of high school. More than 25% of Hispanic youths drop out of high school, and those in low-income households are most likely to drop out (MCHB, 2002, p. 13). The breastfeeding rate in the United States is 68.4%, the highest since recording began (MCHB, 2002, p. 18). In the United States, 7.6% of all babies are born with low birth weights, the same rate as 30 years ago, although some of this is attributable to the increase in multiple births. Very low birth weights (under 3.3 pounds) account for 1.4% of all live births (MCHB, 2002, pp. 20–21). The United States is 28th in the world for rates of infant mortality and often this statistic has been related to the number of women who are poor and have not received prenatal care for various reasons, including poverty (MCHB, 2002, p. 22). Fortunately, vaccine-preventable disease rates are all down, but pertussis, hepatitis A, and H. influenza remain common. However, achieving high rates of immunization before age 2 in all states continues to be a challenge; and often the major barrier involves parents' mistaken belief that immunizing agents can produce developmental problems later in childhood, which is contrary to numerous research findings (Hviid, Wohlfahrt, Stellfeld, & Melbye, 2005).

In 2000, disease of the respiratory system, injuries, and digestive problems accounted for the majority of hospitalizations. There were 12,282 deaths among children, mostly from injuries such as motor vehicle accidents, drowning, and homicide, representing a slight decline from previous years (MCHB, 2002, p. 32) Unfortunately, 879,000 children are reported victims of abuse and neglect, a rate of 12.2 per 1,000, among boys and girls from all income brackets, races, and cultures (MCHB, 2002, pp. 27–28). Thus, serious gaps in disease prevention and health promotion services remain to be filled especially among the poor and vulnerable families.

Throughout the history of pediatric nursing and pediatrics, the focus has been on anticipatory guidance, lifestyle habits, and initiation of services based on children's developmental progress. Parents as well as pediatric health care practitioners have been shown to place a high value on health supervision and well-child care. In 2001, more than 30% of visits to physicians by children up to age 15 were for well-child care, representing an increase of 10% since 1994. Both regulators and health plans use the provision rate of preventive services as a measure of quality (Moyer & Butler, 2004).

A study was conducted to determine parents' satisfaction with basic preventive services, including developmental assessment, injury prevention counseling, screening for parental smoking, and parental guidance on various topics. Results showed that most children received excellent or good care, according to their parents, but almost one third indicated fair or poor care. Higher satisfaction was reported for longer well-child visits, more counseling on family and community risk factors, and lower rates of delayed or missed care (Zuckerman, Stevens, Inkelas, & Halfon, 2004).

There is a more evident satisfaction gap among lower-income parents. A 2002 survey of families with young children insured by Medicaid found that only about 20% of parents thought their children received the full range of recommended preventive and developmental services. Two out of five parents expressed at least one concern about their child's social, behavioral, or cognitive development, but were not routinely asked by their pediatric practitioner about these concerns. The survey looked at such topics as nutrition, sleep, nurturing, injury prevention, communication, discipline, and language development. It also examined whether counseling was available to parents of developmentally at-risk children, or whose home life may include mental health problems, substance abuse, violence, or other problems. The study recommends more efforts to combine evidence-based pediatric care guidelines with practice (Bethel et al., 2002).

There have been additional attempts in the past two decades to measure the health and development of infants, children, and youths using different yardsticks. Three of these approaches are described here because of their usefulness in measuring continuous quality improvement efforts in well-child care: (1) The first of these measurement approaches (and perhaps the most long-standing) is known as the assets/strengths approach. (2) The second is known as the population and selected (high risk) approach. These approaches rely on traditional epidemiological methods, wherein the effort and resources are either concentrated on the pediatric population as a whole or identification of, and intervention with, the most vulnerable or at-risk segment of this population. (3) The community indicators movement measures the health of the population in terms of the social and economic conditions of the community.

The Assets/Strength Approach

The Assets for Health and Development (AHDP) initiative originated at the World Health Organization during the 1980s. Its working definition was "any factor (or resource) which enhances the ability of individuals, communities and populations to maintain and sustain health and well being" by operating at individual, family, and community levels to protect against life stress. When implemented, some of these asset projects have come to be known as Healthy Cities demonstrations throughout Europe. Flynn brought this concept to the United States with the support of the W. K. Kellogg Foundation and established models throughout Indiana (Flynn, 1996).

In attempts to firm the evidence base around what keeps people healthy, various organizations including the Search Institute (www.search-institute.org/assets) have conducted community-based programs throughout the country, advocating family and individual assets (values) related to health and development. Another example comes from McKnight and Kretzmann (1996), codirectors of the Asset-Based Community Development Institute at Northwestern University in Illinois, which has set out primary and secondary building blocks that couple individual strengths of residents with cultural practices, religious affiliations, and linkages with private and nonprofit organizations. Among their investigations, community connectedness, resilience among young people, and access to health systems are viewed as special assets that contribute to the health of individuals, families, and communities. Most recently, Vermont has invested considerable energy and resources into the assets approach for measuring health. Table 11.2 provides further resources and information ("Vermont's Indicator Evolution," 2004). The Steps to Healthier US initiative is a federal level program to further strengthen communities (see http://www.healthierus.gov/steps).

Population and Selected (High Risk) Approaches

According to Starfield and Vivier (1995), there are two approaches to the delivery of disease prevention and health promotion services to infants, children, and youths. One strategy is a population approach in which every child is targeted to receive a recommended unit of care, regardless of the probability of the child's acquiring the problem that is the focus of the preventive service. The other strategy is the selective or high-risk approach wherein a secondary prevention approach prevails and only those at risk for developing the health condition are targeted for attention. Both the population and the high-risk approaches have potential advantages and disadvantages as service delivery models and measurement approaches for determining well being. Although discussion of these issues is beyond the scope of this chapter, Starfield and Vivier, as described in Rose (1992), have outlined and discussed this topic in depth. Feetham (1999) also provides additional analysis of characteristics of successful community programs.

The Community Indicators Movement

Community indicators are social and health measures of child and family well-being that are tied to local community areas (Coulton, 1995). For example, the rate of children entering school ready to learn has been used to help gauge the progress of early childhood education (Gibbs & Brown,

TABLE 11.2 National Studies, Surveys and Reports Using Positive Indicators

	National Studies, Surveys, and Reports	Sample Positive Indicator Areas
National Longitudinal Studies Studies following single cohort over time	**National Survey of Families & Households** 1987 www.ssc.wisc.edu/nsfh/home.htm	Family relationships, rules and interactions, out-of-school and religious activities, academic expectations
	National Longitudinal Survey of Adolescent Health 1995 www.cpc.unc.edu/addhealth	Family and peer relationships, school environments, out-of-school and religious activities
	National Longitudinal Survey of Youth 1997 www.bls.gov/nls/nlsy97.htm	Employment information, parent relationships and expectations, out-of-school activities
	National Education Longitudinal Surveys (88&02) www.nces.ed.gov;surveys/nels88; www.nces.ed.gov/surveys/els2002	School effectiveness, structural and climate issues, expectations and achievement, parent involvement, school-to-work transition
	4-H study of Positive Youth Development 2002 www.ase.tufts.edu/4hstudy_pyd	Competence, confidence, character, connection, caring and contribution

National Trend Data Surveys Ongoing surveys with representative data	**Monitoring the Future** (1975–) www.monitoringthefuture.org	Citizenship, activism, academics, jobs, future goals, media use, out-of-school activities, parental-involvement, religious involvement
	US Census Bureau, Survey of Income and Program Participation (1994–) www.sipp.census.gov/sipp	
	National Household Education Surveys (1996–) http://nces.ed.gov/nhes	Family rules and interactions, out-of-school activities, academic expectations and achievement
	National Survey of Children's Health (2003–) www.cdc.gov/nchs/about/major/slaits/nsch.htm	Civic involvement, family involvement Emotional health, family rules and interactions, out-of-school activities, media use, perceptions of neighborhood
National Reports	**Trends in the Well-Being of America's Children and Youth** (2003) www.aspe.hhs.gov/hsp/03trends/	Life goals, religious involvement, voting behaviors, parental involvement, academicproficiency
	A Child's Day: 2000 www.census.gov/prod/2003pubs/p70-89.pdf	Family interactions, support and expectations, out-of-school activities

Note: From "Vermont's Indicator Evolution," 2004 (November), *Youth Today,* p. 24. Used with permission.

2000). Another example of the use of community health indicators cited by Simmes, Lim, and Dennis (2003) involved tracking the prevalence rates of asthma by measuring changes in the rate of children hospitalized with asthma. In school health, some evaluators are investigating the return-to-class rates of students seen in school nurse offices and by nurse practitioners in school-based student health centers as a measure or indicator of the influence of nursing services may have on lowering student dismissal rates (Igoe, 2002). Much of Milio's (1996) research reflects a community-indicators approach and has aided in the growing awareness of the importance of this approach in studying and enhancing children's health.

At the beginning of the twentieth century, the formation of the Children's Bureau, now the Maternal and Child Health Bureau, used indicators as a primary strategy to document the relationship of family earnings, maternal employment, and access to primary care on the health and survival of children (Skocpol, 1991).

According to Brown and Corbett (1998), indicators are commonly used for the following five purposes: (a) to describe circumstances in the community with the potential to influence health and social well being, (b) to monitor health and social trends evolving in communities over time, (c) to assist organizations in goal setting for their programs, (d) to operationalize outcome-based accountability, and (e) to evaluate programs for their effectiveness in fostering the development of a healthier America.

With the growing importance and use of outcome measures, the emphasis is on performance and results. In the minds of proponents, the presence of indicators provides the public with understandable information needed to hold community organizations and the government responsible for programs and activities developed and implemented with either tax-supported resources or donations or both.

The potential importance of community indicators in promoting social change cannot be overstated. Only with information provided by indicators can a community measure its baseline data, follow its progress toward new social norms, and access what it needs to develop healthier lifestyles.

INFLUENCE OF DISEASE PREVENTION AND HEALTH PROMOTION SERVICES FOR INFANTS AND CHILDREN

Throughout the history of pediatric nursing, the focus has been on anticipatory guidance, lifestyle habits, and initiating services depending on the developmental progress of children. Parents as well as pediatric health care practitioners have been known to place a high value on health supervision and well-child care. Consequently, preventive services are being recommended with increasing frequency at expert consensus conferences and by professional organizations and parent groups (Hardy et al., 1997). In addition, as some screening interventions become more economical and efficient with technological advances, it is possible a growing variety of screening procedures will be included in routine health examinations in the future (Moyer & Butler, 2004).

As popular and valued as preventive interventions are and have been historically, recent studies on their effectiveness have found limited direct evidence to support them. Rigorous evaluation of these interventions is hampered due to the difficulty of accurate cost accounting and the lengthy time from incidence to outcome. There is also a high risk of bias due to noncompliance and individual differences in motivation and participation. In addition, the potential adverse effects of well-child health supervision have not been evaluated (Moyer & Butler, 2004).

A recent study tabulated the well-child recommendation of seven organizations in three categories: behavioral counseling, screening, and prophylaxis. Immunization was not considered. More than 40 preventive interventions were recommended by some of the organizations and these were subject to systematic review and clinical trials for effectiveness. Results showed that although brief counseling can be shown to modestly decrease some tobacco smoking behaviors, others—such as parental smoking and alcohol consumption—have been found to actually increase slightly after counseling. There may also be adverse effects on practitioner-patient relations when sensitive subjects are brought up in counseling. The study found that intensive repeated counseling was most likely to be effective (Moyer & Butler, 2004).

The traditional criteria for screening programs are (a) conditions should be an important health problem; (b) tests should be accurate, simple, and acceptable; and (c) conditions should be improved with early treatment. Very few screening interventions have actually been supported by clinical trials. Although some screening interventions may be mandated by payers or used to assess provider quality, they do not address potential harmful effects or require proof of effectiveness (Moyer & Butler, 2004).

Future priorities that have been suggested by the Moyer and Butler (2004) study include establishing how best to implement interventions that are already known to be effective, setting research priorities in an explicit and scientifically supportable manner, and investigating how systems of care may influence the effects of individual interventions. In its Translating Research Into Practice initiative, the Agency for Healthcare Research and Quality (AHRQ) has begun research on how to implement interventions already known to be effective. Moyer and Butler (2004) suggest that these efforts should focus on children's preventive services, and address how individual preventive services may function when bundled with other interventions. They also recommend studying the systems of care and settings that may be best for patients, and using only evidence-based preventive interventions that address potential consequences. Regulations that mandate the use of specific but unproven interventions should be reassessed.

Schor (2004) calls for a "major revision of well-child care" (p. 210). He argues for the need to return to a holistic approach to promoting children's health, encompassing both the promotion of children's health and development as well as the treatment of childhood diseases. Well-child care today applies to fewer children. Many of the morbidities such as acute illness and premature birth that were common in the early part of the century have been substantially reduced, but there is now an increasing prevalence of new morbidities. These include obesity, attention deficit/hyperactivity disorder, behavior disorders, depression, and adolescent risk behaviors.

Schor (2004) points out that although well-child care is a core service of pediatrics and covers a wide variety of health promotion and disease prevention services, it has been all but ignored by research, professional education, and payers. Quality, effectiveness, and outcome measures are lacking, all of which provide a major rationale for insurance reimbursement. According to Schor, it may be that the heavy emphasis on disease and critical care that has been predominant in many teaching programs for nursing and medical students and residents has actually contributed to this lack of an evidence-based rationale for preventive and developmental services.

The recommendations of the U.S. Clinical Prevention Task Force (Coffield et al., 2001) that preventive services must be evidence-based has been a step in the right direction for the Clinical Prevention Guidelines for ages 0–18 (U.S. Preventive Services Task Force, 1996). These guidelines offer pediatric nurses a basic structure from which to develop their practice plans, realizing of course the need to draw on the growing body of child and family health research findings available from the National Institute of Nursing Research.

Other leaders in the field of health promotion have confirmed similar difficulties in demonstrating the permanence of healthy lifestyle habits over time. Renslow's critique of theoretical models of health behavior change, especially Bandura's social cognitive theory, is especially informative (Resnicow, 1997). Green's essay, "Ecological Foundations of Health Promotion" (Green, Richard, & Potvin, 1996), reflects on Brofenbenner's constructs and is long familiar to health professionals working with infants, children, youths, and their families. It offers an equally helpful understanding of the opportunities and challenges researchers now face in trying to document the relationships between new or modified lifestyles and specific disease prevention and health promotion interventions.

One less theoretical but practical framework for planning, implementing, and evaluating health promotion and disease prevention programs is the Spectrum of Prevention (Table 11.3) (Cohen & Swift, 1999).

Inherent in this framework is the assumption that healthy behaviors will evolve provided there are social norms to support them; and many other individual and community conditions prevail to produce this kind of behavior change. According to this perspective, individual health lessons, appealing as they may be, do not independently produce results. Two successful examples of the Spectrum of Prevention framework in action would be Mothers Against Drunk Driving (MADD) and Project Northland (Perry et al., 1996).

INFLUENCE OF DISEASE PREVENTION AND HEALTH MAINTENANCE AND PROMOTION ON THE FAMILY

Healthy Steps (HS) represents an advanced evidence-based primary care model of well-child care for infants and toddlers and their family. A profile of the program is presented here as an example of the effect this

TABLE 11.3 Spectrum of Prevention

Level of Spectrum	Definition of Level
1. Strengthening Individual Knowledge and Skills	Enhancing an individual's capability of preventing injury or illness and promoting safety
2. Promoting Community Education	Reaching groups of people with information and resources to promote health and safety
3. Educating Providers	Informing providers who will transmit skills and knowledge to others
4. Fostering Coalitions and Networks	Bringing together groups and individuals for broader goals and greater impact
5. Changing Organizational Practices	Adopting regulations and shaping norms to improve health and safety
6. Influencing Policy Legislation and policies to influence outcomes	Developing strategies to change laws

Note: From "The Spectrum of Prevention: Developing a Comprehensive Approach to Injury Prevention by L. Cohen and S. Swift, 1999, *Injury Prevention, 5,* 203–207.

interdisciplinary program has had on families of various income and education levels and cultural backgrounds throughout the United States. The Healthy Steps (HS) program has numerous funders nationally and locally. The Commonwealth Fund has been the major source of support for this program from its inception.

Based on the standards and principles of *Bright Futures* (Green & Palfrey, 2002) and the American Academy of Pediatrics Health Supervision Guidelines and adapted by Crowly and Magee (2003) for advanced practice nurses in pediatric nursing, HS services include (a) evidence-based health promotion and prevention-oriented well-child visits up to 30–45 minutes in length, (b) instructional home visits, (c) a telephone information line to exchange ideas, reinforce key points about growth and development, and answer questions, (d) attractive and informative instructional videotapes and guidelines for parents and, (e) more seamless linkages to community resources and parent support groups.

Healthy Steps is based on a set of assumptions that are vastly different from the beliefs that framed and supported the need for these disease prevention, health maintenance, and health promotion services in the nineteenth century (Brodie, 1986). Consider these four assumptions upon which the Healthy Steps program has been developed:

1. Extended family and neighborhood support for young parents around child rearing has declined over the past decades. A number of recent surveys support this assumption. Commonwealth Fund reported that 4 out of 5 parents expressed a need for assistance with sleep issues, toilet training, discipline, coping with parenthood, and concern with the child getting on their nerves (Young et al., 1998). Beyond basic child rearing, the findings from a survey conducted by Zero to Three: National Center for Infants, Toddlers, and Families (1997) revealed parents had a limited understanding of developmental stages of young children.

2. To a significant degree, the structure of the adult brain is influenced by early experiences. Consequently, early childhood activities that influence neurodevelopment and school readiness activities such as reading and talking to children at young ages are of significant importance to development and school readiness.

3. Teachable moments are important to parents and enhance family life. Visits for pediatric well-baby care are significantly important teachable moments.

4. Maternal health influences children's health and development. Consequently, postpartum depression places infants as well as mothers at risk (Minkovitz et al., 2005).

At present, the emphasis countrywide is on community-based family-focused programs to support infants and children and their development, academic achievement, and growth into adulthood and eventual employment. The California Comprehensive Vision (see Figure 11.1) provides an excellent example of a framework for Healthy Steps and other related community developments. As this model illustrates, in order to translate vision into results there must be integrated health, education, and social systems within which high-energy creative interagency teams work closely together with families.

On a different level, the Logic Model Framework (Figure 11.2) (W. K. Kellogg, 2004) is a more detailed planning and evaluation framework favored by many health planners to operationalize and evaluate the visions shown in Figure 11.1).

This model has been widely disseminated, implemented, and evaluated in the past decade with support from the Kellogg Foundation (W. K. Kellogg Foundation, 2004). The framework not only encourages planners and evaluators to move beyond outputs to outcomes; it also sets the expectation that someone will identify and test for measured improvements when new interventions are implemented. Finally, logic models have opened the doors and encouraged families to join the professionals in a collaborative effort to design, develop, and evaluate community projects. This type of "buy-in" from the public has a positive effect on the sustainability of programs that work.

COMPONENTS OF NURSING
EXCELLENCE IN PRACTICE

In providing disease prevention, health maintenance, and promotion services, what can nursing science contribute to health promotion for infants, children, youths, and their families? As the largest segment of health service providers, nurses have more opportunities to prevent children's illnesses and promote their well-being than any other group of health professionals. By virtue of their clinical skills and health education, contact with the pediatric population, credibility, visibility, and diversity, nurses are a critical component of the interdisciplinary health team for infants, children, and youths and their families.

The field of nursing adds a special breadth and depth to health promotion by bringing an understanding of developmental changes and transitions and their effects on health and lifestyle, and the integration of this knowledge into appropriate health interventions (Pender, Murdaugh, & Parsons, 2006).

Daily disease prevention and health promotion guidelines, strategies, programs, and services are used by pediatric and maternal- and child-health nurses worldwide to improve the health and well-being of children and families (Frey & Naar-King, 2001; Glascoe & Sandler, 1995).

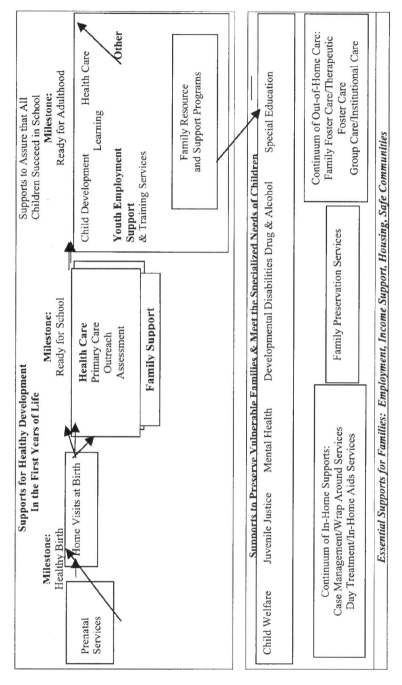

FIGURE 11.1 California Comprehensive Vision. A strategy for change: Communities supporting families and children.

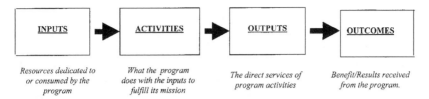

FIGURE 11.2 Logic model.

From *Logic Model Development Guide*, by W. K. Kellogg Foundation, 2004, Battle Creek, MI: W. K. Kellogg Foundation. Used with permission.

Officially described as Standards of Nursing Practice, Guideline #9 is highly valued by pediatric and child health specialty professional organizations and is reflected throughout the position statements and policies of our professional organizations (Betz et al., 2004).

The overall goals for nurses providing disease prevention, health maintenance, and health promotion services and programs for infants, children, and youths and their families have been described as follows: The nurse (a) recognizes developmental immaturity and distinguishes these normal characteristics from disease processes, (b) identifies threats to well-being related to physical, intellectual, and emotional-social developmental processes, (c) directs nursing strategies to support the unique response of this child to issues of health and illness, and (d) supports parental advocacy and initiates professional advocacy for the child within the health care system and within the community (Betz et al., 1994).

In the early 1990s, National Institute of Nursing Research (NINR) and National Institutes for Health (NIH) convened a number of Priority Expert Panels to examine the state of the science and make recommendations for an agenda for nursing research. The Health Promotion for Older Children and Adolescents Panel convened in 1993 and for the first time the state of the science in children's health promotion and the needs, opportunities with recommendations for nursing research were identified. The report focused on the role of nurses and the contributions of nursing science. The recommendations were intended to strengthen nursing science and improve nursing practice. Subsequently, NINR has funded child health promotion research projects at several university schools of nursing within centers for nursing research. These activities continue today and have broadened in scope over the years.

The NIH Nursing Science: Children and Families (NSCF) Study Section was established and regularly reviews applications related to health promotion, nursing diagnosis, and treatment of human responses to actual or potential health problems, and patient outcomes responsive to nursing interventions. Nursing research findings from research applications reviewed in this study section and funded by NINR or other NIH institutes have led to improvements in the health habits of children, re-duced childhood lead exposure, and reduced adolescent suicide risk be-haviors by enhancing self-esteem, family integration, and problem-solving and decreasing depression (NIH, 2005). Other interdisciplinary research investigations supported by NSCF are related to caregiving, health pro-motion, and disease prevention, including normal growth and develop-ment, maturational processes, and lifestyle behavior changes. Examples of the type of applications reviewed by NSCF have included stress, adap-tation, coping training, social support, diet, exercise, and smoking cessa-tion. As is clearly evident, the science of health promotion as developed, practiced, and evaluated by nurses is well under way.

Several classification systems have evolved within nursing for the purpose of identifying, tracking, and measuring the nursing outcomes from preventive and health promotion nursing care. These are expensive and complex endeavors that have required decades to develop and test. Now these demonstrations must move forward into a world where pro-fessionals from many different disciplines work together with families to achieve results. Everyone is expected to be accountable for meaningful re-sults. It is hoped that as these nursing classification systems become easier to understand, use, and teach to others, their practical value will become apparent; and that the benefits to be derived from their use in answering questions related to the effectiveness, efficiency, and cost benefits of care would be clarified. When this happens, changes in coding policies from a strictly disease-oriented approach could follow and the illness-oriented U.S. system (with 97% of its resources invested in disease) might begin to shift and adjust itself in the direction of health.

Compiling a practice formula for nursing excellence in the areas of disease prevention, health maintenance, and health promotion is compli-cated, especially given the controversies surrounding well-child care de-scribed earlier in this chapter. Theories of health promotion are not being supported by research and it is not uncommon for promising creative in-terventions to produce only weak and time-limited results in terms of lifestyle behavior changes. While there are advances in the science and in-tervention research, continued progress is needed in order for research to demonstrate the outcomes of prevention interventions. Even *Healthy People 2010* findings have been disappointing (USDHHS, 2000). For these reasons, it is especially important that pediatric nursing be well or-ganized, focused, and clear in terms of the direction in which it is headed with its well-child research agenda and demonstration models.

A solid evidence-based foundation of services, programs, and strategies must develop that can be regionally disseminated for repli-cation through practice-based research networks (PBRNs) such as the one Grey and Melkus have established at Yale University (http://nurs-ing.yale.edu/research/initiatives/apn/grey_5.html). Through such efforts, advanced practice nurses not only field test a practice protocol but also provide feedback for its refinement so that eventually improvements in the outcomes of this care are evident and measurable and the protocol's effectiveness in enhancing infant and child health is demonstrated. It is hoped that more uniform as well as evidence-based practice patterns from one nurse to the next will finally emerge; and it will be much more feasible to design and demonstrate well-child services ideally suited to nursing for delivery to individual children, families, and the rest of the pediatric and adolescent segment of the community.

MULTIDISCIPLINARY INTEGRATION AND PARTNERSHIP

In 1976, sociologist Lois Pratt identified active consumer participation, self-care, and a sense of empowerment as valuable to health and well-being:

Consumers need to approach health care as a problem-solving endeavor that requires an active coping effort, rather than as a situation calling for passivity and submission. This involves seeking out health information from various sources, making rational choices among alternative services and practitioners, plotting out the implications of actions for long-term well-being, evaluating the results of health services, and striving for increasingly greater mastery of personal health needs (Pratt, 1976).

From a policy perspective, active consumer involvement is now acknowledged as an important *Healthy People 2010* focus area called "health literacy." The health literacy component (HLC) is administered by the National Center for Educational Statistics (NCES) and the U.S. Department of Education as a part of the larger literacy agenda for children and adults.

Under objective 11-2, Improvement of Health Literacy, there are three types of health information and services targeted for attention: clinical, prevention, and navigation of the health care system (Nielsen-Bohlman, 2004). The clinical type includes interactions between health care providers and consumers, clinical encounters, diagnosis and treatment of illness, and medication. Examples include understanding and completing a health history for an office visit and understanding self-care measures for managing acute and chronic illness.

The prevention type of health information and services includes those activities associated with maintaining and improving health, preventing disease, and intervening early in emerging health problems. Examples of this type of care include following evidence-based guidelines for age-appropriate preventive health services and changing eating and exercise habits to decrease health risks.

The navigation of the health system type of health information and service includes activities to teach consumers how the health system works and teaching individual rights and responsibilities. Examples include knowing medical terminology, understanding health insurance plans, and knowledge of informed consent policies (Rudd, 2004).

In other words, the "patient as partner" era has arrived. Providing effective, efficient, and economical disease prevention, health maintenance, and health promotion services takes special planning efforts, coordination, and commitment from consumers as well as providers. Relationships between these two parties need to reflect a sense of affiliation, two-way communication, mutual problem solving, and negotiation. Then the health plan developed works for the family involved, healthier lifestyle habits evolve, satisfaction grows, and adherence to new behaviors is possible and more frequently realized.

The development of new roles and functions for health consumers begins in early childhood, continues during adolescence and throughout adulthood, and extends beyond the health care delivery system. Developing healthy lifestyle habits, the practice of self-care, and a sense of commitment to healthy public policies are equally compelling reasons for consumers to pursue actively their own health affairs beyond the organized community health care delivery system.

CASE STUDY AND EPILOGUE

Self-reliance is the name of the game in Center City. Everywhere one looks, it is evident that residents of this town place a high value on being responsible for themselves.

At school, students are learning how to navigate the community health care delivery system starting with the school health facilities. Here, the generalist school nurses' health room is the gateway into a school health system that offers disease prevention, health promotion, environmental health and safety services, and health education to all students; and for some students, access to school-based or school-linked student health centers

In both settings, students are often oriented to their roles and responsibilities as health consumers by school nurses, nurse practitioners, consulting physicians, and mental health teams. A simple communication code serves as the vehicle for introducing students at their level of understanding to the concept of patient as partner (Igoe, 1991). Talk, listen and learn, ask, decide, and do (TLADD) is the social norm for visits for health care throughout the school district as well as in the rest of Center City's health facilities.

Developed as a consumer health education program for school-age children in the 1970s at the University of Colorado at Denver and Health Sciences Center School of Nursing Office of School Health, HealthPACT was intended to assist children and youths in developing a set of social skills and a communication code for use during appointments for health care. The acronym TLADD (talk, listen and learn, ask, decide, do) served as a memory cue for the four basic consumer rights and responsibilities: to be informed, to choose, to be heard, and to be safe.

School health professionals are adept at teaching students of all ages how to adopt these communication skills, using a variety of educational materials (also including, one hopes, high-tech simulations in the not too distant future) to encourage students to actively participate in their care. Coupling these approaches with self-monitoring exercises during visits for health care also helps students become consciously aware of their use of the TLADD behaviors during their encounters with school health providers. When students receive plenty of positive reinforcement as they become involved as active health consumers, the TLADD behaviors appear, resulting in greater satisfaction with the visit as well as better follow-through in terms of the students' health care plans.

The TLADD skill set is considered to be consistent with the type of classroom behavior that enhances learning, and it is assumed to contribute to positive family functioning in the opinion of many child health experts (Feetham, Meister, Bell, & Gillis, 1993). For these reasons, its diffusion has been relatively smooth, provided adults believe in this style of student participation not only in health settings but also at school and home as well. Obviously, schools, homes, and communities in which the organizational culture fosters active student participation and self-reliance are ideally suited to the introduction of this role-development program for health consumers of school age—and the sooner the better.

If encouraged throughout the rest of the community health facilities in Center City, within a generation these same HealthPACT lessons for school age-health consumers will significantly improve the consumer's ability to understand, navigate, and influence this community's health care system. Here is a futurist's description of what lies ahead, from a recent issue of the *Center City Times:*

> Twelve years from now we will graduate our first class of students who will have been continually exposed to the "patient as partner" concept throughout their elementary and secondary school years. What influence will these lessons have on these students and what demands will they make on Center City's health care delivery system and all the other health systems they will encounter in their lifetimes? Only time will tell. However, here are some assumptions we can make about this attempt to establish a new set of social norms for navigating the health care system:

1. Students will enter their adulthood and their careers with a similar view of the health care system. Consequently whether they chose to become nurses, psychologists, hospital administrators; or they chose fields other than health; or they go on to become city council members or hospital board members, they will indeed expect to be treated as partners when they use the health care system; and there will be no conflict with one another as consumers and providers over this point of view. Once this period of mutual understanding arrives, the future of the health care industry will be decided mutually by the partnership, namely, the providers and the consumers at all levels of business and government with full support of their professional and civic organizations.

2. TLADD will become an acceptable set of social norms; and indeed may even become known in some circles as a disruptive innovation capable of resolving a number of the health literacy problems now facing many health systems and delaying progress toward a more health-oriented approach to care.

3. Encounters for health care will become mutual problem-solving sessions during which providers will facilitate decision making with consumers instead of directing these efforts. Consequently, the outcomes of this care will improve because people will be more likely to adhere to health plans in which they actually have ownership.

SUMMARY

Over the years, a number of instructional HealthPACT demonstrations have been conducted in schools and other community settings (clubs, after-school programs, camps) and developmentally appropriate videotapes and workbooks have been utilized to depict children of all ages actively communicating with their health care providers using the TLADD code. These demonstrations have been reported as successful (Igoe, 1993). That is, students could and did adopt the TLADD behaviors, experienced a greater sense of control and comfort during appointments for health care, and parents were highly satisfied. On the other hand, there have been difficulties in translating this concept into reality and disseminating this type of role-development instruction for consumers of all ages (Lewis & Lewis, 1990). For example, the HealthPACT program currently is being updated and revised one more time to be compatible with simulations via technology that are now being widely adopted not only in K–12 education but also in nursing education. The hope is that we are finally about to enter an era in which this notion of self-reliance, health literacy, and consumerism will catch on.

Students with chronic diseases and special health needs and disabilities utilize the health care system far more frequently than their classmates do, and they will need these services, in many cases for a lifetime. Therefore, students with chronic health conditions will not only need evidence-based interventions that address their condition of being overweight, or diabetic, or having asthma, but they will also need health literacy strategies like HealthPACT so that they might learn how to communicate effectively with their health care providers, as well as how to navigate the complex health care system skillfully. Without these opportunities, it is unlikely these students and others will be motivated to adhere to disease prevention and health promotion guidelines and actually to change and enhance their lifestyle habits.

What remains a mystery and a challenge for every maternal- and child-health and pediatric nurse is how to combine these communication skills and evidence-based practice protocols into PBRNs, so that students with special health needs eventually receive the life skills package they need to become self-reliant in caring for themselves while also learning how to make their way around the health care system. Therein lie the research questions nursing has to address if we are to lead this effort in designing new kinds of disease prevention health maintenance and health promotion services, so that students eventually become their own care managers.

Finally, as the information in this chapter suggests, there is every reason to believe that the child health teams of providers and consumers are well prepared and positioned to assume this challenge. The special affiliations that are developing from these emerging efforts will soon become transformative in the sense that interdependence will replace dependency in terms of the style of consumer/provider relationships, and soon these changes will occur with greater frequency and on a wider scale. Then, members of many communities will begin together to plan, develop, implement, and evaluate wellness-oriented services that are not only effective but also efficient and economical.

ACKNOWLEDGEMENT

The author gratefully acknowledges the review and contributions to this chapter by Dr. Suzanne L. Feetham, Senior Program Manager, Center for Quality Health Resources and Services Administration.

REFERENCES

Bethel, C., Peck, C., Abrams, M., Halfon, N. Sareen, H., & Collins, K. S. (2002). *Partnering with parents to promote the healthy development of young children enrolled in Medicaid.* New York: The Commonwealth Fund, Program on Child Development and Pediatric Care.

Betz, C. L., Cowell, J. M., Lobo, M. L., & Craft-Rosenberg, M. (2004). American Academy of Nursing Child and Family Expert Panel health care quality and outcomes guidelines for nursing of children and families: Phase II. *Nursing Outlook, 52,* 311–316.

Betz, C. L., Hunsberger, M. M., & Wright, S. (1994). *Family-centered nursing care of children* (2nd ed.). Philadelphia: Saunders.

Brodie, B. (1982). Children: A glance at the past. *MCN: American Journal of Maternal Child Nursing, 7,* 219–220.

Brodie, B. (1986). Yesterday, today, and tomorrow's pediatric world. *Children's Health Care, 14,* 168–173.

Brown, B., & Corbett, T. (1998). *Social indicators and public policy in the age of devolution.* Madison, WI: Institute for Research on Poverty.

Coffield, A. B., Maciosek, M. V., McGinnis, J. M., Harris, J. R., Caldwell, M. B., Teutsch, S., et al. (2001). Priorities among recommended clinical preventive services. *American Journal of Preventive Medicine, 21,* 1–9.

Cohen, L., & Swift, S. (1999). The spectrum of prevention: Developing a comprehensive approach to injury prevention. *Injury Prevention, 5,* 203–207.

Coulton, C. (1995). Using community-level indicators of child well being in comprehensive community initiatives. In J. Connell, A. Kubisch, L. Schorr, & C. Weiss (Eds.), *New approaches to evaluating community initiatives: Concepts, methods and contexts* (pp. 173–200). Washington, DC: Aspen Institute.

Craft-Rosenberg, M., Krajicek, M. J., & Shin, D. (2002). Report of the American Academy of Nursing Child-Family Expert Panel: Identification of quality and outcome indicators for maternal child nursing. *Nursing Outlook, 50,* 57–60.

Crowley, A. A., & Magee, T. K. (2003). Integrating healthy steps into PNP graduate education. *Journal of Pediatric Health Care, 17,* 232–239.

Feetham, S. L. (1999). Families and health in the urban environment. *International Journal of Child and Family Welfare, 4,* 197-227.

Feetham, S. F., Meister, S. B., Bell, J. M., & Gillis, C. L. (Eds.). (1993). *The nursing of families. Theory, research, education, practice.* Newbury Park, CA: Sage.

Flynn, B. C. (1996). Healthy cities: Toward worldwide promotion. *Annual Review of Public Health, 17,* 299–309.

Frey, M. A., & Naar-King, S. (2001). The challenge of measuring adherence in children and adolescents. *Journal of Child and Family Nursing, 4,* 296–300.

Gibbs, D., & Brown, B. (2000). *Community-level indicators for understanding health and human service issues: A compendium of selected indicator systems and resource organizations.* Office of the Assistant Secretary for Planning and Evaluation, U.S. Department of Health and Human Services. Retrieved June 6, 2005 from http://aspe.hhs.gov/progs ys/Community/intro.html

Glascoe, F. P., & Sandler, H. (1995). Value of parents' estimates of children's developmental ages. *Journal of Pediatrics, 127,* 831–835.

Green, L. W., Richard, L., & Potvin, L. (1996). Ecological foundations of health promotion. *American Journal of Health Promotion, 10,* 270–281.

Green, M., & Palfrey, J. S. (2002). *Bright futures: Guidelines for health supervision of infants, children and adolescents* (2nd ed.). Arlington, VA: National Center for Education in Maternal and Child Health.

Hardy, J. B., Shapiro, S., Mellits, E. D., Skinner, E. A., Astone, N. M., Ensminger, M., et al. (1997). Self-sufficiency at ages 27 to 33 years: Factors present between birth and 18 years that predict educational attainment among children born to inner-city families. *Pediatrics, 99*(1), 80–87.

Hutchins, V. L. (1994). Maternal and Child Health Bureau: Roots. *Pediatrics, 94,* 695–699.

Hviid, A., Wohlfahrt, J., Stellfeld, M., & Melbye, M. (2005). Childhood vaccination and nontargeted infectious disease hospitalizations. *Journal of the American Medical Association, 294,* 699–705.

Igoe, J. B. (1991). Empowerment of children and youth for consumer self-care. *American Journal of Health Promotion, 6,* 55–56.

Igoe, J. B. (1993). Healthier children through empowerment. In J. Wilson-Barnett & J. M. Clark (Eds.), *Research in health promotion and nursing* (pp. 145–153). London: Macmillan Press.

Igoe, J. B. (2002). *An evaluation of the Missouri Department of Health School-Age Children's Health Services Program.* Springfield, MO: Department of Health and Human Services, Bureau of Family Health

Iverson, D. C., & Kolbe, L. J. (1983). Evolution of the national disease prevention and health promotion strategy: Establishing a role for the schools. *Journal of School Health, 53,* 294–302.

Laffrey, S .C. (1990). An exploration of adult health behaviors. *Western Journal of Nursing Research, 12,* 434–447.

Lewis, M. A., & Lewis, C. E. (1990). Consequences of empowering children to care for themselves.*Pediatrician, 17*(2), 63–67.

Maternal and Child Health Bureau. (2002). *Child health USA 2002.* Washington, DC: U.S. Department of Health and Human Services.

McKnight, J. L., & Kretzmann, J. P. (1996). *Mapping community capacity.* Evanston, IL: Northwestern University Institute for Policy Research.

Milio, N. (1996). *Engines of empowerment: Using information technology to create healthy communities and challenge public policies.* Chicago: Health Administration Press.

Minkovitz, C. S., Strobino, D., Scharfstein, D., Hou, W., Miller, T., Mistry, K. B., et al. (2005). Maternal depressive symptoms and children's receipt of health care in the first 3 years of life. *Pediatrics, 115,* 306–314.

Moyer, V. A., & Butler, M. (2004). Gaps in the evidence for well-child care: A challenge to our profession. *Pediatrics, 114,* 1511–1521.

National Institutes of Health, National Institute of Nursing Research. (2005). *Center for Scientific Review. Nursing Science: Children and Family Study Section (NSCF).* Retrieved June 6, 2005 from http://cms.csr.nih.gov/PeerReviewMeetings/CSRIRG Description/HOPIRG/NSCF.htm.

Nielsen-Bohlman, L. (2004). *Health literacy: A prescription to end confusion.* Washington, DC: National Academies Press.

Olds, D. L., Robinson, J., Pettit, L., Luckey, D., Holmberg, J., Ng, R. K., et al. (2004). Effects of home visits by paraprofessionals and by nurses: Age 4 follow-up results of a randomized trial. *Pediatrics, 114,* 1560–1568.

Palfrey, J. S. (1997). Keeping children and families in the center of our concern: Ambulatory Pediatric Association presidential address. *Archives of Pediatric and Adolescent Medicine, 151,* 337–340.

Pender, N. (1994). Nursing roles in health promotion. In C. L. Betz., M. M. Hunsberger, & S. Wright (Eds.), *Family centered nursing care of children* (2nd ed., p. 385) Philadelphia: Saunders.

Pender, N. J., Murdaugh, C. L., & Parsons, M. A. (2006). *Health promotion in nursing practice* (5th ed.). Upper Saddle River, NJ: Pearson/Prentice Hall.

Perry, C. L., Williams, C. L., Veblen-Mortenson, S., Toomy, T. L., Komro, K. A., Anstine, P. S. et al. (1996). Project Northland: Outcomes of a community-wide alcohol use prevention program during early adolescence. *American Journal of Public Health, 86,* 956–965.

Pratt, L. (1976). Reshaping the consumer's posture in health care. The doctor-patient relationship in the changing health scene. In E. Gallagher (Ed.), *Proceedings of an international conference sponsored by the John F. Fogarty Center for Advanced Study in the Health Sciences.* National Institutes of Health, Geographic Health Studies, DHEW Publication No. (NIH)78-183. Bethesda, MD: National Institutes of Health.

Resnicow, K. (1997). Appendix C. Models of health behavior change used in health education programs. In D. Allensworth, E. Lawson, L. Nicholson, & J. Wyche (Eds.), *Schools and health: Our nation's investment* (pp. 356-364). Washington, DC: National Academies Press.

Rose, G. (1992). *The strategy of preventive medicine.* New York: Oxford University Press.

Rosenbaum, S., Hughes, D., & Johnson, K. (1988). Maternal and child health services for medically indigent children and pregnant women. *Medical Care, 26,* 315–332.

Rudd, R. (2004). *Communicating health: Priorities and strategies for progress. Objective 11-2. Improvement of health literacy.* Retrieved June 6, 2005 from http://adphp.osophs.dhhs.gov/projects/HealthCOMM/objective2.htm

Schor, E. L. (2004). Rethinking well-child care. *Pediatrics, 114,* 210–216.

Simmes, D. R., Lim, L. F., & Dennis, K. (2003). Documenting child health: The community indicators movement. In E. J. Sobo & P. S. Kurtin (Eds.), *Child health services research: Applications, innovations, and insights* (pp. 121–154). San Francisco: Jossey-Bass.

Skocpol, T. (1991 Summer). Politically viable policies to combat poverty. *Brookings Review, 9,* 29–33.

Smith, T. W., Orleans, C. T., & Jenkins, C. D. (2004). Prevention and health promotion: Decades of progress, new challenges, and an emerging agenda. *Health Psychology, 23,* 126–131.

Stachtchenko, S., & Jenicek, M. (1990). Conceptual differences between prevention and health promotion: Research implications for community health programs. *Canadian Journal of Public Health, 81,* 53–59.

Stanhope, M., & Lancaster, J. (2004). *Community and public health nursing.* St. Louis, MO: Mosby.

Starfield, B., & Vivier, P. M. (1995). Population and selective (high-risk) approaches to prevention in well-child care. In M. R. Solloway & P. P. Budetti (Eds.), *Child health supervision: Analytical studies in the financing, delivery and cost-effectiveness of preventive and health promotion services for infants, children, and adolescents* (pp. 205–226). Washington, DC: George Washington University, Center for Health Policy Research.

Thompson, R. H. (1986). Where we stand. Twenty years of research on pediatric hospitalization and health care. *Children Health Care, 14,* 200–210.

U.S. Department of Health and Human Services, Public Health Service. (1991). *Healthy people 2000: National health promotion and disease prevention objectives* (PHS 91-50212). Washington, DC: U.S. Government Printing Office.

U.S. Department of Health and Human Services. (2000). *Healthy people 2010* (PHS 99-1256). Washington, DC: U.S. Government Printing Office.

U.S. Department of Health and Human Services. (2004). Steps to a healthier us. Retrieved August 11, 2005, from http://www.healthierus.gov/steps/index.html

U.S. Department of Health, Education and Welfare. (1979). *Healthy people: The surgeon general's report on health promotion and disease prevention* (DHEW PHS 79-55071). Washington, DC: Government Printing Office.

U.S. Department of Health, Education and Welfare. (1978). *Disease prevention and health promotion: Federal programs and prospects (PHS 79-55071B).* Washington, DC: Government Printing Office.

U.S. Preventive Services Task Force. (1996). *Guide to clinical preventive services* (2nd ed.). Washington, DC: U.S. Department of Health and Human Services, Office of Disease Prevention and Health Promotion.

Vermont's indicator evolution. (2004). *Youth Today, 2*(5), 25.

W. K. Kellogg Foundation. (2004). *Logic model development guide.* Battle Creek, MI: W. K. Kellogg Foundation.

Young, K. T., Davis, K., Schoen, C., & Parker, S. (1998). Listening to parents: A national survey of parents with young children. *Archives of Pediatric and Adolescent Medicine, 152,* 255–262.

Zero to Three: National Center for Infants, Toddlers, and Families. (1997). *Key findings from a 1997 nationwide survey among parents of zero to three years old.* Washington, DC: Author, Retrieved October 28, 2003 from http://www.zerotothree.org

Zuckerman, B., Stevens, G. D., Inkelas, M., & Halfon, N. (2004). Prevalence and correlates of high-quality pediatric care. *Pediatrics, 114,* 1522–1529.

CHAPTER TWELVE

Care for Children and Youth With Disabilities or Special Health Care Needs

Wendy M. Nehring

This chapter focuses on the quality indicator that addresses the provision of a full range of health care services for children and youth with disabilities or special health care needs (D/SHCN). I will argue that the literature basically supports the premise that, in general, children and youth with D/SHCN receive a full range of health care services, but inequalities exist for those who are poor and minorities. Controversies over definitions and their measurement will be discussed. I will further include a review of the literature to support my premise and follow this with a discussion of existing standards of care and policies for practice in different settings. The chapter will conclude with a discussion and case study illustrating interdisciplinary collaboration, which is essential for successful comprehensive health care for children and youth with D/SHCN. There is no doubt that all children, regardless of intelligence or ability to perform activities of daily living, including physical capabilities, deserve equal quality health care from health care providers. Most important, such care must be available across the life span.

DEFINITIONS AND THEIR MEASUREMENT

Definitions

Terminology used to address or identify persons that do not fit an "ideal" or "normal" perception is most often derogatory and carries stigma. This is no less true for children and youth with D/SHCN. Each of these current terms that are used in this chapter are "umbrella" terms in that they represent a wide range of diagnoses. It is important to provide some background to the terminology that is used today.

A number of terms have been used over the years to describe an individual with subnormal intelligence, and various permutations have occurred to define the criteria by which to identify someone with that characteristic. Terminology often changes due to societal attitudes and advocacy from different constituencies, such as parent or self-advocate groups. There are many references in which this history is described (e.g., Nehring, 1999; Scheerenberger, 1983, 1987). Currently, the most common labels include mental retardation, developmental disabilities, and special health care needs. They do not mean the same thing.

Mental Retardation

Mental retardation is the term that has been used for the longest period of time. There are three main sources for finding a definition of mental retardation today: the American Association on Mental Retardation (Luckasson et al., 2002), the American Psychological Association (APA) (Editorial Board, 1996), and the American Psychiatric Association (APA. 2000) in which their definition appears in the *Diagnostic and Statistical Manual–IV–TR*. In addition, each state may choose to use one of the above definitions, or it may choose to use its own. The American Association on Mental Retardation definition is the most recognized definition and is as follows (Luckasson et al., 2002):

> Mental retardation is a disability (not a diagnosis) characterized by significant limitations both in intellectual functioning and in adaptive behavior as expressed in conceptual, social, and practical adaptive skills. This disability originates before age 18. (p. 19)

Developmental Disabilities

The term *developmental disabilities* was first coined in the late 1970s as an alternative term to mental retardation so that President Nixon would sign into legislation sources of funding and programming for individuals with such conditions (Nehring, 1999). The primary definition of developmental disabilities currently appears in the Individuals with Disabilities Education Improvement Act of 2004 (Public Law 108-46, 1148 Stat. 2647). This definition identifies those conditions that constitute a child with a disability, such as mental retardation, visual and hearing impairments, or autism.

The World Health Organization (WHO) also discusses disability in its *International Classification of Functioning, Disability, and*

Health (ICIDH-2) (WHO, 2001). The U.S. government also uses the term *disability* in a very broad sense by defining it as the degree of limitation that a person experiences. In *Healthy People 2010* (U.S. Department of Health and Human Service, 2000), the authors call for a more succinct and descriptive definition of disability. Disability alone is a broader term, which can originate at any point in the life span, and it is important that intellectual and developmental disabilities that begin in childhood are included so that these children's needs are met and not forgotten in the broader context when such disabling conditions as arthritis are discussed.

Special Health Care Needs

The term *children with special health care needs* originated with the Maternal and Child Health Bureau's Division of Services for Children with Special Health Care Needs, and the American Academy of Pediatrics (AAP). Children with special health care needs are those who have or are at increased risk for a chronic physical, developmental, behavioral, or emotional condition and who also require health and related services of a type or amount beyond that required by children generally (McPherson et al., 1998). There is no comparable definition for adults.

It is important to note that all terms have three criteria in common: age, intelligence, and adaptive behavior. Other minor differences separate the definitions. In recent years, professionals from many disciplines in this field, governmental officials, and self-advocates gathered to find a positive and politically correct term to use. After several years of meetings, a consensus had not been reached. A controversy exists because different individuals and groups use different definitions to meet funding and eligibility criteria for services such as special education, and they also use terms that are less negative. The latter is the reason that the United Kingdom uses the term *learning disability*. Even so, such terminology will change in the future due to continued advances in genetic knowledge and diagnostic technologies.

For example, the National Research Council and Institute of Medicine, Committee on Evaluation and Children's Health (2004) stressed that "there are growing numbers of children in the United States with serious chronic diseases, including many emerging disorders that reflect the interaction of genetics, behavior, and the environment" (p. ES-1). After many years, early and accurate identification of children and youth with D/SHCN will be essential.

Measurements

Disabilities and special health care needs are often caused by brain dysfunction due to malformation of or damage to the developing brain.

These etiologies are most often prenatal and due to genetic causes (Handmaker, 2005). Unfortunately, they are not always diagnosed at birth. In other situations, the symptomatology is not present until the school years. Therefore, a variety of screening and diagnostic measures must be available to the primary health care provider in order to identify cognitive, behavioral, emotional, and physical deficits.

Identification of Disabilities and Special Health Care Needs

When suspected, the first step in identifying a disability or special health care need in a child is a comprehensive prenatal and birth history from the mother and a medical history from both parents, listing any hereditary, genetic, or familial health problems. This family history should also be represented in a three-generation pedigree. Next, the primary care provider should conduct a thorough physical examination and order serology, cytogenetic analysis, metabolic testing, and any neuroimaging studies that are necessary to assess the symptomatology or dysmorphology in the child. Recent genetic discoveries now warrant early and comprehensive genetic testing to ascertain identification of genetic etiologies that only a few years ago had not been identified, such as mitochondria diseases. Battaglia and Carey (2003) provide a useful algorithm to evaluate the child with a possible disability or special health care need.

It is important that the primary care provider refer the child and family to a pediatric specialist at the earliest sign of abnormalities. Such collaboration is necessary to provide the child with an optimal prognosis (AAP Committee on Children with Disabilities, 2001). A primary care provider should never wait to see if the child will "grow out of the problem." Palfrey and colleagues (1987) found that fewer than 30% of children with behavioral or developmental disabilities are identified by their primary care provider.

Bright Futures (Green & Palfrey, 2002) offers the primary care provider a set of guidelines for the health supervision of children from birth through age 21 years including (a) questions to ask the parents to ascertain parenting practices and concerns, (b) questions to ascertain the child's developmental levels and normal developmental milestones, (c) physical examination parameters and physical conditions to observe for, (d) parent-child interaction patterns to observe, (e) necessary immunizations, if applicable, (f) sensory screening measures, such as vision and hearing, and (g) anticipatory guidance pointers to share with the parents based on the child's age at designated times for well-child visits.

Screening and Diagnostic Testing: Developmental

The primary care provider may also choose to conduct developmental screening tests, such as the Denver Development Screening Test II, to ascertain if the child is at risk or shows a delay in age-appropriate behaviors. If such a finding is identified, then referral for diagnostic developmental testing is warranted. Vessey and Rumsey (2003) provide a list of instruments commonly used in screening and diagnostic assessment of intelligence, adaptive behavior, temperament, vision, speech and language, hearing, behavior, stress anxiety, and self-concept. In many cases, an individual must obtain specialized training in the conduct of specific instruments, such as the Bayley Scales of Infant Development-II. The AAP Committee on Children with Disabilities (2001) provides recommendations for developmental screening and surveillance of infants and young children for primary care providers.

Physical Health Problems

As symptoms arise, the primary care provider may decide to order serology tests, x-rays, or neuroimaging tests as appropriate.

Guidelines for Specific Conditions

Guidelines have been developed for specific D/SHCN. Most of these guidelines have been developed by American Academy of Pediatrics committees and include achondroplasia, Down's syndrome, Fragile X, Marfan syndrome, neurofibromatosis, Turner syndrome, and Williams syndrome (see the AAP Web site, http://aappolicy.aappublications.org/policy_statement/index.dtl). These guidelines list specific history questions, aspects of the physical assessment, and diagnostic tests that should be run at specific ages to assess for common secondary conditions. In some cases, such as Down's syndrome (Cohen, 1999), specific height and weight charts have been developed.

In their book, *Primary Care of the Child with a Chronic Condition*, Allen and Vessey (2003) provide valuable information for the primary care provider on the etiology, incidence and prevalence, clinical manifestation at diagnosis, treatments, associated secondary problems, and primary care management for a variety of childhood D/SHCN. Another handbook that provides similar information for early childhood personnel is the *First Start Program Handbook for the Care of Infants, Toddlers, and Young Children with Disabilities and Chronic Conditions* (Krajicek, Hertzberg, Sandall, & Anastasiow, 2004).

INFLUENCES ON THE PROVISION OF COMPREHENSIVE HEALTH CARE: PRIMARY, SECONDARY, AND TERTIARY CARE

It is interesting that although children and youth with D/SHCN have received health care for centuries, it is only recently that such health care has been systematically evaluated and this research was focused on primary care. This body of research is medically based.

Primary Care Practices

Pediatric Practices

The American Academy of Pediatrics Council on Pediatric Practice first discussed the concept of the "medical home" in 1967. This concept was originally coined to describe the need for a central location of a child's medical records, but has evolved to define pediatric medical care (AAP Medical Home Initiatives for Children with Special Needs Project Advisory Committee, 2004).

McPherson and colleagues (2004) detailed the results of the 2001 National Survey of Children with Special Health Care Needs and National Health Interview Survey in which the elements of the medical home were evaluated for children with special health care needs. The following are some of the key findings. Approximately 84.3% of children with special health care needs had nurses or doctors who made the parents feel like partners in their child's care. The majority of children with special health care needs (89%) are estimated to have a primary care provider who is either a doctor or an advanced practice nurse. About three quarters (78.1%) of children with special health care needs received needed referrals to specialty care. Only 39.8% received appropriate care coordination. An even smaller percentage (15.3%) of children with special health care needs aged 14 through 17 years obtained necessary advice and support for a successful transition to adulthood.

Strickland and associates (2004) described the same survey results in more detail. For example, not only did 11% of the sample of greater than 373,000 children not have a primary care provider that was either an advanced practice nurse or doctor, but also the percentages decreased as poverty increased (17.9%). Children with special health care needs who were also members of a minority also experienced decreased percentages, with non-Hispanic children of other ethnic and race backgrounds having the lowest percentage of an identified primary care provider (14.2%). Similar results were also found for obtaining needed referrals: only 66.7% of poor children and 68.9% of Hispanic children (the lowest percentage among the ethnic groups) did not have difficulty getting needed specialty referrals. Another factor discussed in this article was communication among doctors, and the results of the survey indicated that only 54.4% of the parents who responded felt that the communication was very good or excellent. In terms of the communication between doctors and other programs, only 37.1% of the respondents felt this communication was very good or excellent. Last, two thirds of the parents felt that doctors provided appropriate family-centered care. This aspect also decreased as the poverty level increased (50.2%) and was lowest for Hispanic children (53.2%).

Pediatricians have listed many reasons over the past few years to address these outcomes: a lack of training and preparation, lack of understanding about specialists and specialty clinics for children and youth with D/SHCN, reimbursement, time (Cooley, 1999; Dobrez et al., 2001; Sia, Tonniges, Osterhus, & Taba, 2004); lack of training or experience in prescribing therapies and durable medical equipment (Sneed, May, & Stencel, 2001); concerns about labeling children, lack of access to specialists, especially in rural areas (Gupta, O'Connor, & Quezada-Gomez, 2004; Kelleher & Rickert, 1994), variability in screening practices (Sices, Feudtner, McLaughlin, Drotar, & Williams, 2003); and lack of health care staff in the office, and lack of specialists and specialty programs in rural areas (Gupta et al., 2004). Such deficiencies have caused problems with access, necessary referrals, and timely and comprehensive care.

No research articles were found to describe the quality of nursing care in primary care settings to children and youth with D/SHCN, nor was there any evidence of child or parent satisfaction with nursing care in the primary care setting. Instead, one can find well-written descriptions of roles and interventions for pediatric nurse practitioners in primary care settings or in managed care environments (Lindeke, Krajicek, & Patterson, 2001; Lindeke, Leonard, Presler, & Garwick, 2002; Rhoades Smucker, 2001).

School Settings

It is important that the primary care provider of a child or youth with D/SHCN coordinates the child's health plan with the school if the child or youth is in school and that the child's health needs are part of the individualized education plan (IEP). Such care coordination is part of the medical home concept.

Again, no studies were found to evaluate the nursing role in coordinating the care of children and youth with D/SHCN. The AAP Committee of Pediatric Workforce (2001) issued a policy statement on the role of the school nurse in providing school health services and a section is included on the care of schoolchildren with special health needs. The roles and responsibilities of the school nurse in this setting are discussed. The list of authors for this document only appears to list one nurse who was a representative of the National Association of School Nurses.

Little is written about the care of children with D/SHCN during the preschool years or during child care experiences. Fortunately, the American Academy of Pediatrics, the American Public Health Association, and the National Resource Center for Health and Safety in Child Care (2002) have published *Children With Special Needs. National Health and Safety Performance Standards: Guidelines for Out-of-Home Child Care Programs.*

Emergency Care

Researchers evaluating emergency medical services (EMS) for children with special health care needs have emphasized the need for protocols relating to emergency transport and treatment (Spaite, Conroy, Karriker, Seng, & Battaglia, 2001). This is especially true in low-income neighborhoods where families use the emergency department for the majority of their health care needs, even when the child has a disability or special health care need.

Secondary Health Care

Hospital Care

Few evidence-based research articles were found on the evaluation of health care in hospital settings with children and youth with D/SHCN. One qualitative study told the story of pediatric nurses' experiences in caring for children with special needs and their families in the hospital (Ford & Turner, 2001). The four themes that emerged from the data were special relationships, development of trust between the nurses and the families, multiple dimensions of who the expert in the care was, and frustration and guilt. The data did not reflect child and parent satisfaction or an evaluation of the nurse's care.

Evaluation of managed care programs for children with special health care needs have been completed. In one survey study conducted in Virginia, researchers found that when the managed care case manager was based in the clinic or hospital, and not in a private practice, the quality and comprehensiveness of the health care improved (Grossman, Rich, Michelson, & Hagerty, 1999).

Tertiary Health Care

Mental Health

Mental health services for children and youth with D/SHCN is one of the most needed services for this population and one of most scarce resources. The only research study found on this topic was a cross-sectional needs assessment of 30 physicians, in which less than half were pleased with the mental health services available to them for referral. They were also unhappy with access to community resources, availability of written information on special health care needs, and transition services (Davidson, Silva, Sofis, Ganz, & Palfrey, 2002).

Dental Care

The second area of need for children and youth with D/SHCN is dental care. It has been only in the past few years that attention has been given to increasing the access and quality of dental care to this population of children. A national survey of dentists in 2001 found that only approximately 10% of dentists commonly care for children with special health care needs and about 25% had any experience with this population when they were in dental school (Casamassimo, Seale, & Ruehs, 2004).

Early Intervention

Early intervention services should be considered for any infant, birth to 3 years, with a disability or special health care need or who is at risk for such. Such programs offer interdisciplinary assessment and interventions to enhance the child's developmental potential and the parent's skills at meeting their child's developmental needs and culminate in the Individualized Family Service Plan (IFSP) (Cooley, 1999). Evaluation studies have not been published recently, but reviews of the literature can be found that summarize past research indicating moderate positive effects (Guralnick, 1991; Majnemer, 1998).

Nurses have been involved in early intervention programs since their onset in the 1980s, but the effectiveness of the nursing role has not been evaluated. Again, the publications center on the roles and responsibilities of nurses (Stepans, Thompson, & Buchanan, 2002).

Therapies

Managed care plans often do not support early intervention programs. Instead, they support needed therapies and equipment as needed by the child, piecemeal rather than comprehensive. It is important that in Arkansas therapists have worked to develop clinical practice guidelines for occupational therapy, physical therapy, and speech and language therapy for children and youth with D/SHCN (Mooney et al., 2000). Evidence-based research on the efficacy of, satisfaction with, and access to, therapists in each of the three areas was not identified.

Telemedicine

An area of emerging importance in the care of children and youth with D/SHCN is telemedicine. When brought to rural areas, inner cities, and areas with scant numbers of specialists, such technologies allow children to be assessed by specialists from a distance (Robinson, Seale, Tiernan, & Berg, 2003). In a study by Marcin and associates (2004), access, quality of care, and satisfaction were found with the use of telemedicine to obtain needed medical specialty consultation and services.

In conclusion, the research concerning primary, secondary, and tertiary care of children and youth with D/SHCN is in its infancy. Descriptive articles on the roles and responsibilities of nurses and other health care professionals are plentiful. Now is the time for evaluation studies that get to the heart of the disparities in access, quality, cost, and satisfaction.

INFLUENCES FOR THE FAMILY

There is an abundance of literature about the effects on the family of a child or youth with a disability or special health care need, but this literature does not focus on aspects of the child's health status and health care. In the past, if a question on health was covered in the research, it was nominal and usually the respondents were asked if they had health concerns about their family member.

In recent years, health and health care of persons with D/SHCN has been a focus of discussion, presentations, and research. Yet, only one research article was found that examined caretaker or parental knowledge of their child's medical problems (Carraccio, Dettmer, duPont, & Sacchetti, 1998). The researchers found that only 53% of the caretakers could identify the child's specific diagnosis(es), 29% could not list the child's medications, and 25% could not name the subspecialist or provide a phone number of the specialty clinic.

It is clear that family research must include health-related variables, such as satisfaction with health care, information needed and received, referrals, and other services and resources, such as needed equipment, therapies, school-based services, transition services, and respite care. Such research must include the evaluation of each of the health care disciplines involved in the child's care. It is time for nurses to step forward to conduct the research that can indicate their worth to the delivery of health care for the child or youth with D/SHCN.

NURSING CARE EXCELLENCE IN THE PROVISION OF COMPREHENSIVE CARE

As previously noted, nurses have been active in describing their roles and responsibilities in the area of children and youth with D/SHCN for many years. The most substantial efforts have been in the delineation of standards of practice and educational materials.

Standards of Practice

Nurses have long realized the importance of having standards of practice for the care of persons with D/SHCN. The first mention of such standards was in 1964 when the American Association of Mental Deficiency (now AAMR) published *Standards for State Residential Care*. In this document, the role of the nurse was described along with recommended nurse-patient ratios and criteria for the position of director of nursing. A few years later, nurses gathered under the leadership of Una Haynes to write *The Guidelines for Nursing Standards in Residential Centers for the Mentally Retarded* (Haynes, 1968). This document was the first of its kind for a specific discipline in this field. This set of standards remained in place for 20 years.

In 1984, nurses in the New York Office of Mental Retardation and Developmental Disabilities wrote *Standards of Nursing Practice in Mental Retardation/Developmental Disabilities* (Aggen & Moore, 1984). This document was the standard of practice for nurses with basic education and was last revised in 1995 (Aggen et al., 1995).

Nursing leaders from AAMR and the American Association of University Affiliated Programs (AAUAP) jointly wrote *Standards for the Clinical Nurse Specialist in Developmental Disabilities/Handicapping Conditions* in 1987 (Austin, Challela, Huber, Sciarillo, & Stade, 1987). This was the standard of practice for advanced practice nurses.

A decade later, a group of nursing leaders from AAMR, together with the American Nurses Association (ANA), wrote the *Statement on the Scope and Standards for the Nurse Who Specializes in Developmental Disabilities and/or Mental Retardation* (Nehring et al., 1998) which became the gold standard for both basic and advanced practice nurses.

This document has been revised in a second edition, entitled *Scope and Standards for the Nurse Who Specializes in Intellectual and Developmental Disabilities* (Nehring et al., 2004). The new document includes an extended discussion of the scope of this nursing specialty with information on the definition of nursing, integration of the art and science of nursing, roles and responsibilities of basic and advanced practice nurses, settings for practice, commitment to the specialty, and trends and issues for nurses in the specialty of intellectual and developmental disabilities.

The standards of nursing practice are then divided into standards of practice and standards of professional performance. ANA's new format is followed for these standards and includes specifics on basic, advanced, and specialty practice. For example, "planning" is a standard under the standards of practice and includes the statement that "the registered nurse who specializes in I/DD develops a plan that prescribes strategies and alternatives to attain expected outcomes" (Nehring et al., 2004, p. 22). Measurement criteria are divided by the registered nurse, the advanced practice nurse, and the specialist nurse. Measurement criteria for the registered nurse for planning includes developing an individualized plan of care; providing person-centered care; collaborating with the interdisciplinary team; considering federal laws, statutes, regulations, and so forth; integrating current research; and using person-first language. The advanced practice nurse designs and uses advanced strategies for care, considers optimal care for the complex patient with D/SHCN, and synthesizes the interdisciplinary care plan along with the patient's values and beliefs. The nurse who is a specialist in D/SHCN has specific measurement criteria depending on whether he or she is a registered nurse or an advanced practice nurse. The registered nurse in the specialty participates more fully in the interdisciplinary care process; contributes actively to the implementation and follow-up of the interdisciplinary plan; involves outside agencies; and considers a wide variety of resources, including financial, that could enhance the health and quality of life of the patient with D/SHCN. Finally, the advanced practice nurse in the specialty serves in the advanced role of consultant to registered nurses (specialty and nonspecialty) and other members of the interdisciplinary team, partners with community partners to enhance the health and quality of life of the patient with D/SHCN, and acts as a care coordinator for patients with D/SHCN and their family members.

The revised standards will provide the field of intellectual and developmental disabilities with specific and comprehensive parameters of practice by which to evaluate nursing practice. Such standards remain unique in the field of intellectual and developmental disabilities.

It should be noted that over the years, specific states and regions wrote their own standards. It is not known if any of these standards remain in force today.

Nursing Education Materials

Nurses have been consistent over the years in documenting their care of children and youth with D/SHCN. This has taken the form of charting, letters, articles, pamphlets, books, and conference proceedings. A discussion of these contributions over the past century can be found in Nehring (1999). More recently, Hahn (2003) summarized curricula from the past decade written by nursing leaders in the Midwest Alliance in Nursing (MAIN), Developmental Disabilities Nurses Association (DDNA), and AAMR. Current nursing leaders have agreed that nursing curricula can contain only so much information and didactic and clinical experiences with children and youth with D/SHCN can be rare. Therefore, recent efforts have focused on materials for continuing education and postdegree learning using a variety of formats, including written and Internet.

Former U.S. Surgeon General Dr. David Satcher convened a national conference on the health disparities affecting persons with mental retardation in 2001. The resulting document, *Closing the Gap: A National Blueprint for Improving the Health of Individuals with Mental Retardation. Report of the Surgeon General's Conference on Health Disparities and Mental Retardation* (U.S. Public Health Service, 2002) identified recommendations for eliminating these disparities, and as a result set the stage for enhancing the health care available to this population of children, youth, and adults. Increased and focused education for physicians and dentists was a prominent recommendation. The AAP has answered with their Future of Pediatric Education II initiative, which includes establishing guidelines for educating physicians to care for children and youth with D/SHCN. Nehring (2005) convened a prominent group of interdisciplinary leaders in the field to write the first interdisciplinary core curriculum for nurses and health professionals specializing in intellectual and developmental disabilities. Yet nursing, as a single discipline, has not responded in general to enhance the general nursing curriculum, even at the advanced practice or graduate level in pediatrics. The exception, perhaps, is in nursing programs located in universities where a university center of excellence in developmental disabilities (UCEDD) is located and where one of the nursing faculty has a joint appointment with the UCEDD.

Nurses can and should continue to document what they do on a daily basis in the care of children and youth with D/SHCN in a variety of settings. The case study that follows will provide an illustration of this important nursing specialty.

MULTIDISCIPLINARY INTEGRATION
AND PARTNERSHIP: CASE STUDY

Juan is 8 years old and has quadriplegic cerebral palsy. He is not ambulatory, uses a motorized wheelchair, uses equipment that assists
him to speak, and participates in inclusion in his elementary school.
Juan's parents are divorced. His mother, Maria, speaks little English
and does not know where Juan's father is. He left when Juan was
born because he "couldn't take having a son who would not be normal." Juan has been admitted to the hospital for heel cord lengthen-
ing surgery due to contractions and increasing pain. Juan is on SSI
and his health care is taken care of by a managed care plan.

Debbie is assigned as Juan's primary care nurse because she has
taken care of Juan in the past and speaks Spanish. After her initial
assessment of Juan and his mother, Debbie confers with Juan's primary care physician; an initial team meeting of all of the health care
professionals who will take part in Juan's care takes place in the first
24 hours of his admission. Maria is a part of this meeting and an interpreter is present to assist her in understanding what is being said
about her son. On the second day of admission, Juan has surgery and
does well. Because his surgeon wants Juan to stay in the hospital for
at least 1 week, Debbie calls Juan's school, speaks to the school
nurse, and together they make plans for Juan's educational needs.
His teacher is going to come and visit him later in the week. Debbie
also asks Maria if she would like other calls made, such as to their
church or other community organizations in which they participate.

Although simplified, this case study offers an illustration of how a
pediatric nurse can provide family-centered, compassionate, culturally
sensitive, coordinated, continuous, and comprehensive care. It is important that such nursing care continues across a child's life span and that the
elements of this quality indicator are consistently met.

SUMMARY

Increased focus on the care of children and youth with D/SHCN has
taken place in the past 5 years across many health disciplines, not just
nursing. Nurses have written about their roles and responsibilities and
have implied that they meet this particular quality indicator related to
children and youth with D/SHCN. Only recently have physicians nationally and systematically begun to evaluate the quality and access to care of
children and youth with D/SHCN, and although the results are positive,
there are health disparities present. Nurses also need to evaluate their efficacy, especially with this population of children and youth. The first step

in this process may be to identify and describe some best practices and these best practices should be from different settings. Next, survey research should take place. It is interesting to note that although the characteristics of a medical home include having an identified pediatrician, the survey asked about either a pediatrician or nurse. It appears that a discussion of the medical home should include a team of a pediatrician and an advanced practice nurse. As nurses, we need to take control of our destiny. Having a good set of standards of practice and various curricula will help, but nurses must continue to represent their comprehensive and unique practice to both an interdisciplinary professional audience and to the public. Now is the time to take the next steps.

REFERENCES

Aggen, R. L., & Moore, N. J. (1984). *Standards of nursing practice in mental retardation/developmental disabilities.* Albany, NY: New York State Office of Mental Retardation and Developmental Disabilities.

Aggen, R. L., DeGennaro, M. D., Fox, L., Hahn, J. E., Logan, B. A., & Von Fumetti, L. (1995). *Standards of developmental disabilities in nursing practice.* Eugene, OR: Developmental Disabilities Nurses Association.

Allen, P. J., & Vessey, J. A. (2003). *Primary care of the child with a chronic condition* (4th ed.). St. Louis, MO: Mosby.

American Academy of Pediatrics, American Public Health Association, and National Resource Center for Health and Safety in Child Care. (2002). *Caring for mentally retarded children. National health and safety performance standards: Guidelines for out-of-home child care programs* (2nd ed.). Bethesda, MD: Maternal Child Health Bureau, Health Resources and Services Administration, and Department of Health and Human Services.

American Academy of Pediatrics, Committee on Children with Disabilities. (2001). Developmental surveillance and screening of infants and young children. *Pediatrics, 108,* 192–196.

American Academy of Pediatrics, Committee on Pediatric Workforce. (2001). The role of the school nurse in providing school health services. *Pediatrics, 108,* 1231–1232.

American Academy of Pediatrics, Council on Pediatric Practice. (1967). Pediatric records and a "medical home." In American Academy of Pediatrics. *Standards of child care.* Evanston, IL: Author.

American Academy of Pediatrics, Medical Home Initiatives for Children with Special Needs Project Advisory Committee. (2004). The medical home. *Pediatrics, 113*(Suppl. 5), 1545–1547.

American Association on Mental Deficiency. (1964). *Standards for state residential care.* Washington, DC: Author.

American Psychiatric Association. (2000). *Diagnostic and statistical manual of mental disorders* (text rev.). Washington, DC: Author.

Austin, J., Challela, M., Huber, C., Sciarillo, W., & Stade, C. (1987). *Standards for the clinical nurse specialist in developmental disabilities/handicapping conditions.* Washington, DC: National Maternal and Child Health Clearinghouse.

Battaglia, A., & Carey, J. C. (2003). Diagnostic evaluation of developmental delay/mental retardation: An overview. *American Journal of Medical Genetics, Part C: Seminars in Medical Genetics, 117C,* 3–4.

Carraccio, C. L., Dettmer, K. S., duPont, M. L., & Sacchetti, A. D. (1998). Family member knowledge of children's medical problems: The need for universal application of an emergency data set. *Pediatrics, 102,* 367–370.

Casamassimo, P. S., Seale, N. S., & Ruehs, K. (2004). General dentists' perceptions of educational and treatment issues affecting access to care for children with special health care needs. *Journal of Dental Education, 68,* 23–28.

Cohen, W. I. (Ed.). (1999). Health care guidelines for individuals with Down syndrome: 1999 revision. *Down Syndrome Quarterly, 4,* 1–16.

Cooley, W. C. (1999). Responding to the developmental consequences of genetic conditions: The importance of pediatric primary care. *American Journal of Medical Genetics, 89,* 75–80.

Davidson, E. J., Silva, T. J., Sofis, L. A., Ganz, M. L., & Palfrey, J. S. (2002). The doctor's dilemma: Challenges for the primary care physician caring for the child with special health care needs. *Ambulatory Pediatrics, 2,* 218–223.

Developmental Disabilities Assistance and Bill of Rights Amendment Act of 2000, Pub. L. No.106-402, 114 Stat. 1677 (2000).

Dobrez, D., Lo Sasso, A., Holl, J., Shalowitz, M., Leon, S., & Budetti, P. (2001). Estimating the cost of developmental and behavioral screening of preschool children in general pediatric practice. *Pediatrics, 108,* 913–922.

Editorial Board. (1996). Definition of mental retardation. In J. W. Jacobson & J. A. Mulick (Eds.), *Manual of diagnosis and professional practice in mental retardation* (pp. 13–41). Washington, DC: American Psychological Association.

Ford, K., & Turner, D. (2001). Stories seldom told: Paediatric nurses' experiences of caring for hospitalized children with special needs and their families. *Journal of Advanced Nursing, 33,* 288–295.

Green, M., & Palfrey, J. S. (Eds.). (2002). *Bright futures: Guidelines for health supervision of infants, children, and adolescents* (2nd ed., rev.). Arlington, VA: National Center for Education in Maternal and Child Health.

Grossman, L. K., Rich, L. N., Michelson, S., & Hagerty, G. (1999). Managed care of children with special health care needs: The ABC program. *Clinical Pediatrics, 38,* 153–160.

Gupta, V. B., O'Connor, K. G., & Quezada-Gomez, C. (2004). Care coordination services in pediatric practice. *Pediatrics, 113*(Suppl. 5), 1517–1521.

Guralnick, M. J. (1991). The next decade of research on the effectiveness of early intervention. *Exceptional Children, 58,* 174–183.

Hahn, J. E. (2003). Addressing the need for education: Curriculum development for nurses about intellectual and developmental disabilities. *Nursing Clinics of North America, 38,* 185–204.

Handmaker, S. D. (2005). Etiology of intellectual and developmental disabilities. In W. Nehring (Ed.), *A core curriculum for specializing in intellectual and developmental disabilities: A resource for nurses and other health care professionals* (pp. 33–46). Boston: Jones and Bartlett.

Haynes, U. (1968). *An ad hoc committee project—Sub-committee on nursing, American Association for Mental Deficiency: Guidelines for nursing standards in residential centers for the mentally retarded.* Washington, DC: United Cerebral Palsy Association.

Kelleher, K., & Rickert, V. (1994). Management of pediatric mental disorders in primary care. In J. Miranda, A. Hohmann, C. Attkisson, & D. Larson (Eds.), *Mental disorders in primary care.* San Francisco: Jossey-Bass.

Krajicek, M. J., Hertzberg, D. L., Sandall, S. R., & Anastasiow, N. (2004). *First Start program handbook for the care of infants, toddlers, and young children with disabilities and chronic conditions* (2nd ed.). Austin, TX: Pro-Ed.

Lindeke, L. L., Krajicek, M., & Patterson, D. L. (2001). PNP roles and interventions with children with special needs and their families. *Journal of Pediatric Health Care, 15,* 138–143.

Lindeke, L. L., Leonard, B. J., Presler, B., & Garwick, A. (2002). Family-centered care coordination for children with special needs across multiple settings. *Journal of Pediatric Health Care, 16,* 290–297.

Luckasson, R., Borthwick-Duffy, S., Buntinx, W. H. E., Coulter, D. L., Craig, E. M., & Reeve, A. (2002). *Mental retardation: Definition, classification, and systems of support.* Washington, DC: American Association on Mental Retardation.

Majnemer, A. (1998). Benefits of early intervention for children with developmental disabilities. *Seminars of Pediatric Neurology, 5,* 62–69.

Marcin, J. P., Ellis, J., Mawis, R., Nagrampa, E., Nesbitt, T. S., & Dimand, R. J. (2004). Using telemedicine to provide pediatric subspecialty care to children with special health care needs in an underserved rural community. *Pediatrics, 113,* 1–6.

McPherson, M., Arango, P., Fox, H., Lauver, C., McManus, M., Newacheck, P. W., et al. (1998). Commentaries: A new definition of children with special health care needs. *Pediatrics, 102,* 137–140.

McPherson, M., Weissman, G., Strickland, B. B., van Dyck, P. C., Blumberg, S. J., & Newacheck, P. W. (2004). Implementing community-based systems of services for children and youths with special health care needs: How well are we doing? *Pediatrics, 113*(Suppl. 5), 1538–1544.

Mooney, D. M., Clark, M. D., Mele, N. C., Schulz, E. G., Lewis, W. C., Jenkins, L. F., et al. (2000). KIDSCARE: A network for children with special health care needs. *Critical Reviews of Biomedical Engineering, 28,* 421–427.

National Research Council and Institute of Medicine, Committee on Evaluation and Children's Health. (2004). *Children's health, the nation's wealth: Assessing and improving child health.* Washington, DC: National Academies Press.

Nehring, W. M. (1999). *A history of nursing in the field of mental retardation and developmental disabilities.* Washington, DC: American Association on Mental Retardation.

Nehring, W. M. (Ed.) (2005). *A core curriculum for specializing in intellectual and developmental disabilities: A resource for nurses and other health care professionals.* Boston: Jones and Bartlett.

Nehring, W. M., Roth, S. P., Natvig, D., Betz, C. L., Savage, T., & Krajicek, M. (2004). *Scope and standards for the nurse who specializes in intellectual and developmental disabilities* (2nd ed.). Washington, DC: American Nurses Publishing and the American Association on Mental Retardation.

Nehring, W. M., Roth, S. P., Natvig, D., Morse, J. S., Savage, T., & Krajicek, M. (1998). *Statement on the scope and standards for the nurse who specializes in developmental disabilities and/or mental retardation.* Washington, DC: American Nurses Publishing and American Association on Mental Retardation.

Palfrey, J. S., Singer, J. D., Walker, D. K., & Butler, J. A. (1987). Early identification of children's special needs: A study in five metropolitan communities. *Journal of Pediatrics, 111,* 651–659.

Rhoades Smucker, J. M. (2001). Managed care and children with special health care needs. *Journal of Pediatric Health Care, 15,* 3–9.

Robinson, S. S., Seale, D. E., Tiernan, K. M., & Berg, B. (2003). Use of telemedicine to follow special needs children. *Telemedicine Journal and E-Health, 9,* 57–61.

Scheerenberger, R. C. (1983). *A history of mental retardation.* Baltimore: Brookes.

Scheerenberger, R. C. (1987). *A history of mental retardation: A quarter century of promise.* Baltimore: Brookes.

Sia, C., Tonniges, T. F., Osterhus, E., & Taba, S. (2004). History of the medical home concept. *Pediatrics, 113*(Suppl. 5), 1473–1478.

Sices, L., Feudtner, C., McLaughlin, J., Drotar, D., & Williams, M. (2003). How do primary care physicians identify young children with developmental delays? A national survey. *Journal of Developmental and Behavioral Pediatrics, 24,* 409–417.

Sneed, R. C., May, W. L., & Stencel, C. (2001). Physicians' reliance on specialists, therapists, and vendors when prescribing therapies and durable medical equipment for children with special health care needs. *Pediatrics, 107,* 1283–1290.

Spaite, D. W., Conroy, C., Karriker, K. J., Seng, M., & Battaglia, N. (2001). Improving emergency medical services for children with special health care needs: Does training make a difference? *American Journal of Emergency Medicine, 19,* 474–478.

Stepans, M. B., Thompson, C. L., & Buchanan, M. L. (2002). The role of the nurse on a transdisciplinary early intervention assessment team. *Public Health Nursing, 19,* 238–245.

Strickland, B., McPherson, M., Weissman, G., van Dyck, P., Huang, Z. J., & Newacheck, P. (2004). Access to the medical home: Results of the National Survey of Children with Special Health Care Needs. *Pediatrics, 113*(Suppl. 5), 1485–1492.

U.S. Department of Health and Human Services. (2000). *Healthy People 2010* (2nd ed.). Washington, DC: U.S. Government Printing Office.

U.S. Public Health Service. (2002). *Closing the gap: A national blueprint to improve the health of individuals with mental retardation. Report of the Surgeon General's conference on health disparities and mental retardation.* Washington, DC: Author.

Vessey, J. A., & Rumsey, M. (2003). Chronic conditions and child development. In P. J. Allen & J. A. Vessey (Eds.), *Primary care of the child with a chronic condition* (4th ed., pp. 23–43). St. Louis, MO: Mosby.

World Health Organization (WHO). (2001). *International classification of functioning, disability, and health (ICIDH-2).* Retrieved September 25, 2002, from http://www.who.int/classifications/en

CHAPTER THIRTEEN

Palliative Care for Children and Families

Margaret M. Mahon

INTRODUCTION, DEFINITIONS, AND MODELS

Palliative care is one of the newest formalized areas of health care. Palliative care is distinct from hospice and different from solely end-of-life care, though it includes elements of each. For most of history, few diseases could be cured by human intervention, and yet there have long been attempts to make the patient feel better, to relieve suffering, especially in the face of dying.

The word "palliative" comes from the Latin *palliare*, meaning to cloak. In the context of health care, this refers to alleviation of the symptom burden, to making the patient feel better. This is distinct from efforts towards cure or disease management. The term *palliative care or palliative medicine* was first used in this context by Lord Balfour Mount to describe the work he and his team were doing at the Royal Victoria Hospital in Montreal in the 1970s.

Palliative care is an approach that improves the quality of life of patients and their families facing the problem associated with life-threatening illness, through the prevention and relief of suffering by means of early identification and impeccable assessment and treatment of pain and other problems, physical, psychosocial and spiritual (World Health Organization, 1990).

That is, palliative care encompasses aggressive symptom management across disease trajectories. Children who will recover from their injuries or illnesses, as well as children who might or will die, deserve palliative care.

Palliative care has recently been recognized as a distinct specialty within nursing and medicine. Its precepts, however, are, or should be, a part of the management of children with any condition that imposes a symptom burden on the child. There are three primary areas of palliative care interventions: symptom management, decision making, and end-of-life care. Each of these will be described in turn within this chapter.

Models of Palliative Care

WHO Model

Perhaps the most widely known model of palliative care is that of the World Health Organization (1990). It has been adopted and adapted by many authors since it was developed (see Figure 13.1). The WHO model had several advantages. First, it was an attempt to describe a newly formalized area of health care in a way that would be widely understood. In so doing, it broadened legitimacy of palliative care as a distinct field, though some still believe it is equivalent to hospice. Second, the WHO model established a framework for discussion about, and analysis of, the components, process, and timing of palliative care. That is, the WHO model provided a forum for common understanding and further development within the field. In addition, it remains the most widely recognized model of palliative care. There are, however, several disadvantages to the WHO model. First, it is built on an understanding of cancer treatment and cancer deaths that existed at the time of the model's development. Two things have happened to make a cancer-based model less than optimal. Though most adults who get cancer will eventually die from

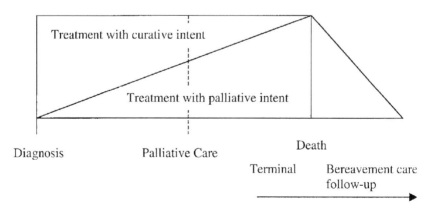

FIGURE 13.1 World Health Organization model of palliative care.

Reprinted from *Handbook of Palliative Care in Cancer* (2nd ed.), by A. Waller & N. L. Caroline, 2000, Boston: Butterworth Heinemann, Copyright (2000), with permission from Alexander Waller, MD and Nancy L. Caroline, MD.

their disease, many people will live with the disease for years. Those years may include periods of remission and relative health. Therefore, continuous deterioration no longer describes most patients' experiences of cancer. In addition, the life expectancy of adults in developed countries continues to increase. Adults die from a wide range of diseases other than cancer, including cardiac, pulmonary, and neurologic diseases and other causes; greater numbers of older adults are contracting and living with HIV. Whereas the average time between diagnosis of cancer and death was 4 days in 1900, the time between diagnosis and death has expanded to greater than 4 years in 2000 (Lynn, Schuster, & Kabcenell, 2000). Although the individual's general health declines, extended period of remissions may occur. It is these diseases typified by periods of remissions and exacerbations that are not described by the WHO model.

Sheffield Model

In part because of the work done by the authors of the WHO model, and based on their vast experiences, there is a model that better captures the complexities of palliative care. Professor Sam H. Ahmedzai and the Sheffield Palliative Care Studies Group of the University of Sheffield in the United Kingdom have developed an evolution of the WHO model (Ahmedzai & Walsh, 2000). There are several strengths to the Sheffield model. First, there is no dichotomy between curative and palliative care. This is especially important, because if palliative care is to be recognized as first addressing symptom management, it must apply across diseases and disease trajectories. In other words, people who will be cured of their diseases or injuries, or those for whom the outcome is unknown, are no less entitled to optimal symptom management than those who will probably or definitely, sooner or later, die from their diseases (see Figure 13.2)

Of note, the Sheffield model recognizes the importance of the time of screening and investigation. This is not only a time of uncertainty for families, especially in pediatrics, but also it is not uncommonly a time that later becomes one of self-recrimination. Families castigate themselves for not recognizing signs and symptoms as harbingers of serious illness. Providers' awareness of the significance of this process and families' reactions to it are a foundation for providing support related to the time preceding diagnosis or injury. This understanding leads to recognition of the dimension of the model that separates the management of the disease from the care of the person. The former is likely to evolve as the disease changes in each person. The latter is based on the needs of the individual (understanding, developmental stage, concurrent life events) as well as those of the family. Both the individual and the family are targets of care.

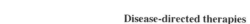

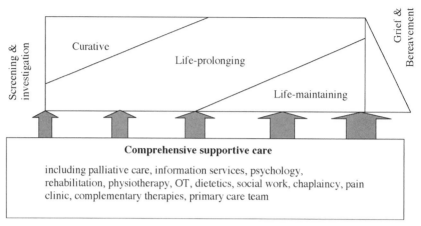

FIGURE 13.2 Sheffield model of palliative care.

From "Palliative Medicine and Modern Cancer Care," by S. H. Ahmedzai and T. D. Walsh, 2000, *Seminars in Oncology,* 27(1), p. 4. Copyright 2000 by S. H. Ahmedzai. Reprinted with permission.

The Sheffield model also challenges providers to specify the goals of therapy. This should include explication of the goal of treatment as curative, life prolonging, or life maintaining. Specificity matters, because "there is probably a discrepancy between the professional's and the patient's definition of 'cure'; the former tending to rely on percent probably of surviving 5 or 10 years, while the latter imagining a return to normal lifespan" (Ahmedzai & Walsh, 2000).

Another important area of palliative care, also embodied in the Sheffield model, is the recognition that each patient will have a unique team addressing palliative care needs. Most children will be referred to palliative care by another medical service. This referral to palliative care does not imply the exclusion of other medical teams. One reason why some providers do not make palliative care referrals is physician fear of abandoning a patient, or of being perceived as abandoning a patient (Abrahm, 2000). The providers who compose the palliative care team for each child are based on the child's disease or injuries, as well as the unique needs of the child and family. The palliative care team is interdisciplinary, comprising nurses, physicians, social workers, nutritionists, chaplains, child life workers, teachers, pharmacists, volunteers, and others. Team members come from across medical specialties, based on the child's illness or injuries. The child and family are also considered essential members of the pediatric palliative care team.

Because the composition of the palliative care team is fluid, there is an increased need for coordination of care. In addition, families are often expected to provide direct care, for example, respiratory or physical therapies, medication administration, dietary modification or supplementation, blood testing, and record keeping, When the palliative care team becomes involved in a child's case, it is an opportunity to unburden the family from this dimension of care, as well as to evaluate whether therapies that are currently a part of the child's regimen are appropriate and whether any can be discontinued.

The Center to Advance Palliative Care (CAPC) is perhaps the leading organization in the United States dedicated to facilitating the development of palliative care services and professionals. CAPC has developed a leveled model of palliative care based on the recognition that different patients and families will need different palliative care services over time. The premise is that much of the knowledge that comprises palliative care should be a part of all health care providers' skill sets. Perhaps the primary example of this is pain management. Few nurses or physicians receive substantive education about pain management, despite the fact that most patients have some degree of physical pain.

CAPC's model (von Gunten, Ferris, Portenoy, & Glajchen, 2001) is an attempt to identify knowledge and skills appropriate for different providers. *Primary palliative care* refers to a set of skills that all providers should have. *Secondary palliative care* is the palliative care team, an institution-based interdisciplinary team "available for consults on difficult palliative care issues" (von Gunten et al, 2001). *Tertiary palliative care* is yet a more advanced level of expertise, a team well versed in all aspects of palliative care. This tertiary team is likely to be based at academic medical centers, and thus likely to be "involved in educational and research activities related to hospice and palliative care." The CAPC model at once challenges all providers to have some level of palliative care knowledge, and to identify and utilize resources for more complex cases. Because there are fewer palliative care resources for children, it is necessary to be aware of all the palliative care services offered for children in a specific geographic area. "It is [also] necessary that programmers have flexibility—the capacity to respond to the varying needs of the patient and to respond quickly" (Davies, 1998, p. 1098).

Pediatric Palliative Care

WHO has defined pediatric palliative care as that which is active total care of the child's body, mind and spirit, and also involves giving support to the family. It begins when illness is diagnosed, and continues regardless of whether or not a child receives treatment directed at the disease. To understand the population of children likely to need palliative care services, one must understand the prevalence of chronic conditions of childhood, as well as causes of death for children (see Table 13.1).

TABLE 13.1 Top Ten Causes of Death, Numbers of Deaths in the United States by Cause and Total, and Total Death Rates, by Age Group (1999)*

Rank	Infant (<1)	Age Group (years)		
		1–4	5–14	15–24
1	Congenital anomalies[a] 5,437	Accidents[b] 1,898	Accidents 3,091	Accidents 13,656
2	Short gestation and LBW[c] 4,392	Congenital anomalies 549	Malignant 1,012	Homicide 4,998
3	SIDS 2,648	Malignant neoplasm 418	Homicide 432	Suicide 3,901
4	Complications of pregnancy 1,399	Homicide 376	Congenital anomalies 428	Malignant neoplasm 1,724
5	Respiratory distress syndrome 1,110	Diseases of the heart 183[d]	Diseases of the heart 277	Diseases of the heart 1,069
6	Complications of placenta, cord, and membranes 1,025	Pneumonia and influenza 130	Suicide 242	Congenital anomalies 434
7	Accidents 845	Perinatal period[e] 92	Chronic lower respiratory diseases 139	Chronic lower respiratory diseases 209

8	Newborn sepsis 691	Septicemia 63	Benign neoplasms 101	HIV 198
9	Diseases of the circulatory system 667	Benign neoplasms 63	Pneumonia and influenza 93	Stroke 182
10	Atelectasis[f] 647	Chronic lower-respiratory diseases 54	Septicemia 77	Pneumonia and influenza 179
Total deaths (all causes)	27,937	5,249	7,595	30,656
Death rate per 100,000 (all causes)	705.6[g]	34.7	19.2	81.2

[a]Congential malformations, deformations, and chromosomal abnormalities.
[b]Most vital statistics reports now use the term "unintentional injury" rather than accidents.
[c]LBW = low birth weight.
[d]Deaths related to congenital malformations of the heart are included with congenital anomalies.
[e]Certain conditions originating in the prenatal period.
[f]Pulmonary collapse or, more generally, absence of gas from part or all of the lungs.
[g]Death rate calculated per 100,000 population (under 1 year) rather than per 1,000 live births, which is the infant mortality rate.

From When Children Die: Improving Palliative and End-of-Life Care for Children and Their Families, by M. J. Field and R. E. Behrman (Eds.) 2002. Washington, DC: National Academies Press. Used with permission (2000) by the National Academy of Sciences, courtesy of the National Academies Press, Washington, DC.

*These figures differ from other figures given for deaths by age in this chapter due to different age parameters for childhood.

Patterns of illness differ markedly between children and adults. For example, children may live with the condition that causes their serious illness or even death for much or all of their lives. Examples of this include HIV, cardiac disease, sequelae of prematurity, cystic fibrosis, the muscular dystrophies, and other conditions. James Oleske, who has done seminal work on the management of HIV in children and who has been involved with this population since the recognition of the disease, has developed (with L. Czarniecki) a model for the provision of palliative care to children. Oleske and Czarniecki's model (1999, p. 1288) was based on the management of children with HIV, but it has implications for other pediatric populations. The Pediatric Palliative Care model describes the integration of therapies specifically towards comfort existing concurrently with restorative care, the goal of which is optimizing the child's functioning. This dimension of living as well as possible is at the core of pediatric palliative care (see Figure 13.3).

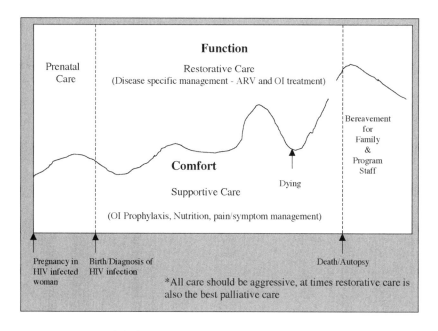

FIGURE 13.3 Model of pediatric palliative care.

From "Continuum of Palliative Care: Lessons From Caring for Children Infected With HIV-1," by J. M. Oleske and L. Czarniecki, reprinted with permission from Elsevier (*Lancet*, 1999, 345, 1287–1291).

INFLUENCES OF PALLIATIVE CARE
ON INFANTS AND CHILDREN

The other variable to be considered when constructing the decision-making process is the extent of the child's involvement. Historically, it has often been the practice not to include children in decision making, usually because of an attempt to protect them, and because of a belief that they are "too young to understand." Researchers have provided important data about children's understanding of their diseases, especially in the context of dying. Children who are dying, even very young children, know they are dying (Bluebond-Langner, 1978). Even healthy children understand death at a much younger age than was previously believed. In one study, 45% of 5–year-olds had an accurate concept of death (Mahon, 1993). Children living with chronic illnesses are acutely aware of the effect of the illness on their daily lives. The implication of children's recognition is that they must at least be informed about, and often involved in, the decision-making process. This does not mean that children should be the ultimate arbiters of their treatments; however, it does mean they should be aware of the process, not just the product, of decision making. *How* to include children must again be a decision of the team. Often, the introduction of the palliative care team is an ideal opportunity to provide a structured process of including children. It is possible, with exquisite teamwork, to have a "no-secrets" philosophy, so information cannot be kept from children. Still, extreme care must be taken in its provision.

INFLUENCES OF PALLIATIVE CARE
ON THE FAMILY

Decisions about children's care are largely understood as the purview of the child's parents. Decision making does not mean, however, an unlimited series of choices for the parents. It is the responsibility of health care providers to construct the options from which parents choose. Often, choices are made without even being acknowledged, or because there is only one option. For example, an atrial septal defect of a certain size must be managed surgically. Certain medications are indicated for the treatment of certain diseases, from HIV to many infections. For most children, immunizations are routine and are not perceived by families as a treatment about which a decision has been made. Across these examples, the foundation for all decision making are the physiologic realities of the child's condition. In turn, physiology establishes the parameters for treatment options. It is only after these treatment options are delineated that the parents have a decision to make.

Decisions made about how a child's condition is managed are often made based on the goals of treatment. Treatment decisions can be categorized by three general goals: treatment to cure the condition, treatment to allow the child to live as well as possible with a chronic or incurable disease or injuries, and treatment that allows the child to die with a minimal symptom burden.

The magnitude of decision making increases with the severity of the child's illness or injuries. Perhaps the two most difficult types of decisions are the point at which treatment goals need to switch from care to comfort, and decisions to withdraw or withhold life-prolonging therapies. In these cases especially, decision making must be structured. Parents should never be asked, "What do you want us to do?" and no parent should hear, "There's nothing else we can do." Though it may not be possible to cure the child, palliative care directs that there is *always* something to be done, not the least of which is aggressive symptom management.

The context and process of structured decision-making is challenging, because few health care providers are educated in this area. In addition, optimal decision-making processes require a collaboration that is not always present in current health care. The model of Jonsen, Siegler, and Winslade (2002) is instructive (see Table 13.2).

Although this model was developed to facilitate the integration of ethics into clinical decision making, it is often useful in family decision-making. In almost all cases, parents are the ideal surrogate decision-makers for their children. There are two caveats that providers must consider to optimize family decision-making. First, parents who are making decisions for or about their child must be choosing between real options. The Jonsen, Siegler, and Winslade model is an appropriate guide in structuring these options. It is the responsibility of the health care team to respect family autonomy. Autonomy, however, is not an absolute right. Rather, autonomy exists only within the context of pathophysiologic parameters. It is the responsibility of providers to structure the options that realistically exist. This also means that providers must use the many good prognostic tools that exist, which often is not something clinicians do well (Christakis, 1999).

NURSING CARE EXCELLENCE
IN PALLIATIVE CARE

In this chapter, the three primary dimensions of palliative care are described: symptom management, family decision-making, and end-of-life care. The overarching goal is to allow the child to live as well as possible, given the physiologic realities of the child's condition.

TABLE 13.2 Decision-Making Model

Medical Indications	Patient Preferences
The Principles of Beneficence and Nonmaleficence	The Principle of Respect for Autonomy
1. What is the patient's medical problem? history? diagnosis? prognosis?	1. Is the patient mentally capable and legally competent? Is there evidence of incapacity?
2. Is the problem acute? chronic? critical?	2. If competent, what is the patient stating about preferences for treatment?
3. What are the goals of treatment?	3. Has the patient been informed of benefits and risks, understood this information, and given consent?
4. What are the probabilities of success?	4. If incapacitated, who is the appropriate surrogate? Is the surrogate using appropriate standards for decision making?
5. What are the plans in case of therapeutic failure?	5. Has the patient expressed prior preferences, e.g., advance directives?
6. In sum, how can this patient be benefited by medical and nursing care, and how can harm be avoided?	6. Is the patient unwilling or unable to cooperate with medical treatment? If so, why?
	7. In sum, is the patient's right to choose being respected to the extent possible in ethics and law?

(continued)

TABLE 13.2 Decision-Making Model (*Continued*)

Quality of Life	Contextual Features
The Principles of Beneficence and Nonmaleficence and Respect for Autonomy	The Principles of Loyalty and Fairness
1. What are the prospects, with or without treatment, for a return to normal life?	1. Are there family issues that might influence treatment decisions?
2. What physical, mental, and social deficits is the patient likely to experience if treatment succeeds?	2. Are there provider (physicians and nurses) issues that might influence treatment decisions?
3. Are there biases that might prejudice the provider's evaluation of the patient's quality of life?	3. Are there financial and economic factors?
4. Is the patient's present or future condition such that his or her continued life might be judged undesirable?	4. Are there religious or culture factors?
5. Is there any plan and rationale to forego treatment?	5. Are there limits on confidentiality?
6. Are there plans for comfort and palliative care?	6. Are there problems of allocation of resources?
	7. How does the law affect treatment decisions?
	8. Is clinical research or teaching involved?
	9. Is there any conflict of interest on the part of providers or the institution?

Note. From *Clinical Ethics: A Practical Approach to Ethical Decisions in Clinical Medicine* (5th ed.), by A. R. Jonsen, M. Siegler, and W. J. Winslade, 2002, New York: McGraw-Hill. Copyright 2002 by The McGraw-Hill Companies.

Symptom Management

The management of chronic and severe illnesses and injuries of childhood has two components. The first is the actual management of the disease or injury, for example, medications and pulmonary treatments to manage asthma or cystic fibrosis; chemotherapy, surgery, and radiation to treat cancer; or therapeutic interventions to optimize functioning in children with neurologic diseases. Existing on a parallel course with disease management is management of the child's symptoms. Symptom management often will not affect the outcome of the disease; however, it has a great impact on how the child lives with the disease. As noted in the American Academy of Pediatrics (AAP) recommendations regarding palliative care, "[t]he goal is to add life to the child's years, not simply years to the child's life" (AAP, 2000, p. 353).

Palliative care is not just for children who are dying, but also for those who are living with chronic conditions and debilitating symptoms. In the United States in 2001, it was estimated that 12.8% of children younger than 18 years of age were living with a chronic condition, more than 9.4 million children (McPherson et al., 2004). There are no good primary data, about the types and numbers of symptoms with which children with chronic disease live, although surrogate data are available (Goldman, 1998). Wolfe and colleagues (2000) investigated parents' perceptions of the symptom burden of children with cancer before the child's death. The breadth of symptoms described by these authors is such that they can be at least somewhat instructive regarding children's symptom burdens across diseases. According to Wolfe and colleagues (2000) "89% of the children experienced a lot or a great deal of suffering from at least one symptom, and 51% from three of more symptoms" (p. 330). In addition, the investigators found notable differences between parents' and physicians' reports of children's symptoms. Although the care of children with chronic and critical illness continues to advance at prodigious rate, management of symptoms has not kept pace. A change in the standards of children's health care necessitates integration of this dimension. For purposes of this chapter, pain will be the symptom addressed.

Pain

Most pain in children can be managed to a satisfactory level. Despite that, many children still live with unacceptably high levels of pain, both acute and chronic. In 1968, McCaffery wrote what has become the most widely used definition of pain: "Pain is whatever the experiencing person says it is, existing whenever he says it does" (McCaffery & Pasero, 1999, p. 16). Within the decade following McCaffery's statement, the newly formed

International Association for the Study of Pain (IASP) put forth the following definition: "Pain is an unpleasant sensory and emotional experience associated with actual or potential tissue damage or described in terms of such damage" (IASP, 1994).

Many factors contribute to the failure of health care providers to manage pain. First, providers rely on objective data; pain is one of the few symptoms that require a diagnosis and treatment based primarily on subjective data. In many cases, pain does not correlate with the nature of the illness or injuries (Baxt, Kassam-Adams, Nance, Vivarelli-O'Neill, & Winston, 2004; Foley, 1998). Second, providers often lack education about pain management, including assessment. The deleterious effects of lack of education are compounded by myths about pain and opioids (Foley, 1998).

Types of Pain

As described by Dame Cecily Saunders (1967), often described as the founder of the modern hospice movement, pain is likely to have physical, psychological, interpersonal, and spiritual components. This multidimensional description of pain is called "Total Pain" (Saunders, 1967). Pain in one of these dimensions affects pain and functioning in other areas. For example, a child with severe physical pain is less able to interact with others. Although nurses, with the palliative care team, have a responsibility to address each of these areas of pain, the focus in this section will be on the management of physical pain.

There are different types of physical pain (see Figure 13.4). First, pain can described as nociceptive or neuropathic. *Nociceptive pain* is the response of an intact nervous system to noxious stimuli. Nociceptors are nerve endings that can distinguish between normal and noxious stimuli. Nociception is the process of perception of pain stimuli (McCaffery & Pasero, 1999). There are two kinds of nociceptive pain: somatic and visceral. *Somatic pain* arises from bone, muscle, soft or connective tissue, or skin. Somatic pain is often described as aching, dull, or boring; it is usually easily localized and easily described. That is, the child can point to where it hurts. Somatic pain is often exacerbated by movement. Often, treating the cause is important in managing somatic pain. Nonsteroidal anti-inflammatory drugs (NSAIDs) and acetaminophen are often appropriate for somatic pain, though opioids may be indicated for more severe pain (Hanks & Cherney, 1998). Bisphosphonates are sometimes utilized for bone pain, and steroids are sometimes an appropriate short-term intervention (Abrahm, 2000).

Visceral pain arises from the structures of the viscera, that is, organs and their supporting structures. Visceral pain is often described as cramp-

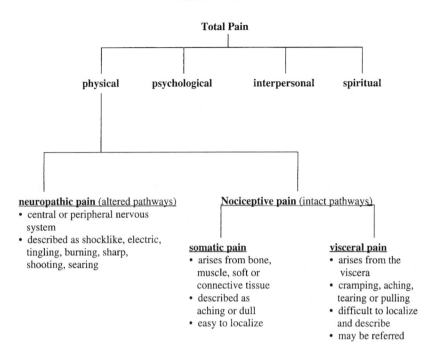

FIGURE 13.4 Types of pain.

ing, aching, tearing, or pulling. Children experiencing visceral pain may naturally draw their knees up towards their abdomen, as this decreases the pressure on the viscera and thus alleviates pain. If a child with visceral pain is asked where it hurts, the description is more vague. This is not a reflection of immaturity, but is rather typical of visceral pain, which is difficult to localize. Visceral pain is often referred to more superficial, larger, or proximal structures (McCaffery & Pasero, 1999). Again, the specific cause of the pain should be addressed. Pain is managed based on its cause. For example, some cramping pain is well treated with NSAIDS. Anticholinergics and prokinetic agents may relieve the pain, and again, a short course of steroids may be helpful (Harrison, 2003; Portenoy, 1998).

Neuropathic pain arises from alteration in structures of the central or peripheral nervous systems. It is often described as "like a shock," tingling, shooting, burning, or sharp (Abrahm, 2000). Neuropathic pain may exist at the site of the disease or injury, or may be referred; it often radiates in dermatomal patterns. Treatments for neuropathic pain vary, based on the cause as well as the sensation of the pain. Tricyclic antidepressants (TCAs) may be useful for burning, tingling, or pain on light touch (McGrath, 1998). TCAs as a group, however, have a high incidence of anticholinergic side effects. Anticonvulsant medications can be effective for shooting or stabbing pain. Gabapentin, for example, is now considered first-line therapy for neuropathic pain. Unfortunately, these medications require slow titration; delayed analgesia is a risk for premature discontinuation. Venlafaxine (Effexor) is increasingly recognized as optimal for certain types of neuropathic pain (Grothe, Scheckner, & Albano, 2004). Venlafaxine is a selective serotonin and norepinephrine reuptake inhibitor. It is both efficacious and economical though its uses in children are still being described. Other medications such as baclofen, local anesthetics, and more invasive procedures can also be used for neuropathic pain with good effect (Portenoy, 1998). Very often, the management of neuropathic pain in children will require a secondary or tertiary palliative specialist.

Pain Assessment

Adequate pain management is founded on comprehensive pain assessments. Largely because of the efforts of the Department of Veterans Affairs to make pain the fifth vital sign, and subsequent efforts by the Joint Commission on the Accreditation of Healthcare Organizations (JCAHO), pain assessment has become better integrated into health care. Though pain assessments are now routine, they are rarely complete.

There are several mnemonics to guide the process of pain assessment. One, OLD CARTS, is ideal because of its comprehensiveness and ease of use. OLD CARTS reminds the provider to assess onset, location, duration, characteristics, aggravating factors, relieving factors, current or prior therapies, and severity. The dimension of pain that is best assessed is typically intensity or severity. Several scales exist for assessing pain intensity in children, including the Beyer Faces Scale, the visual analogue scale (VAS, a 0 to 10 intensity scale), and the FLACC (face, legs, activity, cry, and consolability) scale (Baxt et al., 2004; McGrath, 1998; Willis, Merkel, Voepel-Lewis, & Malviya, 2003; Winston, 2004). Pain assessment scales, too, are too often inconsistently or inappropriately utilized (Foley, 1998; McGrath, 1998).

The pain assessment should also include assessment of whether the pain is acute or chronic. *Acute pain* is a response to injury, illness, or surgery. Acute pain results in vital signs and blood flow changes that, in part, allow the individual to protect the injured area. Procedure pain is one example of acute pain; procedures and therapies and anticipating procedures and therapies, such as IV insertion, blood tests, spinal taps, physical therapy, and others, are often painful and anxiety inducing in children (and adults). Procedure-related pain should be aggressively managed. EMLA (eutectic mixture of localized anesthetics) is excellent for procedures that involve needle sticks; however, because it requires transdermal absorption, it should be applied at least 1 hour prior to any procedures. One of the principles of acute pain management is to treat the sources of pain.

Chronic pain is pain that has lasted longer than 3 months. It has been estimated that at least 15% to 20% of children may experience chronic pain (Goodman & McGrath, 1991). Assessment measures used for children with acute pain are often not valid for children with chronic pain. One cannot assume that a child blithely and intensely playing a video game, interacting animatedly with friends, or successfully completing a day of school is not experiencing severe pain; children develop exquisite self-distraction techniques. Outward appearances, therefore, cannot be taken as complete and valid assessments in children whose pain is chronic. Chronic pain may cause fatigue and stress, and necessitate other changes in lifestyle. Children with acute pain are likely to guard a painful body part, decreasing movement to the area. The same response may be contraindicated for a child in chronic pain. For example, a child with a joint injury that has not healed well may continue to guard the joint. With this guarding, the muscles surrounding the joint are likely to atrophy, and the child is likely to lose range of motion in the joint. Pain management often requires a broad range of therapies including heat, cold, hydrotherapy, physical therapy, and others.

Opioids

Inadequate pain assessment and a lack of understanding of the types of pain both contribute to less than optimal pain management in children. Even late in the twentieth century, myths about children's ability to feel and remember pain impeded appropriate pain management. Myths and misunderstandings about the effects of opioids still contribute to their underutilization. Opioids can be used safely in children, and should be used when indicated. In infants up to 6 months of age, opioids are dosed at 25% to 33% of the mg/kg dose of older children, but titration to relief should be aggressive (Levetown & Frager, 2003, p. 53). Important principles of opioid use include the fact that there is no ceiling on opioid dosages (Hanks & Cherney, 1998). Frequently, the initial dose is not adequate to manage the child's pain, necessitating an increase in dose. Increases in the amount of opioid a child is receiving should not be by number of milligrams, but rather by percentage of the current dose. Dose increases can be in increments of 25% to 50%. Doses should include accommodations for breakthrough pain (usually 10% to 20% of the 24-hour dose) (Abrahm, 2000; Foley, 1998). Though multiple opioids exist, one principle of opioid use is not to add another opioid, but rather to increase the dose of the current opioids.

The clinician should anticipate side effects to opioid therapy. Children develop tolerance to the majority of unwanted opioid side effects; side effects dissipate over varying periods of time. Many side effects can be pharmacologically managed while tolerance develops. The one exception to this observation is constipation. Therefore, constipation should be anticipated and prophylactically treated. In certain cases, the side effect burden necessitates rotation (not adding) opioids, substituting one opioid for another in an effort to minimize side effects.

Opioids used appropriately do not cause addiction (Hanks & Cherney, 1998; McGrath, 1998). Providers must be able to distinguish physical dependence and tolerance (both predictable physiologic responses) from psychological dependence. The danger of respiratory depression is largely restricted to opioid-naïve patients receiving large initial doses. Children who are dying naturally experience respiratory depression. Naloxone should not be used solely for a decreased respiratory rate; there is a danger of reversing analgesia and precipitating withdrawal syndromes. Naloxone should be used for an unexpected respiratory depression (presuming adequate prognostication). If naloxone is used, it should be diluted and administered slowly (McGrath, 1998).

Pain Management Principles

Three principles of pain management include the following:

1. Assess for multiple causes of pain.
2. Treat each type of pain.
3. Reassess continually, especially when pain remains uncontrolled. (Storey & Knight, 2003, p. 16)

The World Health Organization has an analgesic ladder to guide pain management (WHO, 1996). Recommendations of Level I are the use of nonopioids plus adjuvant medications. Acetaminophen or NSAIDs are often appropriate at this level. The recommendations of Level 2 (persistent or increasing pain) include opioids for mild to moderate pain plus nonopioids plus adjuvant medications. If pain is not relieved or continues to increase, the recommendations of Level 3 are opioids for moderate to severe pain plus nonopioids plus adjuvant medications. Nonopioids are often combined with opioids because the former have an opioid-sparing effect, that is, using the two together allows for smaller does of opioids (McCaffery & Pasero, 1999). Also important for pain management are the five concepts of the WHO ladder: medication should be administered by the mouth, by the clock, by the ladder, for the individual, with attention to detail (Storey & Knight, 2003, p. 29). All medications have side effects. Nonopioids have ceiling doses that must not be exceeded. Not only does the risk of harm increase greatly when the ceiling dose is exceeded, but also the efficacy of the medication is not increased.

There are many other principles to pain management that are not addressed here. Several of the many excellent resources for the use of pain medication appear in the reference list for this chapter. Any palliative care provider must anticipate and ensure for the provision of optimal pain management. In addition, a pharmacist is an essential member of the palliative care team and can provide suggestions for information about routes, combinations, and interactions of medications.

End-of-Life Care

Although the death of a child in the United States is much less common than it once was, the reality is that 53,000 children (0 to 19 years) die in the United States every year, 36% from chronic conditions, and the remaining 64% from sudden causes (trauma, homicide, suicide, and SIDS) (Children's Project on Palliative/Hospice Care [ChiPPS], 2001). Children who die from sudden causes may require the symptom management and family decision-making aspects of palliative care. Almost 2% of children (ages 0 to 17) in the United States are living with severe illnesses. Though only about 5,000 children in the United States receive hospice services, it has been suggested that the 2% living with severe illness should be eligible for palliative care services (ChiPPS, 2001). As stated in the AAP recommendations, "If palliative care is reserved for children who are dying or have a terminal condition, other patients who may benefit from these services may not receive them" (AAP, 2000, p. 352). Because palliative care is not just for children who are dying but for all children who are seriously ill, the goals are compatible.

The recognition that a child is dying is arduous, complex, and painful. It causes upheaval in daily living and in the family's worldview (Feeg, Miller-Thiel, & Will, 2001). Interventions, as across palliative care, focus on the child and the family. For the child, the goal is to minimize the symptom burden and allow the child to say good-bye. For the family, the goal not only is to say good-bye, but also to leave them reassured that they have done all that can be done for the child. In addition, the nurses and the remainder of the palliative care team must collaborate to leave the family in the best position possible to adapt to life without the child after the death.

Hospice as a means to organize or frame end-of-life care is available to terminally ill children, although it is relatively rare for hospices to have specific staff to address the needs of terminally ill children. The same principles of caring for adults who are dying cannot apply. The pediatric palliative care team must be aware of those agencies that are qualified to provide care for children and families.

The goals of care must be clear. For children who are dying, it is often either the staff of the emergency department or the team who has been caring for the child across the child's chronic illness who become aware that the child is dying. In other cases, the family or even the child may be the first to confront the reality of impending death. Discussion about this is essential to diminish the child's and family's isolation. The child and family must be reassured that they will not go through the arduous process alone. Furthermore, the child and family are likely to have important ideas about how the child should die. This may include religious or family rituals, and even planning organ donation or the funeral.

In discussing the child's death with the child and family, it is important to find out what the child knows, as well as to convey comfort with the topic. Asking the child, "What do you think is going to happen?" is an ideal child-centered way to start the conversation. As with all serious discussions, those involved in the conversation must sit back and leave the discussion to the child and parents. Although children must be included in discussions, it is appropriate to talk with parents first. At the same time, it is not acceptable to attempt to hide this information from the child. The dying child knows he or she is dying, even as young as age 3 (Bluebond-Langner, 1978). It is appropriate to work with families to plan for the dissemination of information. The plan should also include where the child will die, who will be involved, and how symptoms will be managed.

For some children, death will follow a decision to discontinue life-prolonging therapies, often ventilators. For other children, death will follow the expected decline of a chronic disease, including cancer. For many children, death will be instantaneous. In those cases, the focus of care is first on the safety of the family, and then on helping family members make the first steps towards living without the physical presence of their child or sibling.

Most of the symptoms experienced by dying children are medically manageable. For some children, there is an increase in pain and other symptoms as death nears, such as dyspnea, seizures, or bleeding. There must be a plan to address these and other symptoms as soon as they appear. Utilization of palliative care specialists is essential to minimize the burden on symptoms. As noted by Field and Behrman (2003), "too often children with fatal or potentially fatal conditions and their families fail to receive competent, compassionate, and consistent care that meets their physicals, emotional, and spiritual needs." Not only do children deserve to die with as few symptoms as possible, but families also deserve not to be left with an image of their child's final hours as ones of agony for the child.

In many cases, how the child will die can be predicted. In these cases, pharmacologic and nonpharmacologic means of symptom management must be planned and implemented. In addition, the family must be prepared. If the child is dying at home, the family may be the ones implementing the plan. For example, if the child is likely to have a bleeding death, dark towels should be available to minimize the overwhelming appearance of bleeding that cannot be stopped.

There are some children whose symptoms are beyond traditional means of management. For those children, palliative sedation may be considered. The goal of palliative sedation is to relieve the child of overwhelming symptoms. The goal is not to hasten death (AAP, 2000). Whether or not palliative sedation is warranted must be based on the child's perception of the symptoms. In addition, the plan must be acceptable to the child and parents (Levetown & Frager, 2003).

Each of the models of palliative care described in this chapter has provisions for bereavement care for the family. It is the responsibility of the palliative care team to be aware of services that are specifically geared towards families bereaved by the death of a child. Unfortunately, those who provide bereavement services to families sometimes do not have the qualifications to provide care to this unique population. Palliative care providers should be aware not only of bereavement services for children and families, but also of the quality of those services. Visiting sites, speaking with providers, and asking about specific pediatric education and philosophy can be instructive.

MULTIDISCIPLINARY INTEGRATION AND PARTNERSHIP: CASE STUDY

Frances (Frannie) Williams is a 12-year-old who was diagnosed with cystic fibrosis (CF) when she was 7 months old. Her older brother and younger sister do not have the disease. When she was first diagnosed, Frannie's parents were both surprised and overwhelmed.

Within months, however, Frannie's treatments and medications became a regular part of the family routine.

For the past 3 days, Frannie has been coughing more. She looks pale and tired. Several of the girls in her day-camp group have been sick. Mrs. Williams takes Frannie to the CF clinic that she has been attending her whole life. Frannie is short of breath and wheezing and her appetite has been decreased for several days. She is admitted to the hospital and is diagnosed with Burkholderia cepacia. She is put on oxygen and aggressive antibiotic therapy. Her dyspnea is further relieved when she sits up in bed and leans forward over the bed stand. She continues to have no appetite and has lost weight and is sleeping much of the time. Her secretions are thicker and blood tinged.

Frannie's condition continued to deteriorate. When the health care team approached Mr. and Mrs. Williams with the care plan, the Williams asked to speak with the CF team. Several members of the CF team came to Frannie's room: the attending physician, the clinical nurse specialist (CNS), and the social worker. After the physician examined Frannie, he asked Mr. and Mrs. Williams to meet with him in the conference room. The CNS stayed behind to speak with Frannie. Frannie told the CNS that she was scared, and she asked, "What's going to happen to me?" The CNS replied, "We hope you'll get better, but you're really sick." Frannie nodded and said, "I know. I might die." The CNS then went to join the family meeting.

The physician reiterated what the parents already knew; Frannie's oxygenation was not good, she was continuing to lose weight, and she was still growing cepacia. The physician said that he believed Frannie was not likely to get better. The option of the ICU and the ventilator was still there, but he believed recovery was still unlikely.

The physician described several options: transfer to the ICU, continued care in the hospital, or continued care at home. Each would involve aggressive symptom management. The social worker explained that if Frannie were to go home, she could receive care from the hospital's home care department, but that she recommended hospice care. The physician also explained that if Frannie did go to the ICU, there would be a time-limited trial of ventilatory support, but that if Frannie did not improve, the ventilator would be withdrawn because it was not a comfortable experience. The physician ended the meeting by saying that they still hoped Frannie would recover, but it seemed unlikely at this point.

The next day Frannie was still not responding. After rounds, the CNS and the physician returned to speak with Frannie's parents. Again, they met in the conference room. The physician said that there had been no changes. Given her condition, the physician said, if her heart does stop, we will not do cardiopulmonary resuscitation (CPR). The physician explained that CPR was not likely to benefit

Frannie with the organ involvement she had. The CNS then explained the plan for continued aggressive symptom management. The focus at that point was on Frannie's dyspnea. Frannie's parents had decided they did not want her put on a ventilator.

Mr. and Mrs. Williams decided they didn't want to take Frannie home. The CNS and SW volunteered to meet with the other Williams children as needed, and both stopped by to meet the siblings while they were visiting. Frannie had many secretions, so a scopolamine patch was applied. It was explained that the secretions probably did not bother Frannie, but that this intervention was done for the family.

Though the family did not notice, the CNS pointed out that Frannie had stopped coughing, indicating that death was near. The CNS described other respiratory changes that also indicated death was near. The family was told that even though she didn't respond, she could probably still hear them. They were encouraged to speak with her and to play music that she liked. About 24 hours after the last time she spoke with her family, Frannie died.

SUMMARY

Perhaps more than any other specialty, interdisciplinary collaboration is the sine qua non of palliative care. This is a tremendous strength, a challenge, and an opportunity. Nurses have long striven to have their voices heard as strong, unique, and significant. Palliative care is structured in such a way that nurses must be included. It is structured so that nurses must collaborate with others towards what is best for this child and this family. Because each child and each family are different, each case must be individualized.

There are three dimensions to palliative care: aggressive symptom management, support in the process of patient and family decision-making, and, when appropriate, providing optimal end-of-life care. Palliative care can and should coexist with curative therapies. It must be interdisciplinary, and the team includes the patient and family. All those who care for children are responsible for knowing some level of symptom management. For cases of more complexity, referral to a pediatric palliative care team is essential. If the palliative care team does not have pediatric expertise, then a plan must be made to access that dimension of care.

REFERENCES

Abrahm, J. L. (2000). *A physician's guide to pain and symptom management in cancer patients*. Baltimore: Johns Hopkins University Press.

Ahmedzai, S. H., & Walsh, T. D. (2000). Palliative medicine and modern cancer care. *Seminars in Oncology, 27,* 1–6.

American Academy of Pediatrics Committee on Bioethics and Committee on Hospital Care. (2000). Palliative care for children. *Pediatrics, 106,* 351–357.

Baxt, C, Kassam-Adams, N., Nance, M. L., Vivarelli-O'Neill, C. & Winston, F. K. (2004). Assessment of pain after injury in the pediatric patient: Child and parent perceptions. *Journal of Pediatric Surgery, 39,* 979–983.

Center to Advance Palliative Care. (n.d.). *Primary, secondary, and tertiary models of palliative care delivery.* Retrieved August 27, 2004, from http://64.85.16.230/educate/content/rationale/modelsofcare.html

Bluebond-Langner, M. (1978). *The private worlds of dying children.* Princeton, NJ: Princeton University Press.

Children's Project on Palliative/Hospice Services (ChiPPS). (2001). *A call for change: Recommendations to improve the care of children living with life-threatening conditions.* Alexandria, VA: National Hospice and Pallitative Care Organization.

Christakis, N. A. (1999). *Death foretold: Prophecy and prognosis in medical care.* Chicago: University of Chicago Press.

Davies, B. (1998). The development of paediatric palliative care. In D. Doyle, G. W. C. Hanks, & N. MacDonald (Eds.), *Oxford textbook of palliative medicine* (2nd ed., pp. 1097–1098). New York: Oxford University Press.

Feeg, V. D., Miller-Thiel, J., & Will, J. (2001). Caring for children and with life-limiting illness and their families: Focus on pediatric hospice nursing. In A. Armstrong-Dailey & S. Zarbock, (Eds.), *Hospice care for children* (2nd ed.). New York: Oxford University Press.

Field, M. J., & Behrman, R. E. (Eds.), and Institute of Medicine Committee on Palliative and End of Life Care for Children and Their Families. (2003). *When children die: Improving palliative care services for children and their families.* Washington, DC: National Academies Press.

Foley, K. M. (1998). Pain assessment and cancer pain syndromes. In D. Doyle, G. W. C. Hanks, & N. MacDonald (Eds.), *Oxford textbook of palliative medicine* (2nd ed., pp. 310–331). New York: Oxford University Press.

Goldman, A. (1998). Life threatening illnesses and symptom control in children. In D. Doyle, G. W. C. Hanks, & N. MacDonald (Eds.), *Oxford textbook of palliative medicine* (2nd ed., pp. 1033–1043). New York: Oxford University Press.

Goodman, J. E., & McGrath, P. J. (1991). The epidemiology of pain in children and adolescents: A review. *Pain, 46,* 247–264.

Grothe, D. R., Scheckner, B., & Albano, D. (2004). Treatment of pain syndromes with venlafaxine. *Pharmacotherapy, 24,* 621–629.

Hanks, G., & Cherney, N. (1998). Opioid analgesic therapy. In D. Doyle, G. W. C. Hanks, & N. MacDonald (Eds.), *Oxford textbook of palliative medicine* (2nd ed., pp. 331–355). New York: Oxford University Press.

Harrison, C. M. (2003, May). *A practical approach to nausea and vomiting in terminal illness.* Presented to the University of Maryland Department of Anesthesiology, College Park.

International Association for the Study of Pain. (2003). Pain terminology. Retrieved October 18, 2004, from http://www.iasp-pain.org/terms-p.html#Pain

Jonsen, A. R., Siegler, M., & Winslade, W. J. (2002). *Clinical ethics: A practical approach to ethical decisions in clinical medicine* (5th ed.). New York: McGraw-Hill.

Levetown, M., & Frager, G. (2003). Unipac eight: The hospice/palliative medicine approach to caring for pediatric patients. In P. Storey & C. F. Knight (Eds.), *Assessment and treatment of pain in the terminally ill* (2nd ed.). Larchmont, NY: American Academy of Hospice and Palliative Medicine.

Lynn, J., Schuster, J. L., & Kabcenell, A. (2000). *Improving care for the end of life. A sourcebook for health care managers and clinicians.* Oxford: Oxford University Press.

Mahon, M. M. (1993). Children's concept of death and sibling death from trauma. *Journal of Pediatric Nursing, 8,* 335–344.

McCaffery, M., & Pasero, C. (1999). *Pain clinical manual* (2nd ed.). St. Louis, MO: Mosby.

McGrath, P. A. (1998). Pain control in paedriatric palliative care. In D. Doyle, G. W. C. Hanks, & N. MacDonald (Eds.), *Oxford textbook of palliative medicine* (2nd ed., pp. 1013–1031). New York: Oxford University Press.

McPherson, M., Weissman, G., Strickland, B. B., van Dyck, P. C., Blumberg, S. J., & Newacheck, P. W. (2004). Implementing community-based systems of services for children and youths with special health care needs: How well are we doing? *Pediatrics, 113*(Suppl. 5), 1538–1544.

Oleske, J. M., & Czarniecki, L. (1999). Continuum of palliative care: Lessons from caring for children infected with HIV-1. *Lancet, 345,* 1287–1291.

Portenoy, R. K. (1998). Adjuvant analgesics in pain management. In D. Doyle, G. W. C. Hanks, & N. MacDonald (Eds.), *Oxford textbook of palliative medicine* (2nd ed., pp. 361–390). New York: Oxford University Press.

Saunders, C. (1967). *The management of terminal illness.* London: Edward Arnold.

Storey, P., & Knight, C. F. (2003). *Assessment and treatment of pain in the terminally ill* (2nd ed.). Larchmont, NY: American Academy of Hospice and Palliative Medicine.

von Gunten, C. F., Ferris, F. D., Portenoy, R. K., & Glajchen, M. (2001). *Center to Advance Palliative Care Manual: How to establish a palliative care program.* New York: Center to Advance Palliative Care.

Waller, A., & Caroline, N. L. (2000). *Handbook of palliative care in cancer* (2nd ed.). Boston: Butterworth Heinemann.

Willis, M. H., Merkel, S. I., Voepel-Lewis, T., & Malviya, S. (2003). FLACC behavioral pain assessment scale: A comparison with the child's self-report. *Pediatric Nursing, 29,* 195–198.

Wolfe, J., Grier, H. E., Klar, N., Levin, S. B., Ellenbogen, J. M., Salem-Schatz, S., et al. (2000). Symptoms and suffering at the end of life in children with cancer. *New England Journal of Medicine, 342,* 326–333.

World Health Organization. (1990). *WHO definition of palliative care.* Retrieved February 10, 2005, from http://www.who.int/cancer/palliative/definition/en

World Health Organization (1996). *Cancer pain relief and palliative care.* Technical Report Series 804. Retrieved February 10, 2005, from http://www.wpro.who.int/pdf/pud/84/125.pdf

CHAPTER FOURTEEN

Health and Behavior Risk Assessment

Judith Vessey

INTRODUCTION, DEFINITIONS, AND THEIR MEASUREMENT

This chapter focuses on examining the guideline or indicator stating *that children's, youths' and families' health and risky behaviors and problems [be] identified and addressed* (Craft-Rosenberg, Krajicek, & Shin, 2002). Risky health behaviors (RHB) are of interest to nurses and the broader community, foremost because of the consequences to the individuals involved and the need for intervention but also because of the negative externalities to other members of society. Some of those externalities are the impact of unplanned pregnancies, costs associated with disabilities sustained secondary to using illicit substances, or the consequences of criminality. This chapter will primarily focus on RHB as manifested during adolescence, roughly ages 11 through 21 because it is this age group that most often engages in those activities that are not in their own best interests.

The term *risky health behaviors* is a generic and somewhat amorphous one, without a universally accepted definition, and an agreed upon set of specific behaviors does not exist. For the purposes of this discussion, risky health behaviors are considered to be any group of interactions between an individual's biopsychosocial processes and the environment, in which the activities have a volitional quality and the outcomes remain uncertain but often end in immediate or future harm to the instigator or others.

RHB comprise the major health risk to today's youths, collectively contributing to more than 70% of adolescent morbidity and mortality. Morbidity and mortality patterns begin emerging in late childhood, increase through adolescence, and serve as precursors for the majority of morbidity and mortality that occurs well into adulthood (Grunbaum et al., 2004). The increasing incidence and prevalence in youths' participation in RHB over the last several decades is due in part to an epidemiologic shift created by the successful eradication or management of acute illnesses and the subsequent rise in chronic conditions and concomitant psychosocial comorbidities, changing family compositions, and an era of escalating social and environmental stressors (Kipke, 1999).

The incidence and prevalence of individual youth's participation in RHB is difficult to quantify. The best available information comes from the Centers for Disease Control's Youth Risk Behavior Surveillance System (YRBSS). The YRBSS monitors six categories of priority health-risk behaviors through a national school-based survey of students in grades 9 through 12 (Grunbaum et al., 2004). These categories, the specific risks assessed, and the percentage of youth participation are reported in Table 14.1. The general consensus of health professionals is, however, that the extent of RHB and subsequent morbidity is under-estimated due to inadequate reporting systems and failure to correctly recognize, diagnose, and treat.

The rise of RHB and their sequelae has led to a substantive body of theoretical and empirical work, most of which has been promulgated over the past three decades. Epidemiological and intervention studies began in earnest during the 1980s, with the focus generally on a single deviant or illegal behavior associated with some form of social sanction, such as delinquency or unprotected sex. Collectively, these studies present a fairly inchoate group of findings that failed to provide robust explanatory models or satisfactory interventional frameworks and few of which have been adopted into evidence-based practice (New York Academy of Sciences, 2000). Since the mid 1990s, a complex nexus of developmental, interpersonal, and environmental conditions and their interface with RHB has been recognized. This has led to a significant movement away from studying single variable explanations of risk to investigating multivariate explanations. Today, risk research focuses on the natural history of risk-taking by youths; the structure, organization, and covariation among youths' developmental attributes, environmental conditions, and the development of risk behaviors; and the role of resilience and other protective factors in minimizing youths' participation in risk-taking activities.

TABLE 14.1 YRBSS: Percentage of Youths that Participate in Selected Health Risk Behaviors

Behavior	%
Behaviors that Contribute to Unintentional Injuries	
Rarely or never wore seatbelts	18.2
Rarely or never wore bicycle helmets	85.9
Rode with a driver who had been drinking alcohol	30.2
Drove after drinking alcohol	12.1
Behaviors that Contribute to Violence	
Carried a weapon	17.1
Carried a gun	6.1
In a physical fight	33.0
Injured in a physical fight	4.2
Dating violence	8.9
Forced to have sexual intercourse	9.0
Carried a weapon on school property	6.1
Threatened or injured with a weapon on school property	9.2
Engaged in a physical fight on school property	12.8
Did not go to school because of safety concerns	5.4
Property stolen or deliberately damaged on school property	29.8
Felt sad or hopeless	28.6
Seriously considered attempting suicide	16.9
Made a suicide plan	16.5
Attempted suicide	8.5
Suicide attempt required medical attention	2.9
Tobacco Use	
Lifetime cigarette use	58.4
Lifetime daily cigarette use	15.8
Current cigarette use	21.9
Current frequent cigarette use	9.7
Smoked > 10 cigarettes/day	3.1
Purchased cigarettes in a store or gas station	18.9
Current smokeless tobacco use	6.7
Current cigar use	14.8
Current tobacco use	27.5
Alcohol and Other Drug Use	
Lifetime alcohol use	74.9
Current alcohol use	44.9
Episodic heavy drinking	28.3
Lifetime marijuana use	40.2
Current marijuana use	22.4
Lifetime cocaine use	8.7

(continued)

TABLE 14.1 YRBSS: Percentage of Youths that Participate in Selected Health Risk Behaviors (*Continued*)

Behavior	%
Alcohol and Other Drug Use (con't)	
Current cocaine use	4.1
Lifetime illegal injection-drug use	3.2
Lifetime inhalant use	12.1
Current inhalant use	3.9
Lifetime illegal steroid use	6.1
Lifetime heroine use	3.3
Lifetime methamphetamine use	7.6
Lifetime ecstasy use	11.1
Smoked a whole cigarette before age 13 years	18.3
Drank alcohol before age 13 years	27.8
Tried marijuana before age 13 years	9.9
Cigarette use on school property	8.0
Smokeless tobacco use on school property	5.9
Alcohol use on school property	5.2
Marijuana use on school property	5.8
Offered, sold, or was given an illegal drug on school property	28.7
Sexual Behaviors	
Ever had sexual intercourse	46.7
Had first sexual intercourse before age 13 years	7.4
Had ≥ 4 sex partners during lifetime	14.4
Currently sexually active	34.3
Condom use during last sexual intercourse	63.0
Birth control pill use before last sexual intercourse	17.0
Alcohol or drug use before last sexual intercourse	25.4
Had been pregnant or gotten someone pregnant	4.2
Taught in school about AIDS or HIV infection	87.9
Dietary Behaviors/Nutrition	
Ate fruits and vegetables ≥ 5 times	22.0
Drank ≥ 3 glasses/day of milk	17.1
Physical Activities	
Participated in significant vigorous physical activity	62.6
Participated in sufficient moderate physical activity	24.7
Participated in an insufficient amount of physical activity	33.4
No vigorous or moderate physical activity	11.5
Enrolled in PE class	55.7
Attended PE class daily	28.4
Exercised or played sports > 20 minutes during an average PE class	80.3
Did strengthening exercises	51.9

(*continued*)

TABLE 14.1 *(Continued)*

Behavior	%
Physical Activities (con't)	
Played on ≥ 1 sports teams	57.6
Watched ≥ 3 hours/day of TV	38.2
Overweight and Weight Control	
At risk behavior for becoming overweight	15.4
Overweight	13.5
Described themselves as overweight	29.6
Were trying to lose weight	43.8
Ate less food, fewer calories, or foods low in fat to lose weight or to keep from gaining weight	42.2
Exercised to lose weight or to keep from gaining weight	57.1
Went without eating for ≥ 24 hours to lose weight or to keep from gaining weight	13.3
Took diet pills, powders, or liquids to lose weight or to keep from gaining weight	9.2
Vomited or took laxatives to lose weight or to keep from gaining weight	6.0

Note. Data taken from "Youth Risk Behavior Surveillance—United States, 2003, by J. Grunbaum, L. Kann, S. Kinchen, J. Ross, J. Hawkins, R. Lowry, R. et al., 2004, *Surveillance Summaries, MMWR: Morbidity and Mortality Weekly Report, 53*(No. SS-2), 1–29.

INFLUENCES OF HEALTH AND BEHAVIOR RISK FOR YOUTHS

Related Theoretical Frameworks

In the beginning of the twentieth century, psychoanalysts concluded that engaging in risky behaviors was evidence of a diseased mind (Llewellyn, 2003). Although now discredited, no single theoretical framework has filled this vacuum. A variety of highly disparate theories are used in describing, explaining, or predicting aspects of RHB.

Specific theories based on dispositional personality traits such as sensation-seeking, locus of control, cognitive appraisal, self-efficacy, or temperament may account for a youth's propensity to take risks. Yet, though a number of behavioral correlates have been identified, no causal relationships or specific personality profiles have been explicated (Rolison & Scherman, 2002). Developmental models view risk-taking as a way of meeting normative adolescent developmental tasks, and these models provide explanatory frameworks for studying RHB. Common frameworks used in health promotion research have been applied, such as the health belief model and protection-motivation theory, but they do not fully capture the complexity of risk-taking behavior. Contextualism and ecological models highlight problematic interactions of youths with their environments and are useful in understanding RHB but are of limited help in designing interventions because many of identified risk factors are not easily modified. Biological contributions, including behavioral genetic expressions and neuroendocrine influences on neuroregulation, and behavioral choice also have been posited but remain underinvestigated (Irwin & Millstein, 1992). Finally, social capital theory and behavioral economic theories have been applied to RHB to help estimate and predict the occurrence of specific risky behaviors and their welfare consequences, but to date have met with limited success (Gruber, 2001; O'Donoghue & Rabin, 2000).

Theoretical support for research on RHB is currently undergoing a fundamental paradigm shift away from models that attempt to explain or predict RHB to models that identify protective factors—those conditions that prevent or modify risk factors or improve the familial, sociocultural, and economic circumstances of families and youths—that promote resilience. By helping youths successfully mature in healthy ways despite psychological stressors, adverse social situations, or physical limitations, their participation in RHB will be minimized.

Synthesis of the Literature

Risky behaviors are prevalent in all socioeconomic, racial/ethnic, and cultural subgroups across all geographic locales (Kipke, 1999). Youths are more likely to engage in risky behaviors in the presence of a nexus of individual, familial, scholastic, and community factors; multiple factors are synergistic and not merely additive (Substance Abuse and Mental Health Services Administration/Center for Substance Abuse Prevention [SAMHSA/CSAP], n.d.). These factors are summarized in Table 14.2. Because of the large number of factors that come into play, the distribution of RHB across youths is highly uneven. Variation is due in part to the relative risk youths perceive in any given activity, something that is heavily influenced by cultural norms and beliefs. Moreover, RHB rarely occur singularly but tend to covary within youths, with selected subgroups of youths engaging in multiple problem behaviors. Generally the younger the age and the larger number of risk behaviors a youth exhibits, the more problematic the outlook (Barrios, Everett, Simon, & Brener, 2000; Brener, Krug, & Simon, 2000; Everett, Giovino, Warren, Crossett, & Kann, 1998).

Although learning to take risks is a normal part of the developmental process, selected conditions in the lives of infants and children influence their likelihood for engagement in RHB with maturity. Knowledge, beliefs, and attitudes garnered throughout childhood lay the foundation for both appropriate and inappropriate risk-taking activities. By adolescence, key developmental tasks—identity formation, gaining autonomy

TABLE 14.2 Individual, Familial, Scholastic, and Community Factors Associated with Promoting Risky Behavior in Youths

Individual Risk Factors

- Inaccurate self-appraisal, such as body image, self-esteem, and skill sets
- Gender
- Personality traits
  - Difficult temperament
  - Sensation-seeking and lowered sense for avoiding harm
  - External locus of control
  - Poor impulse control
  - Poor sense of humor
  - Lack of empathy
- Psychopathology, such as conduct disorders
- Internalized negative values
  - Poor social/coping skills; social maladjustment, alienation from family/school
- Underdeveloped communication, critical thinking, and decision-making abilities
- Inability to accept responsibility for one's own actions
- Failure to visualize a positive future

Familial Factors

- Poor parenting and familial connectedness
  - Unsupportive or ambivalent relationships with parents
  - Lack of parental involvement in children's activities
  - Cold or laissez-faire parental attitudes
  - Parental use of guilt as a discipline/behavioral control tactic
  - Parents with mental health problems
  - Inadequate parental-child communication
- Chaotic home environments
  - Poor role-modeling by parents
  - Abuse and neglect
  - Ready access to firearms, alcohol, tobacco, and drugs
- Minimal religiosity or spirituality
- Few opportunities to foster healthy developmental transitions
- Unclear behavioral boundaries and consequences
- Inadequate social support systems, familial isolation
- Poverty

Scholastic Factors

- Dysfunctional educational system and poor school climate
- Academic difficulties, poor achievement
- High absenteeism
- School disconnectedness
  - Little participation in extracurricular activities

(continued)

TABLE 14.2 Individual, Familial, Scholastic, and Community Factors Associated with Promoting Risky Behavior in Youths *(Continued)*

Peer Factors

* A deviant peer group
* High affiliation and peer approval needs

Community Factors

* Impoverished community with a poor health services infrastructure
* Ready access to firearms, alcohol, tobacco, and drugs
* Few community policies or legislation that support prevention

Note. Data on risk factors were primarily drawn from these sources: *Handbook of Health Behavior Research* (Vols. 1–4), by D. S. Gochman (Ed.), 1997, New York: Plenum Press; and *SAMHSA/CSAP Prevention Protocols*, by Substance Abuse and Mental Health Services Administration/Center for Substance Abuse Prevention (n.d.), available online at http://www.ncbi.nlm.nih.gov/books/bv.fcgi?rid=hstat5.part.13409

from parents, and establishing a personal value system—serve as the lenses through which youths pursue opportunities, make decisions, and hopefully learn from the accompanying mistakes (Cowell & Marks, 1997).

For all adolescents, the lack of experience, sense of invulnerability, and limited, romanticized future orientation make it difficult for them to recognize a full array of behavioral consequences (Jessor, 1998; Rolison & Scherman, 2002). Although youths have the capacity for decision making, they value the anticipated consequences of their decisions differently than adults do, more likely choosing to engage in behaviors they believe will bring immediate gratification *from their worldview* (Gruber, 2001). Over time and with experience, youths generally become more competent decision-makers.

Youths who are more heavily influenced by sensation seeking and peer reaction, and who have a heightened sense of invincibility and impulsivity coupled with poor appraisal skills and limited cognitive capacity are more likely to engage in RHB (Greene, Krcmar, Walters, Rubin, & Jerold Hale, 2000; Little, Axford, & Morpeth, 2004; Rolison, & Scherman, 2002; Steinberg, 2004). When a youth's family, school, and larger community environments fail to provide appropriate structure and guidance, peer groups and other external influences such as the media take precedence in the youth's decision making.

INFLUENCES OF HEALTH AND BEHAVIOR RISK FOR THE FAMILY

The first decade of life lays the foundation for the development of health behaviors, risk avoidance, and intrapersonal resiliency (Green & Palfrey, 2002; O'Brien, & Bush, 1997). Therefore, the family plays a pivotal role in helping their children establish lifelong healthy behaviors. Outcomes for children's long-term psychosocial health bode well when parents provide a nurturing environment and protect them from traumatizing events; inversely, poor parenting is the most robust predictor of children's behavioral health issues later in life (Gochman, 1997b).

Family culture helps determine youth participation in RHB. Authoritative parenting, where direction and love are given in ample quantities, is most likely to result in youths who are interpersonally competent and less likely to experiment in RHB. Youths from democratic families are also likely to be competent, but exhibit greater risk-taking potential (Gochman, 1997a). Youths face greater challenges in resisting RHB if they come from families that embrace either an authoritarian or laissez-faire parenting style, lacking in love or supervision, respectively. Other risk factors are family cultures that encourage competition and aggressiveness or promote early-childhood autonomy, particularly if the parents are emotionally detached.

Selected ethnic and cultural beliefs, such as promoting machismo in males or condoning early sexual activity, further influence risk-taking by family members (Gochman, 1997a). Familial attitudes and expectations may vary according to the child's gender, with boys ultimately engaging in greater risk taking and girls exhibiting greater health concerns (Waldron, 1997). Although RHB are thought to occur more frequently in youths from families with low socioeconomic status, it is not family status per se. Rather, a confluence of factors place youths at risk, including multiple family stressors, inadequate parenting skills, living in an impoverished neighborhood with poor connectedness among its residents, and increased opportunities to participate in RHB (Dryfoos, 1990; Gochman, 1997b; Little et al., 2004).

Because participation by youths in RHB are rarely isolated events but rather are embedded in complex familial and societal processes, positive family relationships and the provision of appropriate structure are two powerful determinants of successful outcomes. Both require significant parental or guardian involvement (Baranowski & Hearn, 1997). Modeling appropriate behaviors, restricting inappropriate media exposure, and monitoring their children's free time are powerful predictors of later behaviors (Gochman, 1997b; Tinsley, 1997).

NURSING CARE EXCELLENCE

To maximize success in reducing risky behaviors and subsequent morbidity and mortality in youths, attention must be given to reduce individual risks while enhancing protective factors and building resilience.

Emphasis should be on systematically identifying those intrapersonal, familial, and community factors that can be modified and ensuring that practitioners have the necessary resources and skills to intervene using best practices.

Initially, strategies need to be directed toward guaranteeing that appropriate health services are available. Adolescent health services are likely to be efficacious when they are readily accessible, quality based, coordinated, confidential, affordable, and flexible in meeting diverse needs (Green & Palfrey, 2002). The reality is inadequate adolescent-specific primary health care services, a fragmented mental health system, and insufficient community and school-based resources. Reimbursement structures also are generally inadequate for preventive health care services or those needed by youths engaging in RHB. The situation is further compounded because the cohort of youths most likely to engage in RHB are the least likely to be proactive in seeking out health care services.

Youths feel more welcome to participate or even initiate discussions about RHB when there is an established trusting relationship with their health care provider. This requires that youths feel cared for and listened to, and that their provider is willing to give the time necessary to explore the difficult issues they face. Unfortunately, most primary care providers have limited skills in counseling youths on risky behaviors. Adolescents indicated that only one in five health care providers were successful in creating such a milieu (Foundation for Accountability [FACCT] and the Robert Wood Johnson Foundation, 2001).

Teens are usually unwilling to discuss their participation in RHB with parents present and may be reluctant to seek help independently, fearing confidentiality concerns. They should always be interviewed alone and their privacy respected. Nurses need to be aware of their respective state legislation specific to parental rights in viewing their child's health record. Confidentiality must be ensured within the confines of the law with the proviso that only very serious risks to an adolescent's health would override this commitment. Although every effort should be made to encourage communication between youths and their parents, in selected cases this is undesirable. Specific strategies designed to protect youths' confidentiality can then be employed and may include shredding screening documentation or keeping secondary records separate from the primary chart until the adolescent reaches 18.

Prevention

Nurse-client encounters frequently occur during periods of developmental transitions; providing anticipatory guidance to families and youths during these periods is ideal because health behaviors are in a state of flux. Parental influence is strongest prior to the initiation of RHB behaviors by their children and has been correlated with their children's tobacco use, drug experimentation, sexual initiation, and condom use. After experimentation begins, peer and societal factors exert a greater influence (Kelder, Edmundson, & Lytle, 1997). The media further influences youths' health behaviors by suggesting that the images portrayed are in some way socially acceptable. Strong correlations between food advertisements and poor eating habits and obesity have been shown; weaker correlations have been shown between pharmaceutical advertisements and illicit drug experimentation. Viewing sexual and violent materials are also implicated as correlates to adolescent risk-taking (Gochman, 1997b). For these reasons, nurses and other health care providers need to adopt a dual approach of strengthening family and community supports while reducing or eliminating environmental risk across the developmental trajectory.

For many families, fears and stigma about behavioral health issues makes them reluctant to seek help early, with such problems remaining hidden until their child exhibits frank psychosocial sequelae. Nurses have the responsibility to increase public awareness about health risk behaviors and the behavioral consequences, and provide educational support for preventing or reducing youths' participation in risky behaviors. Emphasis needs to be on creating supportive milieus in schools and communities where youths feel safe and connected (Prakash, n.d.). Both schools and their larger communities can set standards and regulate opportunities that promote health while creating barriers to participation in RHB (Kelder et al., 1997). For example, school and community personnel such as coaches and scout leaders who interface with youths in a variety of settings often have a profound impact on adolescents' behavioral choices (Ungar, 2004). They should be encouraged to exert their influence, identify youths at risk for engaging in RHB, and be provided with avenues of referral.

Assessment

In addition to prevention activities, nurses need to have a healthy skepticism and consider that even the most unlikely youths may engage in RHB—whether from naïveté, ignorance, peer pressure, or rebellion. Coming from a "good" family or community in and of itself does not lessen the risk for participation. Screening for RHB as well as for protective factors should be an integral part of adolescent primary care visits and developmental surveillance. The former identifies areas for immediate intervention, whereas the latter helps nurses identify strengths upon which youths can rely and providers can support and facilitate.

Using simple mnemonics can help ensure that nurses and other providers interview youths about the major risk categories (See Box 14.1). Guides that are more formalized also may be used. The most widely recognized evidence-based guide is *Guidelines for Adolescent Preventive Services* (GAPS) (Montalto, 1998). GAPS was developed by the American Medical Association's Department of Adolescent Health for youths aged 11 to 21 and contains 24 evidence-based health care recommendations. Although not solely designed to address RHB, a substantial portion of the instrument is dedicated to identifying RHB and intervening in order to reduce their occurrence or minimize their sequelae. GAPS provides health care providers with preventive service recommendations and a flow sheet for documenting these services and outcomes. More information is available at http://www.amassn.org/ama/pub/category/1980.html.

A number of standardized screening measures also are available that help identify youths engaging in risky behaviors. They vary significantly in their scope, psychometric adequacy, and clinical utility; many are normed for a narrow population or cultural group. One useful instrument

---

BOX 14.1 Mnemonics Useful in Evaluating Participation in Risky Health Behaviors

HEADS

H   Home, habits
E   Education, employment, exercise
A   Accidents, ambitions, activities, abuse
D   Drugs (tobacco, alcohol, others, diet, depression
S   Sex, suicide

SAFE TEEN

S   Sexuality
A   Accident, abuse
F   Firearms/homicide
E   Emotions (suicide/depression)

T   Toxins (tobacco/alcohol/drugs)
E   Environment (school, home, friends)
E   Exercise
N   Nutrition

Note. Information adapted from "Implementing the Guidelines for Adolescent Preventive Services," by N. J. Montalto, 1998, *American Family Physician, 57,* pp. 2181–2190. Copyright 1998 by American Academy of Family Physicians. Adapted with permission.

that is available in the public domain is the Problem-Oriented Screening Instrument for Teenagers (POSIT). This valid and reliable tool consists of 10 scales, or problem areas (139 questions) primarily designed to screen troubled youths 12 to 19 years of age for RHB that may be amenable to treatment. It has high clinical utility and may be used with individuals or groups. POSIT is available through the National Institute on Alcohol Abuse and Alcoholism (NIAAA, n.d.). Other widely accepted instruments available in the public domain can be found in Table 14.3.

Intervention

Interventions should be prioritized around those RHB that a youth is most likely to engage in and are associated with the most serious sequelae. Although specific interventions such as counseling, behavioral contracting, and referral will vary by type of RHB, severity of risk, and practice setting, interventions should be geared at simultaneously reducing modifiable risk factors while improving protective factors. This two-pronged approach has been shown to be the most efficacious in producing long-term behavior change (Resnick, 2000). Youths should be helped to evaluate trade-offs between short-term thrills and the long-term costs of real situations. They particularly need help in learning how to evaluate the response costs of their actions and building coping skills to manage peer pressure and environmental influences that make avoiding RHB difficult (Gruber, 2001). When there is a good provider-patient relationship, counseling can be highly effective, particularly when combined

TABLE 14.3 Screening Instruments for Specific Cohorts of Risk Factors

Risk Factor and Instrument	Citation
General Behavior	
Pediatric Symptom Checklist	http://psc.partners.org/psc_literature.htm
Eating Disorders	
The SCOFF Questionnaire	http://bmj.bmjjournals.com/cgi/content/full/319/7223/1467
Substance Abuse	
The CAGE Alcohol Abuse Screener	http://chipts.ucla.edu/assessment/Assessment_Instruments/ Assessment_files_new/assess_cage.htm
The CRAFFT	http://www.ceasar-boston.org/studies/crafft.html

with long-term follow-up. Skill-building activities such as role-playing, peer counseling, and support groups are strategies known to be effective. Ongoing, meaningful social support promotes adherence and better outcomes. If possible, parents and school personnel should be involved to ensure that messages and expectations are consistent. Three efficacious approaches are parent and family skills training, in-home family support, and family therapy (Baranowski & Hearn, 1997; Lightfoot, 1997).

Resources

Some nurses and other health care providers may not feel competent in confronting the complex problem of risky behaviors, reporting that they do not routinely screen youths due to inadequate knowledge, skills, time, and reimbursement. However, reducing inappropriate risk-taking and promoting resilience are a paramount to providing quality adolescent health care. Several national prevention programs can help health care providers hone their skills in working with high-risk youths. One such initiative is the KySS campaign, sponsored in part by the National Association of Pediatric Nurse Practitioners (NAPNAP). This campaign emphasizes educational-behavioral interventions to teach youths and their parents about all aspects of physical and emotional safety and to build developmental assets (see http://www.napnap.org/partnerships/programs/kyssprogram.html for a full report of the (Melnyk et al., 2001; Melnyk, Brown, Jones, Kreipe, & Novak, 2003). A core curriculum will be available in the foreseeable future.

A second initiative called Bright Futures is a general health promotion project dedicated to the principle that every child deserves to be healthy and promulgates the need for trusting relationships between the health professional, children and their families, and the community as partners in health practice. Materials for Bright Futures materials were constructed and reviewed by multidisciplinary panels and offer a practical developmental approach to providing health supervision for children and adolescents from birth through age 21. They may be accessed at http://www.brightfutures.org/

A variety of evidence-based RHB prevention protocols designed for providers and community workers published by Substance Abuse and Mental Health Services Administration/ Center for Substance Abuse Prevention (SAMHSA/CSAP) are available at http://www.ncbi.nlm.nih.gov/books/bv.fcgi?rid=hstat5.part.13409. The National Guidelines Clearinghouse, sponsored by the U.S. Agency for Healthcare Quality (AHRQ) and the Department of Health and Human Services, is another public resource. Their Web site (www.guidelines.gov) posts evidence-based guidelines developed by professional organizations and public agencies. Guidelines are available for many specific risk factors, including substance abuse, tobacco cessation, and HIV prevention.

MULTIDISCIPLINARY INTEGRATION AND PARTNERSHIPS: A CASE STUDY

Marie McGuire is a school nurse at a middle school in an affluent community and is a member of her school's Safe Schools initiative. The Safe Schools committee is comprised of the principal, guidance counselor, school nurse, teacher, health safety officer, coach, and parent and community representatives. Collectively, they are responsible for overseeing the climate of the school and working with children identified to be at risk.

Caitlin is a chubby 12-year-old, an only child from an upper-middle-class home, and new to her middle school. She recently transferred because this school offered more supports for students like her who have been diagnosed with attention deficit hyperactivity disorder (ADHD). A "latchkey kid," Caitlin comes home to an empty house each day after school until her parents return from work late in the evening. Her parents worry about her impulsivity but Caitlin thinks she is too old for a nanny; instead, she agrees not to leave the house or to have friends in. Caitlin spends her afternoons munching on snacks while she surfs the Internet. Recently, she has been conversing about music videos and sex in a teen chat room with a boy who says he is 15. He is pressuring Caitlin for her address so he can come over or meet in town; she has already sent him her picture. Caitlin is thinking, "What could be the harm? He's so nice!" Caitlin, who goes to the health suite each day for her medication, shares her excitement about her newfound romance and their plans with Ms. McGuire.

Unfortunately, such situations are all too common and particularly problematic as youths such as Caitlin fly below the radar until something unseemly occurs. Although at first glance Caitlin appears fine, she is dealing with a numerous risk factors including loneliness, impulsivity, poor nutrition leading to obesity, and the possible sexual exploitation resulting from her cyber friendship. Working with members of the Safe Schools team, Ms. McGuire identified and coordinated activities that minimized Caitlin's risk. The school safety officer immediately helped Caitlin recognize the risks of meeting unknown individuals, further suggesting that content be added to the school's health curriculum regarding cyber stalking. While protecting her privacy concerning the aborted affair, the counselor explored supervised after-school activities with Caitlin and her parents. Capitalizing on her computer skills, Caitlin began serving as a mentor in an after-school tutoring program for elementary students and participating in her school's drama club. Her parents also adjusted their schedules so someone would be home by 6 each night. Ms McGuire helped Caitlin chose a healthier diet and developed a plan to increase her exercise.

Multidisciplinary integration and partnerships are required to address diverse challenges such as this. Concepts and knowledge about RHB from diverse fields of study and disciplines are necessary to create new and unique approaches to the problem. The synergies created as a result of such collaborations identify major opportunities and gaps in knowledge development and clinical care that no single discipline alone would likely be successful in addressing.

SUMMARY

Although adolescence is the time for experimentation, a quality parent-child relationship marked by open communication with judicious supervision and structured opportunities to interface within the community help youths successfully navigate these potentially treacherous times. Nurses and other health care providers who work directly with youths can help them recognize potential risks and develop psychosocial competence and emotional resilience. They can further assist parents develop a parenting style that is more likely to result in positive youth outcomes.

REFERENCES

Baranowski, T., & Hearn, M. D. (1997). Health behavior interventions with families. In D. S. Gochman (Ed.), *Handbook of health behavior research* (Vol. 4, pp. 303–321). New York: Plenum Press.

Barrios, L. C., Everett, S. A., Simon, T. R., & Brener, N. D. (2000). Suicide ideation among U.S. college students: Associations with other injury risk behaviors. *Journal of the American College of Health, 48*, 229–233.

Brener, N. D., Krug, E. G., & Simon, T. R. (2000). Trends in suicide ideation and suicidal behavior among high school students in the United States, 1991–1997. *Suicide and Life-Threatening Behavior, 30*, 304–312.

Cowell, J. M., & Marks, B. A. (1997). Health behavior in adolescents. In D. S. Gochman (Ed.), *Handbook of health behavior research* (Vol. 3, pp. 73–96). New York: Plenum Press.

Craft-Rosenberg, M., Krajicek, M. J., & Shin, D-S. (2002). Report of the American Academy of Nursing Child-Family Panel: Identification of quality and outcome indicators for maternal child nursing. *Nursing Outlook, 50*, 57–60.

Dryfoos, J. G. (1990). *Culture of risk taking*. New York: Oxford University Press.

Everett, S. A., Giovino, G. A., Warren, C. W., Crossett, L., & Kann, L. (1998). Other substance use among high school students who use tobacco. *Journal of Adolescent Health, 23,* 289–296.

Foundation for Accountability and the Robert Wood Johnson Foundation. (2001). *A portrait of adolescents in America, 2001.* Portland, OR: Foundation for Accountability.

Gochman, D. S. (1997a). Demography, development, and diversity of health behavior: An integration. In D. S. Gochman (Ed.), *Handbook of health behavior research* (Vol. 3, pp. 325–350). New York: Plenum Press.

Gochman, D. S. (1997b). *Handbook of health behavior research* (Vols. 1–4). New York: Plenum Press.

Green, M., & Palfrey, J. S. (Eds.). (2002). *Bright futures* (2nd ed.). Washington, DC: National Center for Education in Maternal-Child Health.

Greene, K., Krcmar, M., Walters, L. H., Rubin, D. L., & Jerold Hale, L. (2000). Targeting adolescent risk-taking behaviors: The contributions of egocentrism and sensation-seeking. *Journal of Adolescence, 23,* 439–461.

Gruber, J. (2001). *Risky behavior among youths. An economic analysis.* Chicago: University of Chicago Press.

Grunbaum, J., Kann, L., Kinchen, S., Ross, J., Hawkins, J., Lowry, R., et al. (2004). Youth risk behavior surveillance—United States, 2003. *Surveillance Summaries: Morbidity and Mortality Weekly Report, 53* (No. SS-2), 1–29.

Irwin, C. E., & Millstein, S. G. (1992). Risk-taking behaviors and biopsychosocial development during adolescence. In E. J. Susman, L. V. Fegans, & W. J. Ray (Eds.), *Emotion, cognition, health, and development in children and adolescents* (pp. 75–102). Hillsdale, NJ: Lawrence Erlbaum.

Jessor, R. (1998). *New perspectives on adolescent risk behavior.* New York: Cambridge University Press.

Kelder, S. H., Edmundson, R. W., & Lytle, L. A. (1997). Health behavior research and school and youth health promotion. In D. S. Gochman (Ed.), *Handbook of health behavior research* (Vol. 4, pp. 263–284). New York: Plenum Press.

Kipke, M. D. (Ed.). (1999). *Risks and opportunities: Synthesis of studies on adolescence.* Washington, DC: National Academy Press.

Lightfoot, C. (1997). *The culture of risk-taking.* New York: Guilford Press.

Little, M., Axford, N., & Morpeth, L. (2004). Research review: Risk and protection in the context of services for children in need. *Child and Family Social Work, 9,* 105–112.

Llewellyn, D. J. (2003). *Psychoanalytic theory.* Retrieved January 23, 2005, from http://www.risktaking.co.uk/intro.htm#psycho

Montalto, N. J. (1998). Implementing the guidelines for adolescent preventive services. *American Family Physician, 57,* 2181–2190.

Melnyk, B. M., Brown, H. E., Jones, D. C., Kreipe, R., & Novak, J. (2003). Improving the mental/psychosocial health of U.S. children and adolescents: Outcomes and implementation strategies from the National KySS Summit. *Journal of Pediatric Health Care, 17*(Suppl. 6), S1–S24.

Melnyk, B. M., Moldenhauer, Z., Veenema, T., Gullo, S., McMurtrie, M., O'Leary, E., et al. (2001). The KySS (Keep your children/yourself Safe and

Secure) campaign: A national effort to reduce psychosocial morbidities in children and adolescents. *Journal of Pediatric Health Care, 15*(2), 31A–34A.

National Institute on Alcohol Abuse and Alcoholism Problem (n.d.). *Oriented Screening Instrument for Teenagers.* Retrieved December 1, 2004, from http://www.niaaa.nih.gov/publications/publications.htm

New York Academy of Sciences. (2000). *Adolescent brain development. Vulnerabilities and opportunities.* Retrieved December 1, 2004, from http://www.nyas.org/ebriefreps/main.asp?intSubSectionID=328

O'Brien, R. W., & Bush, P. J. (1997). Health behavior in children. In D. S. Gochman (Ed.), *Handbook of health behavior research* (Vol. 3, pp. 49–67). New York: Plenum Press.

O'Donoghue, T., & Rabin, M. (2000). Risky behavior among youths: Some issues from behavioral economics. *Institute of Business and Economic Research,* Paper E00'285. Retrieved November 29, 2004, from http://repositories.cdlib.org/cgi/viewcontent.cgi?article=1028&context=iber/econ

Prakash, L. G. (n.d.). *Preventing substance abuse among children and adolescents: Family-centered approaches (reference guide).* (DHHS Publication No. SMA 3223-FY98). Retrieved December 2, 2004, from http://www.ncbi.nlm.nih.gov/books/bv.fcgi?rid=hstat5.chapter.18271

Resnick, M. D. (2000). Protective factors, resiliency, and health youth development. *Adolescent Medicine, 11,* 157–164.

Rolison, M. R., & Scherman, A. (2002). Factors influencing adolescents' decisions to engage in risk-taking behavior. *Adolescence, 37,* 585–596.

Substance Abuse and Mental Health Services Administration/Center for Substance Abuse Prevention. (n.d.). *SAMHSA/CSAP prevention enhancement protocols.* Retrieved December 1, 2004, from http://www.ncbi.nlm.nih.gov/books/bv.fcgi?rid=hstat5.part.13409

Steinberg, L. (2004). Risk taking in adolescence: What changes, and why? *Annals of the New York Academy of Sciences, 1021,* 51–58.

Tinsley, B. J. (1997). Maternal influences on children's health behavior. In D. S. Gochman (Ed.), *Handbook of health behavior research* (Vol. 1, pp. 223–240). New York: Plenum Press.

Ungar, M. (2004). The importance of parents and other caregivers to the resilience of high-risk adolescents. *Family Process, 43,* 23–41.

Waldron, I. (1997). Changing gender roles and gender differences in health behavior. In D. S. Gochman (Ed.), *Handbook of health behavior research* (Vol. 1, pp. 303–328). New York: Plenum Press.

CHAPTER FIFTEEN

Developmental Transition Care: Children, Youth, and Families Receive Care That Supports Development

Cecily Betz

INTRODUCTION, DEFINITIONS, AND THEIR MEASUREMENT

The word "transition" is derived from the Latin prefix *trans* meaning "across, beyond, to go beyond" (Harper, 2000). According to Meleis, transition refers to "a passage or movement from one state, condition, or place to another" (Schumacher & Meleis, 1994, p. 119). Meleis submits that there are four types of transition: developmental, situational, health/illness, and organizational (Schumacher & Meleis, 1994). Transitions have important cultural and clinical significance. The transition from one period of development to another is viewed as an important rite of passage that is often acknowledged with a formal ceremony, celebration, or both. Some of these transitions include the graduation ceremonies that signify the successful completion of an academic program whether it is at the elementary, middle, high school, and college levels. Other transitions are based on religious or cultural practices such as the coming of age ceremonies of the Jewish Bat or Bar Mitvzah, the Catholic confirmation, and the Mexican Quinceanera (Meleis, Sawyer, Im, Hilfinger Messias, & Schumacher, 2000; Meleis & Trangenstein, 1994; Schumacher & Meleis, 1994).

Situational transitions may be caused by environmental factors such as war, civil disorders, natural disasters, and economic turmoil. Transitions may be brought about by familial circumstances caused by divorce, relocation, unemployment, birth of a sibling, and death of a family member. Situational transitions have role-altering consequences, forcing the child to alter behaviors and attitudes significantly. Organizational transitions refer to the changes a child will experience due to agency or system requirements. For example, transitions are conferred by federal or state legal mandates, such as attaining the age of majority, which enables the adolescent to have greater legal authority and responsibility for accessing and obtaining school and health services. Last, health/illness transitions refer to the circumstances that a child will experience due to a disability or chronic condition, such as recovery from cancer, activity limitations due to a deteriorating neuromuscular condition, or the acquisition of self-care skills that enable the child to become more self-sufficient in managing his or her type 1 diabetes (Grey, Boland, Davidson, Li, & Tamborlane, 2000; Grey & Kanner, 2000).

Although there are a myriad of transitions that most, if not all, children will face as they develop, there are those transitions that will affect a very small number of children such as those associated with a special health care need (SHCN)[1] or the premature death of a parent (McPherson et al., 1998; McPherson & Honberg, 2002). The purpose of this chapter is to explain the relevance for nurses in addressing the transition needs of infants, children, and adolescents, and to provide a clinical example of application for practice. The process of transition from childhood to adulthood for adolescents with special health care needs (ASHCN) will be presented to illustrate the components of the transition planning process that include assessment, diagnosis, planning, intervention, and evaluation of outcomes. Transition is an important area of clinical practice for nurses, and the information provided in this chapter will provide the support for addressing childhood developmental transitions.

ADOLESCENT TRANSITIONS

Every stage of human development involves a process of anticipatory preparation before entering it. The process of preparation will vary, depending on the developmental tasks to be acquired in the upcoming stage,

---

[1]"Children with special health care needs are those who have or are at increased risk for a chronic physical, developmental, behavioral, or emotional condition and who also require health and related services of a type or amount beyond that required by children generally" (McPherson et al., 1998, p. 4). For the purposes of this chapter, this term will be used to describe the population of adolescents and children with chronic conditions and disabilities.

the level of social support from family, and the circle of friends, prerequisite skills, and personal characteristics of the individual. For children who transition from elementary to middle school, the preparation process is considerably less complicated and involved than is the transition process for adolescents who are approaching adulthood. The transition to adulthood is recognized with many rituals and symbols of passage, which include the high-school graduation, obtaining the driver's license, registering to vote, and the signs of emerging fiscal independence such as the first paycheck, credit card, and checking account (Havighurst, 1953).

INFLUENCES OF TRANSITION CARE FOR ADOLESCENTS

For adolescents with special health care needs (ASHCN), their transition to adulthood is fraught with many more concerns and needs compared to those of typically developing adolescents. Their dreams for the future are contingent upon the realistic assessment of the impact of their chronic condition on their choices for the future. These choices include the selection of a job, postsecondary program for additional training or education, and a place of residence in a community of their choosing. For other ASHCN, these choices may not be possible because the severity of their disability or chronic condition results in more restrictive life choices (Davis & Vander Stoep, 1997; Fiorentino et al., 1998; Heal, Khoju, & Rusch 1997; Kohler & Chapman, 1999; Vogel, Klaas, Lubicky, & Anderson, 1998). The research on outcomes of adult individuals who acquired chronic conditions indicates that employment, housing, and social options are more limited for those with more severe levels of involvement (McCauley, Sybert, & Ehrhardt, 1986; Moise, Drotar, Doershuk, & Stern, 1987; Vander Stoep et al., 2000).

As national prevalence reports indicate, the percentage of ASHCN living into adulthood is rising, due in large measure to the advancements in treatment modalities and scientific knowledge. The survival rate of ASHCN has doubled over the past two decades wherein estimates indicate that almost 90% of ASHCN survive into the second decade (Blum, 1995). Although accurate estimates of survival rates for specific childhood-acquired chronic conditions are difficult to obtain, the available data reveal that the numbers of these adults have reached critical mass and their needs for specialized services can no longer be discounted or ignored (Reiss & Gibson, 2002; Rosen, Blum, Britto, Sawyer, & Siegel, and the Society for Adolescent Medicine, 2003). Estimates of adults with congenital heart disease are more than 700,000 and those with childhood acquired cancer number 270,000 (National Cancer Policy Board and National Institute of Medicine, 2003; Warnes et al., 2001).

In response to this growing needs for services, serious attention is being directed to the development and implementation of transition services and programs to ensure that ASHCN continue to have uninterrupted comprehensive health care as they "grow and develop" out of the pediatric model of care (Betz, 2003; Blum, 1995; Reiss & Gibson, 2002; Rosen et al., 2003; Schultz & Liptak, 1998; White, 2002).

INFLUENCES OF TRANSITION CARE
FOR THE FAMILY

The child-rearing practices of parents of ASHCN have a crucial impact on their adolescent's readiness to initiate the transition process to adulthood. As the empirical data have revealed, the psychosocial outcomes of ASHCN are associated with parenting practices that foster self-sufficiency and positive attitudes related to quality of life (Blum, Resnick, Nelson, & St. Germaine, 1991; Brotherton et al., 1988; Camfield, Breau, & Camfield, 2003; Ingersoll, Orr, Herrold, & Golden, 1986; Kirpalani et al., 2000; McDonnell, Wilcox, Boles, & Bellamy, 1985; Sawin, Brei, Buran, & Fastenau, 2002). Parents who endeavor to involve their children with typically developing children in family responsibilities and inclusive community activities (such as school and recreational activities and after-school programs) provide the opportunities for their children to learn the necessary prerequisite developmental competences needed for being better prepared for transition. The developmental tasks associated with the transition to adulthood are less imposing for ASHCN who have been developing the confidence of skill building in the preceding years with the watchful support of their parents.

Parents have an important and changing role during the ASHCN's transition to adulthood. Their parental role transforms from that of primary caretaker to steady and reliable allies. As researcher and clinical experts have noted, this role evolution is not easy and may be fraught with its own set of challenges. Parents may feel ostracized by members of the health care team because they are no longer included in health care decision-making (Boyle, Farukhi, & Nosky, 2001; Geenen, Powers, & Sells, 2003; Patterson & Lanier, 1999). Some parents have described this conflict as a "role blurring" with health care professionals as the control shifts from them to their children (DePoy, Gilmer, & Martzial, 2000). Other parents, supportive of their adolescents' needs for independence and autonomy, may need assistance with the process of letting go. Transition experts have described the need to provide support programs for parents to assist them in coping with these changes in their parental roles and dealing with their anxieties about the challenges, risks, and opportunities their adolescents will encounter as they embark on their own (DePoy et al., 2000; Geenen et al., 2003; Hauser & Dorn, 1999; Patterson & Lanier, 1999; Russell, Reinbold, & Maltby, 1996; Stewart, Law, Rosenbaum, & Willms, 2001).

NURSING CARE EXCELLENCE

The aims of pediatric health care transition programs are to facilitate the transfer to adult health care providers and access to adult health insurance coverage. Other objectives include the teaching of skills needed for SHCN self-sufficiency, and coordinating and referring to transition and adult programs to assist ASHCN achieve their goals for the future in the areas of employment, education, and community living. All of these program objectives are integrated into the common goal of preparing ASHCN to successfully transition to adulthood. The effectiveness of transition-preparation service approaches or programs will be contingent on the extent to which they are based upon the currently accepted principles of best practices advocated by governmental agencies and professional associations (American Academy of Pediatrics [AAP], American Academy of Family Physicians, and American College of Physicians-American Society of Internal Medicine, 2002; National Association of Pediatric Nurse Practitioners [NAPNAP], 2001; Rosen et al., 2003).

For ASHCN transition planning to be successful, it is essential that *formal* preparation begin *early*. Ideally, a formalized process of transition planning should begin in the preadolescence or early adolescent period. During this early phase, the concept of transition planning is raised as an emerging developmental milestone requiring careful preparation. This ongoing process of transition planning that spans a period of several years includes self-assessment, goal setting, strategic planning, implementation, and retooling to accommodate to the changing needs and circumstances of ASHCN. Health care transition preparation will be more successful if it is integrated and coordinated with the transition planning approaches carried out in the middle and secondary schools, state vocational rehabilitation, and youth employment programs, to name a few (Betz, 1999; Betz & Redcay, 2002; Blomquist, Brown, Peersen, & Presler, 1998; Schultz & Liptak, 1998; Wojciechowski, Hurtig, & Dorn, 2002).

Transition planning is a lifelong process beginning at diagnosis. For ASHCN, their diagnosis may have been determined at birth or prenatally or later during childhood. At whatever point the diagnosis was made, it is important that visions and images for the future be integrated within the background of health care and SHCN treatment discussions. Parents, and children if they are old enough, will want to know the long-term implications of the diagnosis. That is, they will have one or more questions about the impact of this special health care need on long-term survival, prospects for employment and living independently, social and intimate relationships, and reproduction. Although these questions cannot be easily answered with direct and specific responses if predictions of outcomes are not possible, providers can offer guidance that outcomes can be enhanced with child-rearing practices that encourage self-reliance, independence, and autonomy (Powers, Singer, & Sowers, 1996; Powers, Sowers, et al., 1996; Sands & Wehmeyer, 1996). Continuous efforts to foster the development of the attitudes, behaviors, and skills needed to become increasingly self-sufficient will enable ASHCN to transition more easily to adulthood once this period of future preparation commences (AAP et al., 2002; Betz, 2000; Blomquist et al., 1998; Schilling, Grey, & Knafl, 2002; Schultz & Liptak, 1998). In essence, transition planning is a lifelong process and not just a period of preparation of brief duration.

Assessment

Nurses who provide nursing care to ASHCN have an important role in preparing them for the transition to adulthood. Whatever the role—as a member of the ASHCN's specialized interdisciplinary team, a nurse practitioner in a primary care setting, a school nurse in an educational setting, or some other community-based setting—the nursing process is an apt frame of reference for transition planning.

Nursing assessment of the ASHCN's transition preparation needs is focused on several components of care. First, the identification of the immediate and long-term needs is made related to managing their SHCN at a developmentally appropriate and reasonably expected level of self-sufficiency. Second, assessment of their service needs for adult medical, dental, and health care providers is performed. Third, determination is completed of when their eligibility for health insurance terminates and what other options are available for health insurance. Fourth, in collaboration with interdisciplinary colleagues, assessment is made pertaining to the health-related accommodations needed to function in school and employment settings and inclusively in the community (AAP et al., 2002; NAPNAP, 2001; Rosen et al., 2003).

The assessment process is an adolescent-centered process, meaning that the ASHCN is the primary respondent in answering questions and sharing information about themselves. Members of the ASHCN's family, teachers, and other adult figures may provide useful input and insights about the adolescent; however, it is essential that the process involve the ASHCN and not rely solely on the perspectives of proxies (AAP, 2002;

NAPNAP, 2001; Rosen et al., 2003). The assessment process involves the identification not only of the adolescent's needs, but also of their willingness, motivation, cognitive, and functional capacity to address or learn to address the needs identified. For example, the adolescent may identify self-catheterization as a learning need, but not have the fine motor capabilities to perform it without some additional assistance or accommodation.

A few tools that are in the preliminary stages of psychometric testing have been developed to measure constructs of importance to transition planning. The 71-item California Healthy and Ready to Work Transition Health Care Assessment Tool (CA HRTW THCA) was developed to identify health care self-care skills of ASHCN as it relates to 14 domains related to transition planning (Betz, Redcay, & Tan, 2003). This tool and other clinical assessment tools or checklists can be used to assess the ASHCN's health care self-care needs. The remaining tools address condition-specific needs. A 55-item tool with 8 subscales was developed by Kennedy and colleagues (1998), with subsequent psychometric testing (Buran, McDaniel, & Brei, 2002) using a 7-point Likert scale (1, highest satisfaction, to 7, highest importance) to assess the medical and nonmedical needs of adolescents and young adults with spina bifida as identified by them and their family members. The 23-item Transition Readiness Questionnaire was developed to assess knowledge and behavioral readiness of adolescents and young adults with cystic fibrosis for transfer from pediatric to adult care (Cappelli, MacDonald, & McGrath, 1989). Although both of these instruments were designed for a condition-specific population, they have application for other conditions in terms of models for developing additional condition-specific transition readiness assessments.

Evidence from the empirical data provides useful guidance that can be integrated into the development of assessment tools and approaches (Betz, 2004). Findings reflect similar thematic issues in the research that explores the challenges and obstacles associated with transition planning. These topics focus on problems associated with care provided by physicians and members of the specialty team, systemic problems encountered in attempting to access health care and social services, and the personal issues associated with ASHCN and their families (Geenen et al., 2003; Hauser & Dorn, 1999; Madge & Byron, 2002; O'Connell, Bailey, & Pearce, 2003; Sawyer et al., 1998; Scal, 2002; Scal, Evans, Blozis, Okinow, & Blum, 1999; Sharp, McNeil, Wales, Cooper, & Dawson, 1994; Telfair, Myers, & Drezner, 1994). Assessment approaches based on the assimilation of available evidence will enhance the gathering of information from ASHCN to develop plans of care that comprehensively address their needs for services.

The specificity of assessing the adolescent's transition needs will be dependent, in part, on the type and the level of involvement of the SHCN. The extent of self-care skills required to manage the daily and ongoing demands of their SHCN will vary considerably. For example, an adolescent with cancer who is in remission may not have any daily treatment regimen to follow, except for the typical primary care guidelines. In contrast, an adolescent with type 1 diabetes will assume or will have assumed many daily responsibilities for disease management. These responsibilities include monitoring serum glucose, titrating insulin dosages, food preparation, and infection control. The nurse, in collaboration with team members, will integrate the particular SHCN guidelines into an assessment template to determine the status of self-care and self-sufficiency.

Other transition assessment components should integrate the best practice guidelines that exist for specialty and primary care. *Bright Futures Guidelines for Health Supervision of Infants, Children, and Adolescents,* developed by the American Academy of Pediatrics, provides clinical guidelines related to primary care health screenings, immunizations, and anticipatory guidance (AAP, 2000). As mentioned earlier, there are a number of transition assessment checklists and tools that are available for use in clinical practice (Adolescent Health Transition Project, 1995; Betz, 1998; Betz et al., 2003). Whatever approach is selected for determining the adolescent's transition needs, the following principles of assessment are necessary: they must be (a) based on best-practice transition guidelines recommended by professionals and policymakers; (b) based on the best-practices primary and specialty pediatric, adolescent, and young adult guidelines; (c) based on the individualized needs of the ASHCN; (d) comprehensive in scope; (e) address both specialized and primary self-care skills; (f) adolescent-centered in terms of language and format; and (g) culturally sensitive.

Nursing Diagnosis

Based on the identification of the ASHCN's transition needs, a number of nursing diagnoses will be generated. Although the list of diagnoses for each adolescent will vary, there are areas of commonalities this group of adolescents will share. Primary among the diagnoses identified for transition-age ASHCN are Ineffective Therapeutic Regimen Management; Delayed Growth and Development; Ineffective Health Maintenance; Impaired Home Maintenance; Self-Care Deficit Syndrome; and Ineffective Community Coping. Other nursing diagnoses will be identified based on the identification of individual needs during the assessment process (Carpenito, 2002).

Planning

The planning process is a pivotal factor of transition preparation. This planning is the next step wherein the ASHCN's needs for services and supports are collectively identified, providing the template for designing a transition plan that will enable the ASHCN achieve goals for the future. During this phase, the nurse is likely to function as the case manager or service coordinator. (The terminology used to describe the nurse's role responsibilities associated with transition planning may differ only in terms of the organizational labels.) In this role, the nurse serves as a liaison between the ASHCN and family and the members of the ASHCN specialized health care team and other service providers who represent other nonhealth service sectors that are critical to the development of a transition plan (Blomquist et al., 1998; Wojciechowski et al., 2002).

The range of needs identified during the assessment process will serve as the starting point for formulating the strategies to achieve the ASHCN's transition goals. The transition plan will identify the referrals to be made, services to be obtained, knowledge and skills to be learned, and coordination to be performed with other agency representatives or multidisciplinary professionals related to health care and postsecondary goals. The transition plan will identify the ASHCN's goals related to the following areas of needs previously identified: (a) current and evolving needs related to long-term SHCN management; (b) identification of adult primary and specialty care physicians and therapists; (c) health and dental insurance options; (d) health-related accommodations for school, work, and in the community; and (e) referral to transition and adult specialists and programs for additional training, education, employment, and other life options such as housing (Blomquist et al., 1998; Lewis-Gary, 2001; Schultz & Liptak, 1998; Wojciechowski et al., 2002).

Members of the transition planning process will offer a number of suggestions to assist ASHCN in achieving their goals. ASHCN and their families may have very different perspectives pertaining to provider recommendations. Their attitude is based on a number of psychosocial factors such as culture, parenting perceptions and child-rearing practices, the ASHCN's self-concept, body image, prerequisite self-care skills, and previous level of experience with practicing the self-care skills. As the service coordinator, the nurse will be responsible for managing the service team recommendations that are sensitive to the preferences, desires, values, and beliefs of the ASHCN and family.

For example, the school nurse may suggest that a student independently perform self-catheterization while at school because during the assessment of transition needs the ASHCN has expressed a desire to do it. However, the parents may initially object to this suggestion because they have consistently performed this task at home. Parents may feel their son or daughter is not ready to perform this self-care responsibility. The process for achieving this goal would be altered by first addressing parental concern about the ASHCN's desire to learn self-catheterization. First, the nursing service coordinator, in collaboration with the adolescent and parents, would explore further the nature of the parental concerns, which would enable greater insight and understanding of the nature of the parental resistance. This additional information could be used to identify interim strategies, such as discussing their concern with the pediatric specialist during the next scheduled visit or speaking with other parents whose children have learned this skill, in order to obtain information about their experience. Serving as the transition team liaison and based on the parents' and adolescent's mutual agreement, the nursing service coordinator would devise a plan to achieve this goal eventually, being sensitive to the individualized concerns of the parents.

Implementation

Implementation of the developed transition plan is based on an integrated, interagency, and adolescent-centered framework. The nursing service coordinator has the major responsibility for following through with the recommendations stated in the plan by the members of the transition health care team. It will be the nursing service coordinator's responsibility to proceed with making the necessary contact with interagency service providers, such as the rehabilitation specialists and special education teacher, to coordinate services and care. Service coordination may include joint consultation with an interdisciplinary colleague from physical therapy, resulting in the formulation of a realistic home plan of therapy with the ASHCN based on family resources, the adolescent's level of motivation, and commitment to continue with the home program. In another instance, the nursing service coordinator would spend time instructing the ASHCN on more specific details about the SHCN. Several studies of selected groups of ASHCN have revealed they have limited as well as primitive concepts about their special health care needs (Bashore, 2002; Kadan-Lottick et al., 2002; Kantoch, Collins-Nakai, Medwid, Ungstad, & Taylor, 1997). Due to their inadequate level of knowledge about their SHCN, ASHCN may not be aware of the health-promoting activities they could engage in to effect better health outcomes and minimize the deleterious effects of the disease. Unknowingly, they will not be vigilant in monitoring for long-term effects or complications of their SHCN, such as the appearance of secondary tumors after achieving remission status when treated for leukemia.

The implementation of the transition plan involves long-term effort. For ASHCN, the delay in observing the concrete outcomes of their hard work may be discouraging and create the incentive to give up. Urging the adolescent to remain persistent in the face of discouragement requires consistent effort. Then again, the task the adolescent is asked to perform may be too difficult and beyond his or her current capabilities. For example, the adolescent's goal is to achieve greater mobility in the community. The transition plan has listed as the service recommendation, "Schedule appointment with paratransit services for transportation to the physician." Upon follow-up, the nursing service coordinator learns the task has not been completed. The ASHCN states that he is uncomfortable with calling paratransit services. There are a number of options available to pursue, depending on the adolescent's preferences. The plan could be revised to include one or more activities such role-playing activities with family members or friends about an imaginary conversation with a paratransit representative; contacting a friend to provide support when calling the agency; talking to a friend who has called paratransit services to schedule an appointments; and rehearing the request prior to making the actual phone call.

Implementation of the transition plan will be focused on putting into operation the plans for attaining goals that the adolescent and the transition team identified. The nursing service coordinator will assist and provide recommendations to the ASHCN and family about available adult primary and specialty care physicians or nurse practitioners, dentists, and therapists who are willing and competent to manage the ASHCN care. The nurse will spend time with the ASHCN and family in reviewing insurance options for both public and private medical and dental care once their pediatric insurance coverage ends. Together with the ASHCN and family, the nurse will assess the approaches for attaining self-sufficiency with self-care skills, whether it requires instruction, reinforcement, or updating of previously learned skills. As mentioned already, the nurse will work closely with interagency partners in making the necessary referrals and coordinating services with them pertaining to their identified needs for education, work, and community living options. Also, working with interagency representatives will involve discussion and recommendations for health-related accommodations as needed in work, school, or community settings.

Evaluation

Evaluation of transition services is an ongoing process. The benchmarks of progress in achieving the goals set forth in the transition plan are evaluated during subsequent scheduled clinic appointments or as a follow-up to a plan recommendation made with the ASHCN. Revisions to the plan are likely, as ASHCN needs will change as circumstances warrant, developmental needs and preferences alter, and life goals are revised. Determining the need to change transition plan goals will not be predicated only on the needs, preferences, and interests of the ASHCN, but will also be raised by the nurse who recognizes that the goals of the transition plan are not being achieved according to the predetermined benchmarks (Betz, 1998; Betz & Redcay, 2002; Blomquist et al., 1998; Schultz & Liptak, 1998).

MULTIDISCIPLINARY INTEGRATION AND PARTNERSHIP: A CASE STUDY

Implementation of the comprehensive transition plan necessitates the involvement of multidisciplinary professionals and interagency providers who can offer the services needed for ASHCN to achieve their goals. Unlike the teams composed of pediatric personnel that are convened to provide integrated interdisciplinary services for children with SHCN, transition teams are composed of both pediatric and adult professionals and providers (Betz, 1998; Betz & Redcay, 2002; Blomquist et al., 1998; Reiss & Gibson, 2002; Schultz & Liptak, 1998; White, 1997, 2002). It is a challenge to assemble a group of professionals who represent not only various disciplines, but also entirely different service systems for segments of the population. Therefore, it is incumbent for transition service professionals, especially service coordinators, to develop partnership with community-based agencies, organizations, and service representatives who provide transition and adult services.

The partnerships include referring adult primary and specialty physicians and nurse practitioners to whom the transfer will be made. Linkages can be sought with representatives from public and private insurance programs. Other interagency partners include transition specialists from school districts, rehabilitation specialists from the state vocational rehabilitation departments, representative from Social Security Administration, counselors from Workforce Investment Agency (WIA) youth programs, youth advocates, representatives from college or university disabled-student services, peer counselors from independent-living centers, and community-based disability specialists (Betz, 1999; White, 1997, 2002). The following case study illustrates the concepts of multidisciplinary integration and partnership.

> T.G. is an advanced practice nurse and a member of a multidisciplinary team that provides specialized services to infants, children, youth, and young adults with developmental disabilities at a major

regional pediatric center. Members of the specialized team include the pediatric neurologist, nutritionist, speech and language specialist, special education educator, physical and occupational therapists, social worker, psychologists, dentist, and audiologist. This team has recently expanded its membership to include transition and adult community providers to provide input on service coordination and referrals that adolescents may need to transition successfully to adulthood.

These community representatives were recruited to participate when it became obvious that the multidisciplinary team did not have the expertise to make referrals to community agencies or adult-services organizations when it conducted transition planning for adolescents. These new team members included representatives from the disabled-student services office at the local community college, a special education transition specialist from a local high school, a vocational rehabilitation specialist, a staff member from the local independent-living center, and a job specialist from the Workforce Investment Agency One-Stop, a publicly financed employment agency. This new team composition enabled the multidisciplinary team to provide more comprehensive and coordinated services to this group of adolescents. Additionally, the blend of pediatric health care professionals and adult providers enabled valuable cross-training to occur, resulting in improved knowledge and understanding of their colleagues' roles and responsibilities in providing transition services to adolescents with developmental disabilities.

During a recent transition team meeting, T.G., the advanced practice nurse, consulted with the team because one of the adolescent girls, R.A.—whom T.G. served as a service coordinator—had expressed a number of concerns about her future plans after high-school graduation in 2 years. R.A. mentioned that during her last individualized education plan (IEP) she was told that enrollment in the home economics class was not possible. In addition, R.A. said she was afraid to say anything else during her IEP because her team members directed their comments about other school options for the upcoming year to her mother rather than to her. In essence, R.A. was dissatisfied with the outcome of her IEP and she did not know what to do.

The team engaged in a thorough discussion about the options available for R.A. and suggested a number of strategies that would enable her to achieve the goals she wanted for her future. The team suggestions included a more thorough transition assessment that fully included R.A. and centered on her preferences, interests, and goals for the future instead of her mother's and that of the IEP team. Community team members provided the contact information on agency representatives who could provide R.A. with suggestions to consider in planning strategies for the future, such as enrollment in the community college summer program for high school students and the summer youth employment program at One-Stop. Another team member suggested that next year R.A. request enrollment in the job-training program offered jointly by the local vocational rehabilitation program and her high school to learn basic job skills. The independent-living center (ILC) representative suggested that R.A. be present for all planning meetings. He added that R.A. should have been at this meeting because it was important that her voice be heard. Additionally, he suggested that R.A. might be interested in coming to the adolescent self-advocacy training group hosted each Saturday morning at the ILC. The other recommendation made during this meeting focused on the scope and availability of community services and programs that R.A. could access to enable her to meet her goals.

As this case study illustrates, creating partnerships with interagency representatives from transition and adult programs will enable the development and implementation of comprehensive and integrated transition service plans. Including interagency partners as transition team members or consultants in health care settings enriches the process of assessment, planning, diagnosis, and implementation by incorporating the divergent views of providers who have essential and important roles in the provision of transition services (Betz, 1999; Blomquist et al., 1998; Schultz & Liptak, 1998; White, 1997, 2002; Wojciechowski et al., 2002).

This chapter has examined the Nursing Care Quality and Outcome Indicator "Children, Youth, and Families Receive Care That Supports Development" (Betz, Cowell, Lobo, & Craft-Rosenberg, 2004) in terms of its implications for practice. Examination of this indicator was presented by focusing on the period of adolescence with a group of adolescents with high needs for services—ASHCN. Strategies for providing nursing support to this group of adolescents were discussed, with examples provided for illustration. Supporting children and adolescents through transition periods is an important nursing role because it is a pivotal time of development.

REFERENCES

Adolescent Health Transition Project. (1995). *Transition timeline for children and adolescents with special health care needs: Chronic illnesses/physical Disabilities*. Seattle, WA: Children with Special Health Care Needs Program, Washington State Department of Health, and University of Washington Clinical Training Unit.

American Academy of Pediatrics. (2000). *Bright futures: Guidelines for health supervision of infants, children and adolescents*. Elk Grove, IL: American Academy of Pediatrics.

American Academy of Pediatrics, American Academy of Family Physicians, & American College of Physicians-American Society of Internal Medicine. (2002). A consensus statement on health care transitions for young adults with special health care needs. *Pediatrics, 110*, 1304–1306.

Bashore, L. (2002). *Childhood and adolescent cancer survivors' knowledge of their cancer treatment and risk for late effects.* Paper presented at the Association of Pediatric Oncology Nurses Conference, Salt Lake City, UT, September.

Betz, C. L. (1998). Facilitating the transition of adolescents with chronic conditions from pediatric to adult health care and community settings. *Issues in Comprehensive Pediatric Nursing, 21*, 97–115.

Betz, C. L. (1999). Adolescents with chronic conditions: Linkages to adult service systems. *Pediatric Nursing, 25*, 473–476.

Betz, C. L. (2000). California healthy and ready to work transition health care guide: Developmental guidelines for teaching health care self-care skills to children. *Issues in Comprehensive Pediatric Nursing, 23*, 203–244.

Betz, C. L. (2003). Nurse's role in promoting health transitions for adolescents and young adults with developmental disabilities. *Nursing Clinics of North America, 38*, 271–289.

Betz, C. L. (2004). Transition of adolescents with special health care needs: Review and analysis of the literature. *Issues in Comprehensive Pediatric Nursing, 27*, 179–241.

Betz, C. L., Cowell, J. M., Lobo, M. L., & Craft-Rosenberg, M. (2004). American Academy of Nursing Child and Family Expert Panel health care quality and outcomes guidelines for nursing of children and families: Phase II. *Nursing Outlook, 52*, 311-316.

Betz, C. L., & Redcay, G. (2002). Lessons learned from providing transition services to adolescents with special health care needs. *Issues in Comprehensive Pediatric Nursing, 25*, 129–149.

Betz, C. L., Redcay, G., & Tan, S. (2003). Self-reported health care self-care needs of transition-age youth: A pilot study. *Issues in Comprehensive Pediatric Nursing, 26*, 159–181.

Blomquist, K. B., Brown, G., Peersen, A. T., & Presler, E. P. (1998). Transitioning to independence: Challenges for young people with disabilities and their caregivers. *Orthopaedic Nursing, 17*, 27–35.

Blum, R. W. (1995). Transition to adult health care: Setting the stage. *Journal of Adolescent Health, 17*, 3–5.

Blum, R. W., Resnick, M. D., Nelson, R., & St Germaine, A. (1991). Family and peer issues among adolescents with spina bifida and cerebral palsy. *Pediatrics, 88*, 280–285.

Boyle, M. P., Farukhi, Z., & Nosky, M. L. (2001). Strategies for improving transition to adult cystic fibrosis care, based on patient and parent views. *Pediatric Pulmonology, 32*, 428–436.

Brotherton, M. J., Turnbull, A., Bronicki, G., Houghton, J., Roeder-Gordon, J., Summers, J., et al. (1988). Transition into adulthood: Parental planning for sons and daughters with disabilities. *Education and Training in Mental Retardation and Developmental Disabilities, 23*, 165–174.

Buran, C. F., McDaniel, A. M., & Brei, T. J. (2002). Needs assessment in a spina bifida program: A comparison of the perceptions by adolescents with spina bifida and their parents. *Clinical Nurse Specialist, 16,* 256–262.

Camfield, C., Breau, L., & Camfield, P. (2003). Assessing the impact of pediatric epilepsy and concomitant behavioral, cognitive, and physical/neurologic disability: Impact of Childhood Neurologic Disability Scale. *Developmental Medicine and Child Neurology, 45,* 152–159.

Cappelli, M., MacDonald, N. E., & McGrath, P. J. (1989). Assessment for readiness to transfer to adult care for adolescents with cystic fibrosis. *Children's Health Care, 18,* 218–224.

Carpenito, L. J. (2002). *Nursing diagnosis: Application to clinical practice* (9th ed.). Philadelphia: Lippincott.

Craft-Rosenberg, M., Krajicek, M. J., & Shin, D-S. (2002). Report of the American Academy of Nursing Child-Family Panel: Identification of quality and outcome indicators for maternal child nursing. *Nursing Outlook, 50,* 57–60.

Davis, M., & Vander Stoep, A. (1997). The transition to adulthood for youth who have serious emotional disturbance: Developmental transition and young adult outcomes. *Journal of Mental Health Administration, 24,* 400–427.

DePoy, E., Gilmer, D., & Martzial, E. (2000). Adolescents with disabilities and chronic illness in transition: A community action needs assessment. *Disability Studies Quarterly, 20,* 16–24.

Fiorentino, L., Datta, D., Gentle, S., Hall, D. M., Harpin, V., Phillips, D., et al. (1998). Transition from school to adult life for physically disabled young people. *Archives of Disease in Childhood, 79,* 306–311.

Geenen, S. J., Powers, L. E., & Sells, W. (2003). Understanding the role of health care providers during the transition of adolescents with disabilities and special health care needs. *Journal of Adolescent Health, 32,* 225–233.

Grey, M., & Kanner, S. (2000). Care of the child or adolescent with type 1 diabetes. *Nursing Clinics of North America, 35,* 1–13.

Grey, M., Boland, E. A., Davidson, M., Li, J., & Tamborlane, W. V. (2000). Coping skills training for youth with diabetes mellitus has long-lasting effects on metabolic control and quality of life. *Journal of Pediatrics, 137,* 107–113.

Harper, D. (2000). *Online etymology dictionary.* Retrieved May 25, 2004, from http://www.etymonline.com

Hauser, E. S., & Dorn, L. (1999). Transitioning adolescents with sickle cell disease to adult-centered care. *Pediatric Nursing, 25,* 479–488.

Havighurst, R. (1953). *Human development and education.* New York: Longmans, Green.

Heal, L. W., Khoju, M., & Rusch, F. (1997). Predicting quality of life of youths after they leave special education high school programs. *Journal of Special Education, 31,* 279–299.

Ingersoll, G. M., Orr, D. P., Herrold, A. J., & Golden, M. P. (1986). Cognitive maturity and self-management among adolescents with insulin-dependent diabetes mellitus. *Journal of Pediatrics, 108,* 620–623.

Kadan-Lottick, N. S., Robison, L. L., Gurney, J. G., Neglia, J. P., Yasui, Y., Hayashi, R., et al. (2002). Childhood cancer survivors' knowledge about their past diagnosis and treatment: A childhood cancer survivor study. *Journal of the American Medical Association, 287*, 1832–1839.

Kantoch, M. J., Collins-Nakai, R. L., Medwid, S., Ungstad, E., & Taylor, D. A. (1997). Adult patients' knowledge about their congenital heart disease. *Canadian Journal of Cardiology, 13*, 641–645.

Kennedy, S. E., Martin, S. D., Kelley, J. M., Walton, B., Vlcek, C. K., Hassanein, R. S., et al. (1998). Identification of medical and nonmedical needs of adolescents and young adults with spina bifida and their families: A preliminary study. *Children's Health Care, 27*, 47–61.

Kirpalani, H. M., Parkin, P. C., Willan, A. R., Fehlings, D. L., Rosenbaum, P. L., King, D., et al. (2000). Quality of life in spina bifida: Importance of parental hope. *Archives of Disease in Childhood, 83*, 293–297.

Kohler, P., & Chapman, S. (1999). *Literature review on school-to-work transition.* Champaign: University of Illinois, Transition Research Institute.

Lewis-Gary, M. D. (2001). Transitioning to adult health care facilities for young adults with a chronic condition. *Pediatric Nursing, 27*, 521–524.

Madge, S., & Byron, M. (2002). A model for transition from pediatric to adult care in cystic fibrosis. *Journal of Pediatric Nursing, 17*, 283–288.

McCauley, E., Sybert, V. P., & Ehrhardt, A. A. (1986). Psychosocial adjustment of adult women with Turner Syndrome. *Clinical Genetics, 29*, 284–290.

McDonnell, J., Wilcox, B., Boles, S., & Bellamy, G. (1985). Transition issues facing youth with severe disabilities: Parents' perspective. *Journal of Association of Severe Handicaps, 10*, 61–65.

McPherson, M., Arango, P., Fox, H., Lauver, C., McManus, M., Newacheck, P. W., et al. (1998). A new definition of children with special health care needs. *Pediatrics, 102*, 137–140.

McPherson, M., & Honberg, L. (2002). Identification of children with special health care needs: A cornerstone to achieving healthy people 2010. *Ambulatory Pediatrics, 2*, 22–23.

Meleis, A. I., & Trangenstein, P. A. (1994). Facilitating transitions: Redefinition of the nursing mission. *Nursing Outlook, 42*, 255–259.

Meleis, A. I., Sawyer, L. M., Im, E. O., Hilfinger Messias, D. K., & Schumacher, K. (2000). Experiencing transitions: An emerging middle-range theory. *Advances in Nursing Science, 23*, 12–28.

Moise, J. R., Drotar, D., Doershuk, C. F., & Stern, R. C. (1987). Correlates of psychosocial adjustment among young adults with cystic fibrosis. *Journal of Developmental and Behavioral Pediatrics, 8*, 141–148.

National Association of Pediatric Nurse Practitioners. (2001). *NAPNAP position statement on age parameters for pediatric nurse practitioner practice.* Retrieved October 26, 2002, from http://www.napnap.org/practice/positions/age.html

National Cancer Policy Board and National Institute of Medicine. (2003). *Childhood cancer survivorship: Improving care and quality of life.* Washington DC: National Academies Press. Retrieved June 14, 2004, from http://www.nap.edu/books/0309088984/html

O'Connell, B., Bailey, S., & Pearce, J. (2003). Straddling the pathway from pae-diatrician to mainstream health care: Transition issues experienced in dis-ability care. *Australian Journal of Rural Health, 11,* 57–63.

Patterson, D., & Lanier, C. (1999). Adolescent health transitions: Focus group study of teens and young adults with special health care needs. *Family and Community Health, 22,* 43–58.

Powers, L., Singer, G., & Sowers, J. (1996). Self competence and disability. In G. Singer, L. Powers, & J. Sowers (Eds.), *Promoting self-competence in children and youth with disabilities: On the road to autonomy* (pp. 4–24). Baltimore: Paul H. Brookes.

Powers, L., Sowers, J., Turner, A., Nesbitt, M., Knowles, E., & Ellison, R. (1996). Take charge: A model for promoting self-determination among adolescents with challenges. In D. Sands &. M. Wehmeyer (Eds.), *Self-determination across the life span: Independence and choice for people with disabilities* (pp. 291–322). Baltimore: Paul H. Brookes.

Reiss, J., & Gibson, R. (2002). Health care transition: destinations unknown. *Pediatrics, 110,* 1307–1314.

Rosen D. S., Blum R. W., Britto, M., Sawyer, S. M., & Siegel, D. M., and the Society for Adolescent Medicine. (2003). Transition to adult health care for adolescents and young adults with chronic conditions: Position paper of the Society for Adolescent Medicine. *Journal of Adolescent Health, 33,* 309–311.

Russell, M. T., Reinbold, J., & Maltby, H. J. (1996). Transferring to adult health care: experiences of adolescents with cystic fibrosis. *Journal of Pediatric Nursing, 11,* 262–268.

Sands, D., & Wehmeyer, M. (1996). *Self determination across the life span: Independence and choice for people with disabilities.* Baltimore: Paul H. Brookes.

Sawin, K. J., Brei, T. J., Buran, C. F., & Fastenau, P. S. (2002). Factors associated with quality of life in adolescents with spina bifida. *Journal of Holistic Nursing, 20,* 279–304.

Sawyer, S. M., Collins, N., Bryan, D., Brown, D., Hope, M. A., & Bowes, G. (1998). Young people with spina bifida: Transfer from paediatric to adult health care. *Journal of Paediatrics and Child Health, 34,* 414–417.

Scal, P. (2002). Transition for youth with chronic conditions: Primary care physi-cians' approaches. *Pediatrics, 110,* 1315–1321.

Scal, P., Evans, T., Blozis, S., Okinow, N., & Blum, R. (1999). Trends in transi-tion from pediatric to adult health care services for young adults with chronic conditions. *Journal of Adolescent Health, 24,* 259–264.

Schilling, L. S., Grey, M., & Knafl, K. A. (2002). The concept of self-management of type 1 diabetes in children and adolescents: An evolutionary concept analysis. *Journal of Advanced Nursing, 37,* 87–99.

Schultz, A. W., & Liptak, G. S. (1998). Helping adolescents who have disabilities negotiate transitions to adulthood. *Issues in Comprehensive Pediatric Nursing, 21,* 187–201.

Schumacher, K. L., & Meleis, A. I. (1994). Transitions: A central concept in nurs-ing. *Image: The Journal of Nursing Scholarship, 26,* 119–127.

Sharp, C., McNeil, R., Wales, S., Cooper, P., & Dawson, K. (1994). Young adults with cystic fibrosis: Social well-being and attitudes. *Australian Nursing Journal, 2,* 38–40.

Stewart, D. A., Law, M. C., Rosenbaum, P., & Willms, D. G. (2001). A qualitative study of the transition to adulthood for youth with physical disabilities. *Physical and Occupational Therapy in Pediatrics, 21,* 3–21.

Telfair, J., Myers, J., & Drezner, S. (1994). Transfer as a component of the transition of adolescents with sickle cell disease to adult care: Adolescent, adult, and parent perspectives. *Journal of Adolescent Health, 15,* 558–565.

Vander Stoep, A., Beresford, S. A., Weiss, N. S., McKnight, B., Cauce, A. M., & Cohen, P. (2000). Community-based study of the transition to adulthood for adolescents with psychiatric disorder. *American Journal of Epidemiology, 152,* 352–362.

Vogel, L. C., Klaas, S. J., Lubicky, J. P., & Anderson, C. J.(1998). Long-term outcomes and life satisfaction of adults who had pediatric spinal cord injuries. *Archives of Physical Medicine and Rehabilitation, 79,* 1496–1503.

Warnes, C. A., Liberthson, R., Danielson, G. K., Dore, A., Harris, L., Hoffman, J. I., et al. (2001). Task force 1: The changing profile of congenital heart disease in adult life. *Journal of the American College of Cardiology, 37,* 1170–1175.

White, P. (1997). Essential components of programs for transition to adulthood. American experience. *Revue du Rhumatisme (English Edition), 64*(Suppl. 10), 198S–199S.

White, P. (2002). Transition: A future promise for children and adolescents with special health care needs and disabilities. *Rheumatic Diseases Clinics of North America, 28,* 687–703.

Wojciechowski, E. A., Hurtig, A., & Dorn, L. (2002). A natural history study of adolescents and young adults with sickle cell disease as they transfer to adult care: A need for case management services. *Journal of Pediatric Nursing, 17,* 18–27.

CHAPTER SIXTEEN

Translating Research Into Practice

Charmaine Kleiber

INTRODUCTION, DEFINITIONS, AND THEIR MEASUREMENT

One of the values put forth in the guidelines or indicators by the Expert Panel on Children and Families from the American Academy of Nursing is that "Quality care is based on scientific evidence, is ethical, safe and economically reasonable." The nursing profession should be proud of its long history of basing care on scientific evidence. Since Florence Nightingale first advocated using data to guide practice (Nightingale, 1863), the process of using research findings to improve the quality of nursing care has been developed and redefined. Pioneer programs in using research findings to guide practice changes include the Conduct and Utilization of Research in Nursing (CURN) project from the University of Michigan (Haller, Reynolds, & Horsley, 1979; Horsley, Crane, & Crabtree, 1983); the WICHEN Regional Program on Nursing Research Development (Krueger, 1978; Lindeman & Krueger, 1977); and the Nursing Child Assessment Satellite Training (NCAST) project (King, Barnard, & Hoehn, 1981). These programs laid the groundwork for the research utilization (RU) movement, a broad interest among nurses to move research findings into practice.

In the 1990s, nursing took a leadership role among the health professions in moving beyond RU, and advancing a more inclusive definition of evidence to guide practice. Nurses in the United States who were skilled with the RU process recognized that the traditional randomized clinical trial was not an appropriate design for answering many nursing research questions. When examining strength of scientific evidence, sometimes the best evidence was found through descriptive or qualitative work. Practicing nurses needed a format to evaluate all forms of evidence, not just experimental research evidence. This experience stimulated the movement toward evidence-based practice (EBP) among U.S. nurses. A broad definition of evidence includes meta-analyses, randomized clinical trials, quasi-experimental studies, observational studies, qualitative studies, case reports, expert opinion, scientific principles, and theory (Goode & Piedalue, 1999).

Nursing also took the lead in defining the process of EBP. Stetler, Bautista, Vernale-Hannon, and Foster (1995) described key proficiencies for beginning the EBP process, such as the ability to gather evidence from numerous sources and the ability to critique the evidence. Models have been published by other nursing scholars that guide the process of implementing evidence-based change, from problem identification through integration of the change throughout an organization (Rosswurm & Larrabee, 1999; Titler et al., 2001).

A brief examination of the evidence-based medicine (EBM) movement demonstrates differences between medical and nursing professional paradigms, and helps to explain some of the difficulty in defining the term "evidence." Concurrent with the RU movement among nurses in the United States, the concept of EBM was forming in Canada. The movement toward evidence-based practice (EBP) in medicine became more formalized with the formation of the Cochrane Collaboration, an international organization that promotes the development and accessibility of systematic reviews of the effects of health care interventions (Jadad & Haynes, 1998). The organization of systematic review topics follows the medical model of physical systems and disease processes such as stroke, tobacco addiction, and wounds. Systematic reviews follow strict criteria for finding and grading evidence. The randomized clinical trial (RTC) is the gold standard for strength of evidence and, until recently, conclusions from other types of research designs were considered to be weak or invalid sources of evidence (Guyatt et al., 1995).

A different definition of EBM is developing over time. Haynes, Devereaux, and Guyatt (2002) acknowledge that the absence of sensitivity to patients' preferences is one criticism of EBM. A new conceptual model of EBM includes clinical expertise, patients' preferences and actions, clinical state and circumstances, and research evidence. A very important shift in EBM is the recognition of patient preference in the application of medical treatment. This shift may hasten multidisciplinary efforts to provide the best evidence-based health care for consumers.

Definitions

Research is the systematic investigation to develop new knowledge or to validate and extend existing knowledge (LoBiondo-Wood & Haber, 2002). Knowledge must be generalizable in order to be moved into evidence-based practice. The effectiveness of an evidence-based intervention or activity is usually tracked through quality improvement (QI) or risk management channels in organizations. QI data are not generalizable, because they lack the rigor and control of research studies. Findings from QI projects are specific to a particular facility or setting. The quality improvement manager in an acute care facility may implement self-scheduling based on research findings, and then track job satisfaction and job vacancy rates to see if the intervention was effective on the local level.

Translation is a word usually meant to describe the movement of meaning between languages. *Translating research* means to move generalizable research-based knowledge into a form that is accessible and useful to the individual practitioner. This is the point at which statistical and clinical significance and relevance must be compared and judged by the clinician. Questions such as the following arise: If the study found one intervention to be significantly superior to another, what was the effect size? Did the intervention make a clinically significant difference for most of the subjects in the study? What risk would be incurred if the study intervention were put into practice? These are questions that can be answered only by clinically knowledgeable nurses who have a background in reviewing and critiquing published research studies.

The clinician must be able to differentiate between *efficacy research* and *effectiveness research* when considering implementation of research-based practices. Efficacy research is done in a tightly controlled environment to establish a causal link between intervention and outcome (Glasgow, Lichtenstein, & Marcus, 2003). Effectiveness research measures the impact of the intervention "when it is tested within a population that is representative of the intended target audience" (Glasgow et al., p. 1262).

For example, consider the efficacy research for using lidocaine gel to decrease the amount of pain associated with nasogastric tube (NGT) placement. A sufficient number of randomized clinical trials demonstrate that in adults, the pain of having an NGT passed is significantly decreased by instilling 5 milliliters of lidocaine gel into the nasal passages 5 minutes before inserting the NGT. Perhaps a staff nurse on a pediatric unit in a hospital would like to have this adopted as routine care. However, before doing so the nurse must examine the evidence in light of children's development and preferences. The only outcome variable addressed in the adult research studies was pain during NGT insertion. The research did not address the potentially noxious side effects of the intervention, such as bitter taste, stinging, and the sensations of having a gel instilled into the nasal passages. These side effects, combined with the inability of young children to understand the intent of the intervention, may cause more harm than good. This is an example of efficacy research that has not been tested for effectiveness in the intended target population: children.

Once research findings have been translated into useful, understandable information for the clinician, the process of implementing EBP can begin. Goode and Piedalue (1999) define evidence-based practice as involving "the synthesis of knowledge from research, retrospective or concurrent chart review, quality improvement and risk data, international, national, and local standards, infection control data, pathophysiology, cost effectiveness analysis, benchmarking data, patient preferences, and clinical expertise" (p. 15).

Another term that is important to this discussion is *best practice*. As explained by Driever (2002), best practice and EBP are differentiated in that EBP usually refers to the adoption of specific evidence-based interventions. Best practice is a broader term that includes an organization's commitment to use evidence for improving care. It encompasses "a level of agreement about research-based knowledge and an integrative process of embedding this knowledge into the organization and delivery of health care" (p. 595).

The meaning of *translation research* is different from "translating research into practice." Translation research is a relatively new field of study in nursing that seeks to discover how research findings are adopted into clinical practice and how to make that adoption happen more effectively. The goal of translational research is to evaluate change interventions for their "effectiveness at changing processes and/or outcomes of care, as well as on whether they are sustainable, reproducible, and generalizable" (Farquhar, Stryer, & Slutsky, 2002, p. 234). Translation research is frequently driven by change theory, adult learning theory, organizational theory, and behavioral theory.

Measurement of Translating Research

Measuring the extent and effectiveness of evidence-based practice is becoming more important as regulatory agencies and the public become more aware of the importance of evidence. As an example, proof that nursing practice is driven by evidence is one of the key elements necessary for achieving the coveted status of "magnet hospital." However, measuring the extent to which EBP has improved the quality of nursing care is difficult for several reasons.

As stated previously, evidence-based change is tracked through quality improvement channels, not through rigorously controlled research studies. Quality improvement data are usually not shared in a public manner, such as through journal articles. This situation can be due to the control of the data enforced by organizational legal counsel, which can make the data off-limits for sharing. It can also be due to journal editors' insistence that institutional review board (IRB) approval be obtained for any article that uses patient data to describe change. Currently there is a lack of agreement among manuscript reviewers and journal editors regarding IRB oversight for quality improvement projects (Lindenauer, Benjamin, Naglieri-Prescod, Fitzgerald, & Pekow, 2002).

Computer discussion lists and conferences that focus on EBP provide a public forum to share and discuss the latest developments in evidence-driven change. These mechanisms are an indication of the evolving nature of information sharing and processing. One of the benefits of these methods of communication is that they provide quick and up-to-date information that is not caught in the prolonged time frame of peer-reviewed journals. On the other hand, findings from conferences that are not published for a wider audience are not retrievable at a later date, and can be easily lost and forgotten. Information posted on computer discussion lists usually does not contain enough detail to be able to judge adequately the effectiveness of the evidence-based change. Comments are often very informal and center on "this is what worked for us." The challenge is to develop new real-time dependable ways of sharing EBP processes, from how the evidence was synthesized to how the change affected patient outcomes.

INFLUENCE OF TRANSLATING RESEARCH FOR INFANTS, CHILDREN, AND FAMILIES

It is the responsibility of all health care professionals to use the best and most recent information to care for those who seek our services. It is especially crucial to provide best-practice services to those who cannot defend themselves, who may not be able to "work the system," who are totally dependent on us for care. Infants, children, and women are over-represented in vulnerable populations, which include low-income families of non-White ethnic backgrounds (Flaskerud et al., 2002). The timely and meaningful translation of research and other evidence into practice is a crucial skill for today's nurses.

Nursing research has had a significant impact on the quality of health care for infants, children, and families. Many nursing scholars have contributed to the science of nursing practice and just a few of their accomplishments are mentioned here. Programs of research have developed interventions for neonates in the areas of feeding (McCain, Gartside, Greenberg, & Lott, 2001), environmental modification (Becker,

Grunwald, & Brazy, 1999), and parent touch (Anderson et al., 2003). Caring for children and adolescents with chronic illnesses has been guided by the work of Grey and her colleagues (2000) and Hinds (2000). Care of the acutely ill child has changed with extensive research on pain measurement (Hester, Foster, & Beyer, 1992). Families have benefited from nursing research with increased family involvement in the intensive care units (Curley & Wallace, 1992). Families also benefit from having nurse practitioners follow their prematurely born infants in the home setting rather than through an extended hospital stay (Brooten et al., 2002). Again, these are just a few of many examples that show the importance of using nursing research to benefit infants, children, and families.

In their review of nursing research on child health and pediatric issues, Miles and Holditch-Davis (2003) suggest that developmental science could provide a framework for evaluating current bodies of research and for guiding future research. The thought is that infants and children, by their nature, are constantly developing and changing. Miles and Holditch-Davis advise researchers to keep this in mind as they design studies. Nurses who put research findings into practice must take development into consideration as well. Interventions that are highly effective for some developmental levels are inappropriate for others. For example, using sucrose-dipped pacifiers can modify neonatal pain. This response gradually disappears after the neonatal period, so it is not effective in older infants. Interventions for families with school-aged children will be different from interventions for families with adolescents. Evidence-based interventions need to be tailored to the specific developmental needs of the children and families. Individualization of nursing care is paramount.

NURSING CARE EXCELLENCE

Once the evidence has been gathered, evaluated, and synthesized, a decision must be made about the strength of the evidence and whether or not to move forward with change. Changing practice in complex organizations with independent-minded practitioners is extremely challenging. In a review of change implementation strategies, Grol and Grimshaw (2003) report that none of the strategies were superior. The authors recommend that change strategies must be individualized for the particular situation and institution. However, there are several helpful models available in the literature for guiding the change process. The Iowa Model of Evidence-Based Practice to Promote Quality Care (Figure 16.1) is shown as an example.

At the very beginning of the process, as nurses think about the possibility of an evidence-based change, they also need to be thinking about

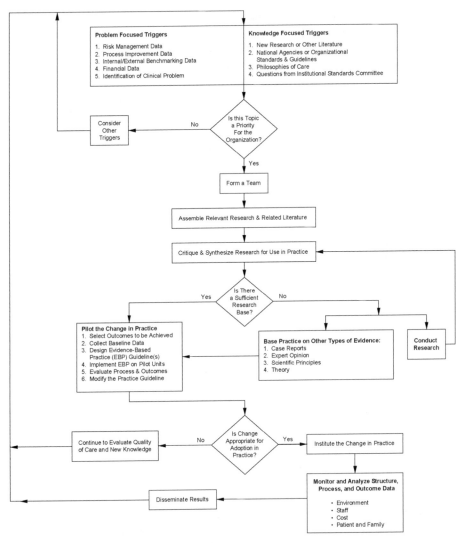

Problem Focused Triggers
1. Risk Management Data
2. Process Improvement Data
3. Internal/External Benchmarking Data
4. Financial Data
5. Identification of Clinical Problem

Knowledge Focused Triggers
1. New Research or Other Literature
2. National Agencies or Organizational Standards & Guidelines
3. Philosophies of Care
4. Questions from Institutional Standards Committee

Is this Topic a Priority For the Organization?

No → Consider Other Triggers

Yes

Form a Team

Assemble Relevant Research & Related Literature

Critique & Synthesize Research for Use in Practice

Is There a Sufficient Research Base?

Yes ← / No →

Pilot the Change in Practice
1. Select Outcomes to be Achieved
2. Collect Baseline Data
3. Design Evidence-Based Practice (EBP) Guideline(s)
4. Implement EBP on Pilot Units
5. Evaluate Process & Outcomes
6. Modify the Practice Guideline

Base Practice on Other Types of Evidence:
1. Case Reports
2. Expert Opinion
3. Scientific Principles
4. Theory

Conduct Research

Is Change Appropriate for Adoption in Practice?

No → Continue to Evaluate Quality of Care and New Knowledge

Yes → Institute the Change in Practice

Monitor and Analyze Structure, Process, and Outcome Data
• Environment
• Staff
• Cost
• Patient and Family

Disseminate Results

= a decision point

FIGURE 16.1 The Iowa model of evidence-based practice to promote quality care.

data elements that can be collected to measure the effectiveness of the change. Examples of outcomes are reduced pain ratings by patients, increased satisfaction scores for families, or decreased costs in care delivery. Data on outcomes can be collected through quality improvement (QI) channels during the development phase of the evidence-based change, so that pre-change and post-change data can be compared. Although it might seem cumbersome to collect baseline data on an EBP project, this step saves time and effort in the long run. For example, many institutions have experience with reinventing the wheel over a period of years. With QI data on file, practitioners can go back to the records and see why a change was made, what data supported the effectiveness of the change, and who approved the change. These data give practitioners the foundation to declare, "This is our rationale for our practice," rather than settling for "It's just the way we do things."

After collecting baseline data, the Iowa model suggests implementing the change on a pilot unit rather than throughout the entire organization. This step in the process has several advantages. First, people need to be educated and convinced that the evidence-based change is a good thing to do. Working with a smaller group of people is easier and might give an indication of potential roadblocks when the change is implemented throughout the organization. Second, it is easier to reverse course of action if the evidence-based change is simply not working. Third, it is more manageable to collect outcome data on a smaller area.

Once the change has been successfully pilot tested and implemented throughout the organization, it is important to monitor evidence-based change periodically to look for practice drift. For example, at one large Midwestern hospital, an evidence-based change was made to allow parents to accompany their children into the operating suite during anesthetic induction. The nurses, physicians, and child life specialists examined the evidence, agreed about the change, and the issue was put to rest. Several years later, however, it was discovered that some of the new physicians did not agree with the practice and it had been abolished.

The lesson learned here is that changes in practice can erode over time. One group in the organization needs to take responsibility for following the integrity of evidence-based change. The evidence supporting the change should be filed along with notes on who attended meetings and signed off on change. Change should be codified as official policy or procedure so that practice cannot be modified without careful consideration.

Every practicing nurse should be responsible for recognizing issues that might trigger the EBP process. These issues can be about specific patient interventions, programs of care, administrative practices, or health policies. For example, a nurse in the pediatric intensive care unit (PICU) might notice that parents are very upset when they are asked to leave the child's bedside during medical rounds. The nurse finds convincing evidence that parents are more satisfied with care and less anxious when allowed to stay at their child's bedside continually. Implementing unrestricted visiting by parents is clearly the right path to take. This fairly minor change in practice can be viewed within the context of a larger philosophy of care called family-centered care. If an organization professes to embrace family-centered care, open visiting hours in all pediatric units in the institution should be encouraged. This is an example of EBP at the administrative level.

Nursing organizations also have the responsibility to promote evidence-based practices. When large influential groups promote evidence-based practices, it is easier to get the attention of administrators and systems managers. For example, the Society of Pain Management Nurses issued a response to the Joint Commission on Accreditation of Hospital and Health Organization's ban on range orders, such as "Morphine, 2 to 4 mg." The society's response (Gordon et al., 2004) eloquently summarized the evidence supporting the need for range orders in order to achieve maximum pain control. Many individual hospitals have used the society's statement as rationale for continuing to have range orders in their organizations.

MULTIDISCIPLINARY INTEGRATION AND PARTNERSHIP: CASE STUDY

Getting the various interested disciplines on board from the very beginning prevents power struggles and promotes a trusting, inclusive model of care. Health care is a complex endeavor, and there are few interventions that do involve only one discipline. For example, there is clear evidence in the nursing research literature that providing sucrose-coated pacifiers to neonates during painful procedures reduces pain. This seems to be a straightforward intervention that has great potential for benefit and little downside. However, neonatologists, hospital epidemiologists, and pharmacists may need to be involved in the decision to bring this simple intervention into a standard of practice. Neglecting to include interested parties can result in backpedaling and lost time and energy.

A case study of multidisciplinary integration is provided here to highlight the process used to successfully implement an evidence-based protocol to minimize the pain of circumcision (Geyer et al., 2002). This process began when an advanced practice nurse found several evidence-based protocols for circumcision pain on the Internet. The protocols recommended a variety of interventions, some of which were not being used at this particular hospital. They included administration of acetaminophen, penile nerve block with buffered lidocaine, eutectic mixture of local anesthetic (EMLA), sucrose pacifier, swaddling, and modification of the environment. The interdisciplinary team that reviewed the evidence for each intervention included nurses from labor and delivery and pediatrics, an obstetrician, a neonatologist, and a pharmacist. Queries were directed to epidemiology for questions about sucrose, and to music therapy for questions about modifying the environment. After reviewing the evidence, the group decided to modify the protocols that were found on the Internet, concluding that penile nerve block is superior to EMLA for pain control.

The dialogue among disciplines proved to be essential for the successful implementation of this protocol for the management of neonatal circumcision pain. The pharmacist was able to work out the details of having buffered lidocaine delivered to the units on a daily basis. Bottles of glycerin had been banned in the nursery for years, based on infection control concerns. However, the nursing staff discovered a method of mixing fresh sucrose slurry for each use, and this was found to be acceptable by the epidemiologists. The support of the physicians was key in the implementation because some of the hospital medical staff refused to use penile nerve block to manage circumcision pain. Change in practice was forced by publicizing this evidence-based protocol as the formal standard of care for the hospital. Physicians who did not choose to follow the protocol were not allowed to perform circumcisions.

As part of the EBP process, the change was monitored through the quality improvement program. Six months after the protocol was put into place, a chart review showed that prior to circumcision, all babies received a dorsal penile block with buffered lidocaine, were swaddled, offered a sucrose pacifier, and had orders for acetaminophen. This is an example of a successful multidisciplinary research based change in practice. This change could not have been made without the agreement and support of each discipline.

SUMMARY

The transfer of new knowledge via electronic sources has revolutionized the way health care providers are made aware of developments in the science. Nursing is so broad in scope and so productive in research that it seems impossible to keep up with new knowledge. New methods for information synthesis need to be developed so that clinical practice can stay up to date with new information.

Many different sources compete to influence nursing practice. Public opinion, local and national policy, and regulatory agencies all make demands on how we spend our time and energies in patient care. It is up to the profession, however, to remain steadfastly focused on improving care through the use of solid evidence. In order to do that, all nurses must accept the responsibility for reading widely and bringing interesting research findings to the forefront. It is only through the constant questioning and challenging of existing practice that change will occur.

REFERENCES

Anderson, G. C., Chiu, S. H., Dombrowski, M. A., Swinth, J. Y., Albert, J. M., & Wada, N. (2003). Mother-newborn contact in a randomized trial of kangaroo (skin-to-skin) care. *Journal of Obstetric, Gynecologic, and Neonatal Nursing, 32,* 604–611.

Becker, P. T., Grunwald, P. C., & Brazy, J. E. (1999). Motor organization in very low birth weight infants during caregiving: Effects of a developmental intervention. *Journal of Developmental and Behavioral Pediatrics, 20,* 344–354.

Brooten, D., Gennaro, S., Knapp, H., Jovene, N., Brown, L., & York, R. (2002). Classic article. Functions of the CNS in early discharge and home followup of very low birthweight infants, 1991. *Clinical Nurse Specialist, 16,* 85–90.

Curley, M. A., & Wallace, J. (1992). Effects of the Nursing Mutual Participation Model of Care on parental stress in the pediatric intensive care unit—A replication. *Journal of Pediatric Nursing, 7,* 377–385.

Driever, M. J. (2002). Are evidence-based practice and best practice the same? *Western Journal of Nursing Research, 24,* 591–597.

Farquhar, C. M., Stryer, D., & Slutsky, J. (2002). Translating research into practice: The future ahead. *International Journal for Quality in Health Care, 14,* 233–249.

Flaskerud, J. H., Lesser, J., Dixon, E., Anderson, N., Conde, F., Kim, S., et al. (2002). Health disparities among vulnerable populations: Evolution of knowledge over five decades in *Nursing Research* publications. *Nursing Research, 51,* 74–85.

Geyer, J., Ellsbury, D., Kleiber, C., Litwiller, D., Hinton, A., & Yankowitz, J. (2002). An evidence-based, multidisciplinary protocol for neonatal circumcision pain management. *Journal of Obstetric, Gynecologic, and Neonatal Nursing, 31,* 403–410.

Glasgow, R. E., Lichtenstein, E., & Marcus, A. C. (2003). Why don't we see more translation of health promotion research to practice? Rethinking the efficacy-to-effectiveness transition. *American Journal of Public Health, 93,* 1261–1267.

Goode, C. J., & Piedalue, F., (1999). Evidence-based clinical practice. *Journal of Nursing Administration, 29*(6), 15–21.

Gordon, D. B., Dahl, J., Phillips, P., Frandsen, J., Cowley, C., Foster, R. L., et al. (2004). The use of "as-needed" range orders for opioid analgesics in the management of acute pain: A consensus statement of the American Society for Pain Management Nursing and the American Pain Society. *Pain Management Nursing, 5*(2), 53–58.

Grey, M., Boland, E. A., Davidson, M., Li, J., & Tamborlane, W. V. (2000). Coping skills training for youth with diabetes mellitus has long-lasting effects on metabolic control and quality of life. *Journal of Pediatrics, 137,* 107–113.

Grol, R., & Grimshaw, J. (2003). From best evidence to best practice: Effective implementation of change in patients' care. *Lancet, 362,* 1225–1230.

Guyatt, G. H., Sackett, D. L., Sinclair, J. C., Hayward, R., Cook, D. J., & Cook, R. J. (1995). Users' guides to the medical literature: IX. A method for grading health care recommendations. *Journal of the American Medical Association, 274*, 1800–1804.

Haller, K. B., Reynolds, M. A., & Horsley, J. A. (1979). Developing research-based innovation protocols: Process, criteria, and issues. *Research in Nursing and Health, 2*, 45–51.

Haynes, R. B., Devereaux, P. J., & Guyatt, G. H. (2002). Physicians' and patients' choices in evidence based practice. *British Journal of Medicine, 324*, 1350.

Hester, N., Foster, R., & Beyer, J. (1992). Clinical judgement is assessing children's pain. In J. H. Watt-Watson et al. (Eds.), *Pain management: Nursing perspective* (pp. 236–294). St. Louis, MO: Mosby Year Book.

Hinds, P. S. (2000). Fostering coping by adolescents with newly diagnosed cancer. *Seminars in Oncology Nursing, 16*, 317–327.

Horsley, J., Crane, J., & Crabtree, M. K. (1983). *Using research to improve nursing practice: A guide*. Philadelphia: Saunders.

Jadad, A. R., & Haynes, R. B. (1998). The Cochran Collaboration—Advances and challenges in improving evidence-based decision making. *Medical Decision Making, 18*, 2–9, 16–18.

King, D., Barnard, K. E., & Hoehn, R. (1981). Disseminating the results of nursing research. *Nursing Outlook, 29*, 164–169.

Krueger, J. C. (1978). Utilization of nursing research: The planning process. *Journal of Nursing Administration, 8*, 6–9.

LoBiondo-Wood, G., & Haber, J. (2002). *Nursing research: Methods, critical appraisal, and utilization* (5th ed.). St. Louis, MO: Mosby.

Lindeman, C. A., & Krueger, J. C. (1977). Increasing the quality, quantity, and use of nursing research. *Nursing Outlook, 25*, 450–454.

Lindenauer, P. K., Benjamin, E. M., Naglieri-Prescod, D., Fitzgerald, J., & Pekow, P. (2002). The role of the institutional review board in quality improvement: A survey of quality officers, institutional review board chairs, and journal editors. *American Journal of Medicine, 113*, 575–579.

McCain, G. C., Gartside, P. S., Greenberg, J. M., & Lott, J. W. (2001). A feeding protocol for healthy preterm infants that shortens time to oral feeding. *Journal of Pediatrics, 139*, 374–379.

Miles, M. S., & Holditch-Davis, D. (2003). Enhancing nursing research with children and families using a developmental science perspective. In M. S. Miles & D. Holitch-Davis (Vol. Eds.), *Research on child health and pediatric issues*. In J. J. Fitzpatrick (Series Ed.), *Annual review of nursing research* (pp. 1–20). New York: Springer.

Nightingale, F. (1863). *Observation on the evidence contained in the statistical reports submitted by her to the royal commission on the sanitary state of the army in India*. London: Edward Standford.

Rosswurm, M. A., & Larrabee, J. H. (1999). A model for change to evidence-based practice. *Image: Journal of Nursing Scholarship, 31*, 317–322.

Stetler, C. B., Bautista, C., Vernale-Hannon, C., & Foster, J. (1995). Enhancing research utilization by clinical nurse specialists. *Nursing Clinics of North America, 30*, 457–473.

Titler, M. G., Kleiber, C., Steelman, V. J., Rakel, B. A., Budreau, G., Everett, L. Q., et al. (2001). The Iowa model of evidence-based practice to promote quality care. *Critical Care Nursing Clinics of North America, 13*, 497–510.

CHAPTER SEVENTEEN

Interdisciplinary Models of Care

Roxie Foster

INTRODUCTION, DEFINITIONS, AND THEIR MEASUREMENT

Interdisciplinary models of health care, which integrate the efforts of a number of professional and lay caregivers, have their roots in much simpler and more intimate approaches. Before the advent of twentieth century advancements in diagnosis and increasingly effective pharmacologic, medical, and surgical treatments, the physician-patient relationship was the dominant force in health care (Chaitin et al., 2003). Sick patients were cared for in the home by the women of the family (Reverby, 1987), not by highly skilled nurses and allied health professionals. Physicians were treated with respect that approached reverence and the bond with their patients has been termed a sacred trust (Chaitin et al., 2003). Contrast that one-on-one relationship with the experience of a modern family. Upon accessing the health care system, they may repeat their child's history to a succession of professionals, including advanced practice nurses, be sent to a number of locations for costly diagnostic tests, and leave hours or days later still unclear about which of these experts is coordinating the child's care.

The fact that health care is no longer simple is both good and bad news: good, in that science and technology are saving lives; bad, in that the burgeoning science and increasing economic, social, and political pressures have created unprecedented complexity. The complex health needs of society now exceed the capability of any single discipline to meet them, necessitating collaboration and cooperation among multiple health care providers (American Association of Colleges of Nursing [AACN], 1995; Hyrkäs & Appelqvist-Schmidlechner, 2003).

Definitions of Interdisciplinary Practice

Collaboration has been defined as "the process of joint decision-making among interdependent parties, involving joint ownership of decisions and collective responsibility for outcomes" (Liedtka & Whitten, 1998, p. 186). The term *collaboration* is often used interchangeably with *interdisciplinary practice*. The definition adopted by the AACN in their 2002 white paper on the professional nursing practice environment specifies, "Interdisciplinary practice or collaboration is defined as a joint decision-making and communication process among health care providers with the goal of satisfying the needs of the patient while respecting the unique abilities of each professional involved in the care" (p. 298).

Interdisciplinary collaboration involves "sharing and is underpinned by teamwork, cooperation, negotiation and establishing partnerships that are client-focused" (McCallin, 2003, p. 364). The concept of teamwork is central to collaborative efforts and, in many ways, distinguishes the terms *interdisciplinary* and *multidisciplinary*. The prefix "inter" implies a mutual or reciprocal sense, whereas "multi" simply signifies many and various components (Hoad, 1986). In an interdisciplinary team, "inputs from a set of interdependent members are jointly planned, coordinated, and integrated so that the work flows efficiently and seamlessly" (Alexander, Lichtenstein, Jinnett, D'Aunno, & Ullman, 1996, p. 38). Thus, while *interdisciplinary* and *multidisciplinary* continue to be used somewhat interchangeably in the literature, multidisciplinary does not imply the same level of teamwork. Both terms are germane to a discussion of interdisciplinary models of care and are used throughout this chapter. As used here, however, interdisciplinary connotes established relationships, reciprocity, and family-focused teamwork, whereas multidisciplinary refers to members of multiple disciplines.

Teamwork is the essence of interdisciplinary collaboration and dictates how well members work together in fulfilling their common responsibilities. "Team functioning characterizes the process of the team's work rather than the team's outputs or effectiveness" (Alexander et al. 1996, p. 38). Teamwork relies on trust, knowledge, mutual respect, good communication, cooperation, coordination, shared responsibility, and optimism (Arcangelo, Fitzgerald, Carroll, & Plumb, 1996).

Measurement in Interdisciplinary Practice

In an extensive review of the literature, Sierchio (2003) identified at least 15 adult studies linking multidisciplinary collaboration with improved patient outcomes. A recent study of 394 professionals in 17 East Coast adult intensive care units provided further evidence of the association between teamwork and desired outcomes (Wheelan, Burchill, & Tilin, 2003). Despite the interest in studying these links, measurement of interdisciplinary practice is in its infancy. Development of an evidence base to guide interdisciplinary teamwork is limited by the diversity of team structure and function; lack of sophistication in evaluating economic indicators; the propensity to study disease-specific outcomes that may overlook more generalizable measures such as patient and caregiver satisfaction (AACN, 2002; Liedtka & Whitten, 1998); and the paucity of valid and reliable instruments to measure collaborative practice.

INFLUENCES OF INTERDISCIPLINARY MODELS OF CARE FOR INFANTS, CHILDREN, AND FAMILIES

Interdisciplinary collaboration has broad implications for the recruitment and retention of pediatric nurses, the expansion of pediatric nursing roles, and actualization of family-centered care. To better understand the influences of interdisciplinary models of care, it is helpful to examine what is known about interdisciplinary practice.

A systematic review of the literature involved searches within the MEDLINE and CINAHL databases using the MeSH headings "patient care team" and "interdisciplinary communication." The patient-care team heading alone produced 12,614 results. When limited to English-language articles within the last 5 years, it yielded 1,822 results. Thus, the search was further limited to review articles, resulting in 223 articles. "Interdisciplinary communication" yielded 226 articles in the last 5 years. Abstracts resulting from these search techniques were reviewed to identify literature that focused on the definition, measurement, or explication of interdisciplinary models of care. Approximately 30 articles were retrieved for examination and additional articles were identified from listed references. National organization Web sites were also searched for relevant position papers on interdisciplinary practice.

Authors have decried the lack of knowledge to support interdisciplinary practice (Alexander et al., 1996; McCallin, 2003) whereas the literature that is available focuses overwhelmingly on the associated challenges. As McCallin (2003) noted, "interdisciplinary team leadership does not occur automatically by assigning a label to a work group" (p. 367). Wagner's (2000) comments amplify McCallin's concerns:

> The delivery of health care by a coordinated team of individuals has always been assumed to be a good thing. Patients reap the benefits of more eyes and ears, the insights of different bodies of knowledge, and a wider range of skills. Thus team care has generally been embraced by most as a criterion for high quality care. Despite its appeal, team care, especially in the primary care setting, remains a source of confusion and some skepticism. (p. 569)

Barriers to Interdisciplinary Collaboration

A number of authors have described barriers to effective interdisciplinary practice (Alexander et al., 1996; Borthwick & Galbally, 2001; Chaitin et al., 2003; Hallas, Butz, & Gitterman, 2004; Henderson, 2003; Hyrkäs & Appelqvist-Schmidlechner, 2003; Lanceley, 1985; National Assembly on School-Based Health Care [NASBHC], 2002; Sierchio, 2003). Alexander and colleagues (1996) surveyed 106 multidisciplinary mental health teams within Veterans Affairs hospitals to identify barriers associated with demographic characteristics. Results indicated that communication and coordination suffer as teams grow in size. Diversity among team members in age, occupation, and organizational tenure were also associated with poorer team function.

Not surprisingly, power struggles and territoriality arose as frequent issues in the literature. Citing previous research, Hyrkäs and Appelqvist-Schmidlechner (2003) concluded that concerns for control, hierarchy, and authority comprised the major impetus for teamwork interventions. In a recent study, Hallas and colleagues (2004) surveyed 24 PNP-MD teams to identify factors associated with effective collaboration. Characteristics identified by PNPs as "red flags" included lack of respect and territorial/control issues. Physician respondents also addressed power struggles by identifying the theme "control/rigid/inflexible."

The history of medicine and nursing as autonomous professions complicates efforts to share power in working relationships. Medicine has long held enviable power and authority in health care, and nursing's history is fraught with attempts to gain acceptance as a discipline and distinguish its practice from the medical model. Ewens (2003) crisply articulated the issue, stating, "The current move towards nurses taking up roles that have previously been the domain of doctors has a certain attraction for a profession dogged by insecurity, low status and gender inequality" (p. 227). Is it any wonder that physician-nurse teams may encounter some bumps in the road toward teamwork?

Others, however, chide nursing toward amicable solutions. Sierchio (2003) suggested that part of being a team player is realizing that individual priorities may not always coincide with team priorities. Perhaps as Borthwick and Galbally (2001) contended, "Nursing needs to go beyond border squabbles with doctors to a true reassessment of functions" (p. 80) and to leadership in health policy.

It is important to note that Alexander and colleagues (1996) suggested "the same qualities that make heterogeneous teams so discordant may create very positive outcomes" (p. 49). They explained that diverse groups might be more innovative and more effective in finding unique solutions to complex issues. Thus, the authors (Alexander et al., 1996) urged managers to focus on team outcomes rather than on process, saying they "may have to accept poor team functioning as a cost of providing care in a team context" (p. 49). Bumpy roads can still lead to the desired destination.

Factors That Facilitate Interdisciplinary Collaboration

Research findings evidence not only barriers to collaboration but also facilitators as well. Key among facilitating factors are mutual trust, respect, and communication (Hallas et al., 2004; Liedtka & Whitten, 1998; NASBHC, 2002; Wetzel & Burns, 2002). Of 24 PNP/pediatrician dyads surveyed by Hallas and colleagues (2004), the majority identified trust, mutual respect, and communication as critical to effective practice. Other facilitating characteristics reported in that study included competence, a similar vision, and "knowing when to seek consultation" (p. 85).

Innovations in Interdisciplinary Collaboration

Shared leadership is an important innovation for future interdisciplinary collaboration. Shared leadership is an "approach to leadership in which all team members carry responsibility for team process and outcomes, thereby accepting formal or informal leadership roles that shift according to situation" (McCallin, 2003, p. 366). Team members "step in and out of the primary leadership role" depending on the expertise needed for that situation (McCallin, 2003, p. 366). Within this model, professional roles may be less distinct. Borthwick and Galbally (2001) went so far as to suggest "the role of nurses may increase, or it may mean that nurses will be moved aside by other groups with different training" (p. 76). Nurses will be challenged to step up to this leadership opportunity and actualize their authority within the interdisciplinary team.

The Attending Nurse Caring Model offers another innovation for interdisciplinary collaboration (Foster, Watson, & Theunissen, 2003).

Based on caring theory, this professional practice model helps nurses and other professionals reconnect with caring values to cocreate caring-healing models of care. The attending nurse "attends to" or focuses on comprehensive nursing care and on the caring-healing relationship with each patient and family. Transdisciplinary in nature, the model draws professionals together through shared values, common goals for patient care, and caring relationships marked by mutual respect and open communication. A pilot study recently completed on a 37-bed postsurgical unit in a large Midwestern children's hospital demonstrated the model's utility in improving interdisciplinary collaboration (Foster, Watson, & Theunnisen, 2004).

Implications for Nurse Recruitment and Retention

Health care excellence for children and families depends on a sustainable, motivated, and progressive nursing workforce. As the largest health care discipline, nursing plays a critical role in interdisciplinary care. Hallmarks of interdisciplinary collaboration are the opportunities for satisfying professional relationships with physicians and other professionals, shared leadership, and expanded nursing roles. There is a striking congruence among the factors affecting nurses' job satisfaction and the opportunities afforded by interdisciplinary collaboration.

Not surprisingly, when nurses are more satisfied with their work, patients are more satisfied with their care (Aiken, Sloane, & Sochalski, 1998). Retention of qualified pediatric nurses is especially important in a time of unprecedented nurse shortages and organizations are increasingly concerned about factors that influence nurses' satisfaction with their work. Aiken and colleagues (1998) demonstrated that autonomy, control over the practice environment, and relations with physicians predicted nurse burnout or emotional exhaustion. Results of a recent pediatric study demonstrated similar results (Ernst, Messmer, Franco, & Gonzalez, 2004). Ernst and colleagues who surveyed 534 pediatric nurses found a relationship among nurses' job satisfaction, organizational work satisfaction, job stress, and recognition in the pediatric setting.

In the emerging context of health care, nurses will have unprecedented opportunities for expanded clinical roles and leadership within interdisciplinary teams. As nurses begin to envision themselves in this way, organizations must keep pace. "If nurses adapting to new roles find themselves constrained and held back by their organizations, they are more likely to either leave their role or move back towards a more traditional view of themselves" (Ewens, 2003, p. 226). Retention of skilled pediatric nurses is paramount to health care outcomes for children and families.

Actualization of Family-Centered Care

Interdisciplinary collaboration also holds the opportunity for pediatric health care professionals to "walk the talk" about family-centered care. Essential elements of family-centered care include facilitating family/professional collaboration at all levels of health care and exchanging complete and unbiased information between families and professionals in a supportive manner (Shelton & Stepanek, 1995). These elements are consistent with the definition of collaboration as "the process of joint decision making among interdependent parties, involving joint ownership of decisions and collective responsibility for outcomes" (Liedtka & Whitten, 1998, p. 186).

It is difficult to understand how informed decision-making could exclude patient and family involvement, yet research has demonstrated some sobering examples. Henderson (2003) found that most of the 33 nurses she interviewed in four Australian hospitals were unwilling to share decision-making power with patients. Simons and colleagues (2001) revealed numerous incidents in which pediatric nurses refused to consider parents' concerns about their children's pain.

Although no published examples were found of family involvement in interdisciplinary care teams, Wetzel and Burns (2002) noted how important it is for interdisciplinary teams to recognize the family's role in their child's care. Madigan and colleagues (1999) reported the successful development of a family liaison model with associated expanded roles for nurses in a cardiac intensive care unit. Melnyk, Small, and Carno (2004) presented a convincing evidence base with guidelines for including parents in the care of their critically ill children. These studies demonstrate how interdisciplinary models of care can significantly expand the patient's and family's role in decision-making.

NURSING CARE EXCELLENCE WITHIN INTERDISCIPLINARY MODELS OF CARE

An interdisciplinary pain service provides a fitting example of teamwork in a tertiary pediatric acute-care setting and will be used here to illustrate elements of mutual respect, trust, and communication; the role of intradisciplinary communication; and a model of interdisciplinary collaboration.

As a construct, pain is uniquely suited to interdisciplinary collaboration. Pain theory specifies that the pain experience is comprised of biological, cognitive, and affective components (Melzack, 1999). Necessarily, then, assessment and treatment are multidimensional and enhanced by collaboration among experts in biological and psychosocial aspects of care. Further, pain necessitates involvement of the child and family. Because pain cannot be measured directly, only the person who has the pain can know the experience. In lieu of a self-report from the experiencing individual, parents can provide reliable proxy reports (Chambers, Finley, McGrath, & Walsh, 2003). Thus, interdisciplinary models of pediatric pain care hold the potential to enfold the child and family.

The Pain Consultation Service at the Children's Hospital in Denver provides an exemplar. From its beginning in 1992 with only two to three patients per week, the Acute Pain Consultation Service now averages more than 2,000 patient days per year, and the Chronic Pain Clinic carries an active caseload of more than 100 families. In keeping with those figures, interdisciplinary staff has increased from 0.25 full-time equivalency (FTE) for nursing and occasional consultation by two physicians, to 3.5 nursing FTEs, a full-time psychologist, nine attending physicians, and collaborating physical and occupational therapists. The ongoing journey of this team's interdisciplinary structure and process provides examples of intra-, multi-, and interdisciplinary collaboration.

Building Trust and Mutual Respect

The primacy of trust and mutual respect that emerged in recent interdisciplinary research (Hallas et al., 2004) was fully operational in our team's beginning work in 1992. As a new PhD graduate and novice pain researcher, I was hired to codirect the Pain Consultation Service with a psychiatrist and an anesthesiologist/intensivist. Developmentally appropriate pain assessment and epidural pain management were the first system-wide changes on our agenda. Looking back, these were ambitious goals for an understaffed, fledgling service.

Even in my naïveté, it was clear to me that success as a change agent depended on establishing credibility with nursing staff across the institution. In an acute care system, credibility is synonymous with clinical competence. With only 10 hours per week for the job in that first year, I divided my time between patient care and spending time with nursing staff, talking with them about pain issues, conveying my respect for their expertise, teaching and role-modeling pain assessment and management, and gently asserting my new role. These activities marked my first experience with intradisciplinary collaboration for pain management.

Although the term *intradisciplinary* is rarely used in published descriptions of teamwork, it plays a significant role. As used here, intradisciplinary refers to communication among members of the same discipline. Change theory evidences the power of communication among "near-peers" (Rogers, 1995, p. 192), people who are likely to respond to innovations in similar ways based on like values and experiences. Rogers contended that near-peers were more effective than anyone else in motivating people to try an innovation. Using this theory, an anesthesiologist would be more successful than a nurse in convincing a surgeon to allow epidural anesthesia/analgesia for a patient's postoperative pain, but another surgeon would be the most influential of all.

The near-peer concept is important because it raises the question of "distant-peers" and things that separate members of a discipline. Factors that have historically distinguished and divided nurses include educational preparation, clinical versus academic practice, competence in high acuity settings, and organizational tenure. Trust and mutual respect are not automatic attributes, even in intradisciplinary relationships.

In those early months and years as the "pain nurse," trust was in short supply. Mistrust among nursing staff stemmed from my PhD preparation, a primary appointment that was academic instead of clinical, unproven clinical competence, and lack of tenure in that setting. In addition to those four strikes against me, I was trying to get staff nurses to change the way they practiced. Although they didn't voice them out loud, challenging questions hung in the air. How could I relate to their clinical reality? Who did I think I was telling them how to assess and manage pain? Why did they have to ask children about pain when they could tell how children felt just by looking at them? How could it be safe to care for a child with an epidural outside the intensive care unit?

As Rogers (1995) cautioned, the change process requires patience. Over time, I became accustomed to the nurses' averting their eyes and assuming that "now-what-does-she-want" posture. That is why I so clearly remember the day I walked onto the pilot unit for children with epidural pain management, and heard one of the senior nurses say, "Oh thank heaven, the Pain Consultation Service is here." It was the watershed moment for intradisciplinary trust and respect. Without that trust, I was a solo force for change; with it, anything was possible.

A dozen years later, I'm convinced that mutual respect is an inviolable aspect of both intra- and interdisciplinary relationships. Extending respect is the surest way to gain it. Mutual respect is a prerequisite to trust, and trust is the cornerstone of collaborative practice.

Communication

Participants surveyed by Hallas and colleagues (2004) named communication as the third critical aspect of interdisciplinary teamwork. Not surprisingly, communication becomes more difficult as the team increases in size (Alexander et al., 1996). With only three codirectors as staff, communications were relatively simple and often informal in the early days of the Pain Consultation Service at Children's Hospital. As the staff grew to include several more nurses and physicians, however, communication became considerably more challenging. Meetings were difficult to schedule because the anesthesiologists were also staffing operating rooms and were rarely, if ever available at the same time. Similarly, nurses' shifts were distributed to provide the broadest possible coverage, and joint meetings required that at least one staff member attend on a day off. Informal or "hallway" communication became a primary interaction mode but these informal encounters began to suffer when departmental growth necessitated offices on three different floors of the hospital. Although we continue to search for an optimal solution, current communication strategies include pagers, e-mail distribution lists, hospital-approved cell phones, an open-door management policy, a shared drive on the hospital's intranet, and a strategy I've termed "trolling." Trolling involves walking through the anesthesia department, which houses some of our Pain Consultation Service offices and all of the attending physician's offices, and through the common surgical services areas to increase the chances of bumping into the people with whom one needs to check in, exchange information, or negotiate a decision. Regularly scheduled interdisciplinary meetings of chronic pain clinic staff and as-needed meetings among the Pain Consultation Service codirectors, other Pain Consultation Service staff, and multidisciplinary consultants extend these informal approaches.

Team communications are essential to effective care for children and families. When communications break down, families hear different opinions from different team members. In the resulting confusion, care suffers along with the declining respect and trust. In our experience, interdisciplinary rounds are among the most effective ways to communicate with inpatient families and to include them in decision-making. Another essential component of care is communication with the child's staff nurse. Rounds always include interaction with staff nurses, respecting their primary relationship in care collaboration, and enfolding their expertise in treatment decisions.

Myriad Components of Interdisciplinary Teamwork

It is important to note that teamwork is not all interdisciplinary. Previous sections of this chapter have emphasized the importance of intradisciplinary nursing collaboration, but the role of multidisciplinary partners is equally important. Multidisciplinary partners provide consultation and collaborate substantively in the provision of care but they are not consistent, ongoing members of the interdisciplinary team and they participate less frequently in decision making. A model for the interdisciplinary

Chronic Pain Service at the Children's Hospital in Denver is depicted in Figure 17.1.

The family-centered interdisciplinary team shown in Figure 17.1 participates directly in the child's assessment and diagnosis. Often, multidisciplinary consultation is sought to rule out previously undetected causes for the pain. With feedback from these specialists, and in consultation with the child and family, the team develops an initial treatment plan. Sometimes interdisciplinary team members, such as the physical therapist, directly implement parts of the treatment and other times the family is referred to treatment closer to their home. The interdisciplinary team continues to see the child for follow-up, coordinates care, and elicits progress reports from multidisciplinary providers. Intradisciplinary communication plays an important part in follow-up. For example, the

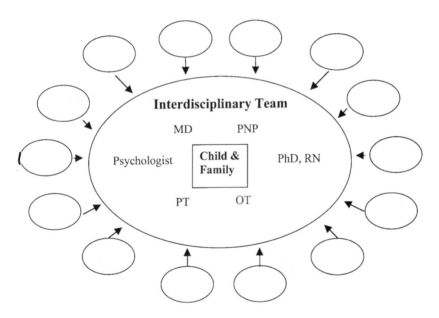

Potential multidisciplinary partners include the child's primary care provider (PCP), insurance provider, school nurse and school officials, therapists in private practice (e.g., psychologist, physical therapist), psychiatrist, interventional radiologist, physiatrist, orthopedist, neurologist, gastroenterologist, rheumatologist, surgeon, acupuncturist, massage therapist, and others. When a child is admitted to the hospital from the Chronic Pain Clinic, physicians and nurses from the Acute Pain Service staff and unit staff (nurses, recreational therapists, respiratory therapists, hospital-based teachers, chaplains, and others) become multidisciplinary partners.

FIGURE 17.1 Example of multidisciplinary collaboration with an interdisciplinary chronic pain team.

PNP usually contacts the school nurse or the advanced practice nurse in a collaborating discipline; the physical therapist usually contacts the collaborating therapist in a satellite clinic, and so on. Not only do near peers tend to speak the same language, but also any existing professional relationships among these individuals greatly enhance communications. Regularly scheduled interdisciplinary team meetings provide a forum for discussion of the progress reports and resulting refinements in the treatment plan.

Although the model in Figure 17.1 categorizes the large number of individuals that may be involved, it also illustrates the complexity of care and the potential for miscommunication among providers and with the child and family. Clearly, the family needs a designated contact. In the Children's Hospital Chronic Pain Program, the point of contact is, increasingly, the team's staff assistant. The staff assistant's role is critical to communication with the family and with the team. The position requires respectful and efficient telephone skills, judgment to triage family requests, consistent follow-through with team members, skill in communicating with insurance providers, knowledge of system operations, and a near-peer network within collaborating departments. As the point of contact, the staff assistant is the family's entrée to care and contributes importantly to their impression of the team's professionalism.

Beyond the point of contact, successful communication requires a designated team leader, the individual who consistently communicates and negotiates the treatment plan with the family. Often, that role falls to the attending physician, but in the team's shared leadership model, the PNP or one of the other members may assume or share leadership for family communications.

MULTIDISCIPLINARY INTEGRATION AND PARTNERSHIP: CASE STUDY

Interdisciplinary collaboration is built on trust and mutual respect, characteristics that are also foundational to relationships with children and families. Some families may display preexisting trust of health care professionals, especially if they have had a previous positive experience in the institution or already have confidence in the health care team (Thompson, Hupcey, & Clark, 2003). Mutual respect is critical in relationships with families and manifests in the health care team's recognition of the family's knowledge of their child and their role in the child's care (Daneman, Macaluso, & Guzzetta, 2003). Mutual respect requires an acceptance of the family's role in decision making. Borthwick and Galbally (2001) described the "contradiction where patients are expected to undertake health promotion and 'responsible' self-care, yet are expected to adopt a passive role in which formal professional care is *administered* to them" (p. 80, emphasis added).

Mutual respect and trust build strong bonds among professionals and those bonds optimize supportive care. A clinical anecdote provides an illustration.

A young child had just arrived on a postsurgical unit after many hours in surgery. Although family members can be expected to be exhausted and impatient after a long day of waiting and worrying, the mother's demeanor in this case could only be described as aggressive and angry. With hands on hips, she challenged, "Who am I going to have to fight with tonight to get what I need for my daughter?" She then demanded that her child be deeply sedated for at least 24 hours, despite the fact the child indicated she was experiencing little pain. I left the child's room to review the medical record, explaining that I would return as soon as I had done so. The attending Pain Consultation Service physician arrived on the unit for rounds at that moment and as I greeted him, the mother approached the nurses' station and angrily engaged the physician. Although the physician and I remained calm, the mother's behavior continued to escalate. After several minutes, we convinced her to return to her daughter's room, promising we would talk with her just as soon as we had reviewed the medical record.

Our subsequent conversation with this family set the stage for successful conflict resolution and a good outcome for the child. The discussion involved active listening, acknowledgement of the mother's distrust and its origins in a previous health care experience, assurance that a doctor or nurse from the Pain Consultation Service was available for consultation 24 hours a day, agreeing on the parameters family and staff would use to assess pain, and a carefully negotiated plan to work together with the family to ensure the child would experience as little pain as possible.

In this clinical scenario, interdisciplinary and intradisciplinary respect and trust were critical to establishing mutual respect and trust with the family. In the absence of a good working relationship, unpleasant encounters like this can fracture the provider team and open the door to splitting and blaming behaviors. For example, unit nurses who witnessed the encounter at the nurses' station could have blamed Pain Consultation Service members for the disruption, placing unit staff and Pain Consultation Service staff in different camps. Based on our history of successfully teaming to support children and families, however, the unit nurses talked with us about how we could mutually support this family and resolve the mother's distrust. When members of the health care team are supportive of one another, they are less likely to be personally threatened by angry behavior. When a family member is disrespectful, a cohesive team is much less likely to respond in kind. Mutual respect begets mutual respect. Extending respect to the child and family is the first step in establishing a trusting, healing relationship.

Advocacy for optimal patient care sometimes involves multidisciplinary, intradisciplinary, and interdisciplinary partnerships that extend beyond institutions and regional affiliations. The issue of range orders for opioid analgesics provides a case example.

In 2002, the Joint Commission for Accreditation of Healthcare Organizations (JCAHO) implemented new Pain Management Standards designed to improve care for patients in pain. Although generally a boon to pain services and individuals advocating for more consistent assessment and treatment of pain, the new standards prompted discussion on JCAHO's Web site about the advisability of range orders for opioid analgesics, with some interpreting this discussion to mean that range orders would no longer be allowed.

In effect, a range order provides for fine titration of an opioid analgesic by providing a range of doses and frequencies, and delegates judgment to the nurse about which dose or frequency is most appropriate in a given situation. For example, a physician may write, "Morphine 1-2 mg IV (0.05-0.01 mg/kg) q2-3 hrs prn." The nurse then chooses the dose and frequency appropriate to the child's pain intensity, pain stimulus, and most recent response to the drug. In the absence of a range of doses and time intervals, the physician must write a specific dose, which may be either too high or too low for the child's situation, and which requires the nurse to call repeatedly for new orders to titrate the analgesic to the desired level of comfort.

By impairing the ability to titrate to comfort, the loss of range orders threatened to erase a decade or more of progress in pediatric pain management. Although the JCAHO clarified that its intent was not to limit nursing judgment or decrease the quality of care but only to ensure patient safety (Gordon et al., 2004), their assurances were met with a groundswell of concern among pain management specialists.

Passionate about the need to preserve nursing judgment in the administration of opioid analgesics, I personally contacted national colleagues and initiated conversations with JCAHO officials. Those interactions led to an invitation to join a task force from the American Society of Pain Management Nurses to develop a position statement on opioid range orders. The position statement incorporated concerns raised by both adult care and pediatric nurses and developed into specific recommendations for prescribers, nurses, and institutions to maintain range orders and ensure their safe use. Because all of us on the task force had ties to the American Pain Society, additional consultation was requested from multidisciplinary experts in that organization and the two groups achieved a consensus statement (Gordon et al., 2004). In this case, multidisciplinary collaboration resulted in policy development and advocacy for patient safety and for optimal pain treatment. The success of this national, multidisciplinary partnership in providing guidelines for practice is a fitting example of the strength in teamwork.

SUMMARY

As the sacred trust of health care moves from the primary provider to the specialty team, nursing will be challenged to assume increasing leadership in intradisciplinary, multidisciplinary, and interdisciplinary teams. Interdisciplinary collaboration contains both challenges and pitfalls. One of nursing's leadership opportunities is in the generation of knowledge and theory to guide successful collaboration and to link interdisciplinary teamwork with patient outcomes. Another opportunity is in the actualization of family-centered care within an interdisciplinary framework. These opportunities will challenge nurses at all levels of practice. Borthwick and Galbally (2001) questioned how far a discipline can stretch before it ruptures. Perhaps the more appropriate question is, How far can nursing go without stretching?

REFERENCES

Aiken, L. H., Sloane, D. M., & Sochalski, J. (1998). Hospital organization and outcomes. *Quality in Health Care, 7,* 222–226.

Alexander, J. A., Lichtenstein, R., Jinnett, K., D'Aunno, T. A., & Ullman, E. (1996). The effects of treatment team diversity and size on assessments of team functioning. *Hospital and Health Services Administration, 41,* 37–53.

American Association of Colleges of Nursing. (1995). *Interdisciplinary education and practice.* Retrieved September 13, 2004, from http://www.aacn.nche.edu/publications/positions/interdis.htm

American Association of Colleges of Nursing. (2002). Hallmarks of the professional nursing practice environment. *Journal of Professional Nursing, 18,* 295–304.

Arcangelo, V., Fitzgerald, M., Carroll, D., & Plumb, J. D. (1996). Collaborative care between nurse practitioners and primary care physicians. *Primary Care: Clinics in Office Practice, 23,* 103–113.

Borthwick, C., & Galbally, R. (2001). Nursing leadership and health sector reform. *Nursing Inquiry, 8,* 75–81.

Chaitin, E., Stiller, R., Jacobs, S., Hershl, J., Grogen, T., & Weinberg, J. (2003). Physician-patient relationship in the intensive care unit: Erosion of the sacred trust? *Critical Care Medicine, 31*(Suppl. 5), S367–S372.

Chambers, C. T., Finley, G. A., McGrath, P. J., & Walsh, T. M. (2003). The parents' postoperative pain measure: Replication and extension to 2-6-year-old children. *Pain, 105,* 437–443.

Daneman, S., Macaluso, J., & Guzzetta, C. E. (2003). Healthcare providers' attitudes toward parent participation in the care of the hospitalized child. *Journal for Specialists in Pediatric Nursing, 8,* 90–98.

Ernst, M. E., Messmer, P. R., Franco, M., & Gonzales, J. L. (2004). Nurses' job satisfaction, stress, and recognition in a pediatric setting. *Pediatric Nursing, 30,* 219–227.

Ewens, A. (2003). Changes in nursing identities: Supporting a successful transition. *Journal of Nursing Management, 11,* 224–228.

Foster, R. L., Watson, J., & Theunissen, B. (2004). [Piloting an Attending Nurse Caring Model with Children in Pain]. Unpublished raw data.

Gordon, D. B., Dahl, J., Phillips, P., Frandsen, J., Cowley, C., Foster, R. L. et al. (2004). The use of "as-needed" range orders for opioid analgesics in the management of acute pain: A consensus statement of the American Society for Pain Management Nurses and the American Pain Society. *Pain Management Nursing, 5,* 53–58.

Hallas, D. M., Butz, A., & Gitterman, B. (2004). Attitudes and beliefs for effective pediatric nurse practitioner and physician collaboration. *Journal of Pediatric Health Care, 18,* 77–86.

Henderson, S. (2003). Power imbalance between nurses and patients: A potential inhibitor of partnership in care. *Journal of Clinical Nursing, 12,* 501–508.

Hoad, R. F. (1986). *The concise oxford dictionary of English etymology.* Oxford, UK: Oxford University Press.

Hyrkäs, K., & Appelqvist-Schmidlechner, K. (2003). Team supervision in multiprofessional teams: Team members' descriptions as highlighted by group interviews. *Journal of Clinical Nursing, 12,* 188–197.

Lanceley, A. (1985). Use of controlling language in the rehabilitation of the elderly. *Journal of Advanced Nursing, 10,* 125–135.

Liedtka, J. M., & Whitten, E. (1998). Enhancing care delivery through cross-disciplinary collaboration: A case study. *Journal of Healthcare Management, 43,* 185–205.

Madigan, C. K., Donaghue, D. D., & Carpenter, E. V. (1999). Development of a family liaison model during operative procedures. *American Journal of Maternal Child Nursing, 24,* 185–189.

McCallin, A. (2003). Interdisciplinary team leadership: A revisionist approach for an old problem? *Journal of Nursing Management, 11,* 364–370.

Melnyk, B. M., Small, L., & Carno, M. A. (2004). The effectiveness of parent-focused interventions in improving coping/mental health outcomes of critically ill children and their parents: An evidence based to guide clinical practice. *Pediatric Nursing, 30,* 143–148.

Melzack, R. (1999). Pain and stress: A new perspective. In R. J. Gatchel & D. C. Turk (Eds.), *Psychosocial factors in pain* (pp. 89–106). New York: Guildford Press.

National Assembly on School-Based Health Care. (2002). *Position statement: Interdisciplinary practice.* Retrieved September 13, 2004, from http://nasbhc.org/app/interdisciplinary_care_policy.htm

Reverby, S. M. (1987). *Ordered to care: The dilemma of American nursing: 1850–1945.* Cambridge, UK: Cambridge University Press.

Rogers, E. M. (1995). *Diffusion of innovations* (4th ed.). New York: Free Press.

Sierchio, G. P. (2003). A multidisciplinary approach for improving outcomes. *Journal of Infusion Nursing, 26,* 34–41.

Simons, J., Franck, L., & Roberson, E. (2001). Parent involvement in children's pain care: Views of parents and nurses. *Journal of Advanced Nursing, 36,* 591–599.

Shelton, T. L., & Stepanek, J. S. (1995). Excerpts from family-centered care for children needing specialized health and developmental services. *Pediatric Nursing, 21,* 363–364.

Thompson, V. L., Hupcey, J. E., & Clark, M. B. (2003). The development of trust in parents of hospitalized children. *Journal for Specialists in Pediatric Nursing, 8,* 137–147.

Wagner, E. H. (2000). The role of patient care teams in chronic disease management. *British Medical Journal, 320,* 569–572.

Wetzel, R. C., & Burns, R. C. (2002). Multiple trauma in children: Critical care overview. *Critical Care Medicine, 30*(Suppl. 11), S468–S477.

Wheelan, S. A., Burchill, C. N., & Tilin, F. (2003). The link between teamwork and patients' outcomes in intensive care units. *American Journal of Critical Care, 12,* 527–534.

Index